# Seafood Nutrition
## Facts, Issues and Marketing of Nutrition in Fish and Shellfish

Joyce A. Nettleton, D.Sc., R.D.

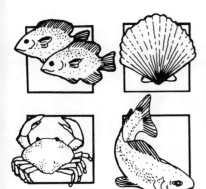

# Seafood Nutrition

## Facts, Issues and Marketing of Nutrition in Fish and Shellfish

Joyce A. Nettleton, D.Sc., R.D.

**VNR** VAN NOSTRAND REINHOLD
New York

Library of Congress Catalog Card Number 85-15297

ISBN 0-943738-12-1

Design by Jean Hammond, Cambridge, Massachusetts.
Composition by New Age Typographers, Inc., Huntington, New York.
Printed and bound by BookCrafters, Inc., Chelsea, Michigan.

Van Nostrand Reinhold
115 Fifth Avenue
New York, New York 10003

Van Nostrand Reinhold International Company Limited
11 New Fetter Lane
London EC4P 4EE, England

Van Nostrand Reinhold
480 La Trobe Street
Melbourne, Victoria 3000, Australia

Nelson Canada
1120 Birchmount Road
Scarborough, Ontario M1K 5G4, Canada

16 15 14 13 12 11 10 9 8 7 6 5 4 3

**Library of Congress Cataloging-in-Publication Data**
Nettleton, Joyce, 1944-
    Seafood Nutrition.

    (Osprey Seafood Handbooks)
    Bibliography: p.
    Includes index
    1. Fish as food — Analysis.   2. Seafood — Analysis.
    3. Diet — United States.   I. Title.   II. Series.
TX556.5.N47 1985      641.3′92      85-15297
ISBN 0-943738-12-1

# Preface

As this book goes to press, there is unprecedented interest in the relationships between seafood and health. The unique fatty acids in fish oils, known as omega-3 fatty acids, appear to have metabolic properties that are associated with a lower risk of heart disease. Much excitement has been generated by the research findings. In order to extend our limited understanding of how these molecules affect health, the National Institutes of Health plans to devote a substantially increased budget to the study of fish oils. Hopes and expectations are very high.

There are several apparent paradoxes in the enthusiasm for fish oils. The most notable of these is that while the virtue of seafood has always been its extraordinarily low fat and cholesterol content compared with other protein foods, omega-3 fatty acids are most abundant in high fat fish and in fish liver oils. Seafood may now be found to be especially healthy *because* of its fat. And high fat species may be particularly advantageous.

Will consumers seeking omega-3 fatty acids eat more seafood or patronize the health food store for a bottle of fish oil capsules? This question is of special concern to nutritionists and health professionals because enchantment with capsules and potions reinforces the myth that refined supplements are necessary for good health. Fish oil preparations may also pose the risk of hazardous levels of fat soluble vitamins, environmental contaminants and cholesterol. Many such preparations on the market today do not give information about the purification procedures used (if any), the vitamin levels or the cholesterol content. And they charge a very high price!

The question is also, of course, of particular concern to the seafood, foodservice and retail food industries, who stand to benefit enormously if eating fish is generally perceived to be a major contributor to good health.

We know that the benefits of regular fish consumption take years to detect, are imperceptible to the consumer and are manifested by health problems avoided rather than by pleasures immediately enjoyed. We do not know how much, or how little, fish oil is needed to confer a benefit; but there is suggestive evidence that even lean fish, which have comparatively small amounts of omega-3 fatty acids, may be useful.

Medical researchers, nutritionists and seafood fanciers are an optimistic lot who are supporting the prospect of seafood being uniquely important for optimum health. The next few years promise exciting and useful advances in our understanding of the part that seafood can play in our health and welfare.

# Seafood Nutrition:
## Facts, Issues and Marketing of Nutrition in Fish and Shellfish

Joyce A. Nettleton, D.Sc., R.D.

## Contents

# Acknowledgements

When the computer screen is empty and deadlines are marching toward you, writing a book seems impossible and ludicrous. Those special people who made sure that it was neither enriched me and this volume with their talents and encouragement. I am truly grateful to them.

Several people provided published and unpublished data for the tables of nutrient composition. The data in turn generated lively discussions which improved my insights into a number of issues. I am especially grateful to Judy Kryznowek, Bob Learson and Jeanne Joseph of the National Marine Fisheries Services laboratories in this regard. Dr. Jacob Exler from the United States Department of Agriculture kindly provided and reviewed some of the nutrient data and had many helpful suggestions for handling some of the fatty acid data. I am most appreciative of his contributions and the conversations we had.

Peter Vlieg of the Department of Scientific and Industrial Research in North Palmerston, New Zealand possesses the magic of shrinking geographical distance with timely and provocative letters. I thank him particularly for the many papers he sent me and the helpful discussions we had by mail. He will recognize his contributions to a number of sections.

Janet Dudeck of the National Food Processors Association, Roy Martin of the National Fisheries Institute, Ken Coons of the New England Fisheries Development Foundation and Caroline Roy of the Massachusetts Nutrition Resource Center shared materials with me that were critical to the development of important parts of the book. We had some enjoyable conversations and I appreciate their help.

Several people in the Washington offices of the National Marine Fisheries Service were most gracious in providing materials and wisdom. Beverly Barton, Betty Hackley and Jim Price deserve many thanks for their inputs and assistance in locating materials.

Others provided materials I surely would have overlooked. Sandy Shimabukuro of the University of Hawaii at Manoa helped a great deal with the names and data for Hawaiian species, while Ted Miller of Wallace Menhaden Products, Inc. kindly sent me many publications I had not seen before.

Many people reviewed sections of the manuscript with thoroughness, perception and mercy. Their suggestions were invaluable and I owe many improvements in the text to their comments. In particular I thank Bob Learson,

Lynne Ausman, Margo Woods, George Giddings, Vincent Ampola, John Kaylor, and Joe Mendelsohn.

Others' work also enhanced the presentation. Terry O'Hara did some careful research for me and Mike Walsh pulled me through more than one computer crisis. Jim and Robin Orr from Memorial University in St. John's Newfoundland, provided data and guided me through more discussions of organic chemistry than I would have thought possible to endure. It turned out to be fun!

Jean Hammond is a talented artist and designer with whom I have worked for several years. Her skills shaped the book and her illustrations enliven it. It is always a pleasure working with her.

Being married to a lipid biochemist who is expert in both platelet and cholesterol metabolism is a distinct advantage in writing a book of this sort. My husband, Arie Derksen, strengthened and polished the material in many parts of the book. In addition to his scholarly contributions, Arie sustained me with frequent surprises from "The Chocolate Box". He also made sure the whole family survived having a writer in the house, a remarkable feat sometimes.

The person who made the entire project possible is Ian Dore. He is the most giving and forgiving of publishers who knows exactly when to exhort and cajole. His mastery of the editing craft is apparent throughout the book and I am most fortunate to have had the opportunity of working with him.

Joyce Nettleton

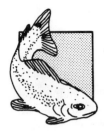

*Chapter One*

# What Is Seafood Nutrition All About?

Excitement and much research activity now mark the quest for understanding about seafood's role in human nutrition. The center of attention is the unique composition of the oil in fish. The excitement stems from the association between the consumption of marine foods and what appears to be a strongly protective effect against the development of heart disease. The original observations were made among Greenland Eskimos, but have been extended to other populations and are currently being investigated among Americans. If fish oil does have the health benefits strongly suggested by current research, the implications for consumers, the seafood industry and health science are enormous:

- the suggestion is that eating seafood regularly can reduce the risk of heart attacks and possibly of other major diseases.

- the demand for seafood will increase.

- the need for nutrition information and consumer guidance for handling and preparing seafood will increase.

- we will extend our understanding of basic metabolic processes and the development of disease.

This book provides basic information about nutrition science with special reference to the nutritive aspects of seafood. The major health problems in America are discussed briefly with emphasis on the ways seafood can promote good health. Tables of nutrient composition are provided which compile the most recent and reliable sources of information in the scientific literature.

Seafood is usually subjected to a variety of processing and cooking procedures before it is consumed. The effects of these processes on nutritive value are discussed. The nutritional merits of new developments such as minced fish and products from surimi are assessed. The book also reviews additives that may be present from both intentional and unintentional processes.

Finally, the book discusses the use of nutrition and health information in the marketing of seafood. Consumers are reluctant about some aspects of handling seafood and suggestions are given for overcoming these consumer worries. Food and nutrition labeling is discussed in relation to seafood. Ideas are proposed for using the health and nutrition benefits of seafood in promoting consumption of fish and shellfish.

Throughout the book care has been taken to document what is being said with evidence from the scientific literature and published resources. Unpublished data are listed as personal communications from the author. References are listed by number in brackets like this (xxx) in order of first appearance in the text. The list of references is at the end of the book, immediately before the index. The references not only document the statements made but give the reader additional sources of information about a particular topic. Assumptions made in interpreting data and arriving at conclusions are defined.

## What Nutrition Means

The simplest definition of nutrition is, "the food you eat and how your body uses it."*(1) Stated differently, nutrition is the partnership between your body and its diet, with each helping the other. Nutrients are those elements and substances the body requires to function and cannot make for itself. Examples are amino acids like tryptophan, vitamins like ascorbic acid and all minerals.

To the body, nutrients are chemicals that are processed for the body's biochemical and physiological needs. They come from the food we eat and from the recycling of tissue products. The breakdown of foods into their chemical parts, the absorption of nutrients from the gut, their transport in the blood to various organs and their ultimate fate in tissue cells are the activities we mean by the term metabolism. We speak of the metabolism of specific nutrients, metabolism in an organ such as liver or, more generally, the metabolism of foods. Each of these uses of the word metabolism implies a different level of detail but each includes the body's handling of substances through its biochemical processes.

Foods may contain other substances that are not actually nutrients, but which affect our well being. We think of nutrients as being essential: that is, the body cannot manufacture them for itself and depends on food for its supply. But there are other substances in food that affect how nutrients are handled and influence health. Examples of such substances are dietary fiber, carbohydrates, cholesterol and certain fatty acids in fish oils. When we include them in the discussion of nutrition, we recognize their importance in body function but do not imply that they are nutritionally essential in the strict sense of the term.

The body's concern is to obtain the nutrients it needs in appropriate amounts so that it can perform both the routine and unusual tasks required of it. These tasks, like providing the energy for muscular contractions, are really a series of biochemical reactions in which various nutrients participate. In its simplest form, nutrition can be reduced to basic biochemistry.

*References are at the end of the book, immediately before the index

Seafood nutrition refers to the relationship between nutrients and other substances in seafood and the body's biochemical needs. How one handles food and its constituent nutrients depends on which foods or food combinations are consumed and on the individual and his requirements. We can describe seafood according to its nutritional merits, but in the end the contribution of seafood toward good nutrition depends not on seafood alone but on the other foods we eat as well. Seafood is a vital spoke in the wheel of nutritious eating.

## What Makes A Food Nutritious?

Determining the nutritive value of a food involves several steps:

- determining which nutrients are present in the food

- evaluating the amounts of nutrients present

- selecting an appropriate serving size so that the quantity of nutrients can be assessed

- considering the effects of processing and cooking on nutrients remaining in the food as it is consumed

- compiling all the information from the above steps into a useful yet relatively simple appraisal of nutritive value

Determining which nutrients are present in food depends on having data about the nutritional composition of the food. This information is found mainly in the United States Department of Agriculture (USDA) Handbooks of Food Composition (2), research findings published in the scientific literature and information made available from private research organizations. One of the most recent compilations of nutrient data for seafood is Sidwell's review of the literature published in 1981 (3). Data from this source as well as more recent publications have been compiled and presented in Chapter Nine.

The use of tables of food composition appears straightforward but it is well to be aware of their difficulties and shortcomings.

- There may be no composition data for the item you are interested in, or there may be no values for certain nutrients.

- There are difficulties with the data themselves, for many assays are not as sound as we would wish; there may be newer, more reliable methods, but no recent analyses for the item you want.

- There may be a wide range of reported values but insufficient evidence for determining which values are most reliable.

- There may be data for the raw form, but not the cooked; or not for the item cooked in the style you seek.

These difficulties are especially relevant to seafood. Clearly, getting the data is seldom a straightforward procedure. The final values often entail making assumptions that may be challenged. The soundness of data in tables of food composition may need careful evaluation. For example, a figure from averaging two widely differing values may be a very poor estimate of the true nutrient level in the food. A basis is needed for determining which of the two values (if either) is likely to be valid. Certainly the average is no more helpful than each of the disparate figures and without knowing something about the two observations and the way they were made, probably both should be discarded.

The analyses for cholesterol in shellfish made several years ago demonstrate another of the problems and pitfalls in the interpretation of nutrient data. The information for cholesterol was based on the analytical results for total sterols. As laboratory techniques became more sophisticated, it turned out that only a small portion of the total sterols present in certain seafoods such as lobster was actually cholesterol (4). Thus, lobster gained a reputation for being relatively high in cholesterol, whereas more recent analyses have shown it to be relatively low in cholesterol, about 70 milligrams per 100 grams on an uncooked basis (5) – virtually the same as for flounder or trout (6).

But let's assume we have data we can trust. Chapter Nine brings together carefully reviewed data from many sources and is intended to be the most comprehensive and accurate data bank of seafood nutrient information to date. The next step is to evaluate the amounts of the nutrients present. No single food, except human milk for young infants, contains all the nutrients we need in adequate amounts. We must eat a variety of foods to get everything we require. That means that we should not expect any one food to be nutritionally complete. What nutritionists try to do is summarize a food's nutritional strengths and limitations. Then we suggest how best it fits into healthful eating.

To make an evaluation of the nutritional content of a food, compare the amount of each nutrient present in the food with the amount of the nutrient we need. Each person's nutrient needs are slightly different, but recommendations of safe and adequate amounts of nutrients that virtually all of us need to consume have been published by the Food and Nutrition Board of the National Academy of Sciences (7). These recommendations are known as the Recommended Dietary Allowances or RDAs and are periodically revised as more information becomes available. The most recent revision is expected to be published late in 1985. The amounts suggested in the RDAs differ according to the age of the populations but for most practical purposes the figures for adult men are used. Dietary needs of children, seniors and pregnant women are different, and those needing the details will find them in reference (7).

It should be observed that the 1980 RDAs were appropriate for use with groups of people, not for individuals. In the 1985 revised edition of the RDAs, the tables are expected to be appropriate for use for individuals. The revised figures are described as "the levels of essential nutrients that are judged to be adequate to protect practically all **healthy** individuals from nutritional deficiencies." (8) The RDAs are set up in such a way as to cover the needs of about 98 percent of the healthy population and include a safety factor to allow for individual variation in nutrient needs. They are not perfect, but they are the best estimates we have for assessing nutritive value.

The RDAs suggest nutrient intakes for some, but not all, of the nutrients we need. No RDA exists where there is not enough data to make a reasonable recommendation. The RDAs are based on estimated total daily nutrient needs. In appraising a food, we consider what a typical serving might provide. The amount of the nutrient present in a serving can be expressed as a proportion of the total day's recommended intake. The RDAs are the most commonly used basis of comparison and one is likely to see statements of nutritional value expressed, for example, as "provides one third of the recommended daily intake for protein".

Another set of figures is also used to appraise nutrient content. These are called the U.S. RDAs and they are based on the numbers in the RDA tables plus a margin to cover variations in the needs of individuals. They are deliberately generous and are expected to meet the needs of practically all healthy people in the United States. The U.S. RDAs are the basis for the nutrition labeling of foods (see Chapter Six).

Sometimes there are features of a particular nutrient that affect how much of it we need. An example is protein – one of the major nutritional features of seafood. Proteins from animal foods are used more efficiently by the body than those from plant foods. That is because most animal proteins contain all the essential amino acids we need for building tissues, while plant proteins may be missing some essential amino acids or may not have them in adequate quantities to meet our needs. As a result, we need less protein for body functions if we derive it from animal foods, more if we consume only vegetable foods. On the other hand, a little seafood consumed with vegetable protein foods such as rice or beans will extend or improve the nutritional value of the meal.

Although certain nutrients may be present in a food, they may not be fully available to the body. By availability, we mean the proportion of a nutrient that is absorbed and utilized (9). Seldom do we fully absorb and utilize the entire amount of a nutrient present in foods. The presence of interfering substances in a food or meal, like phytate and oxalate that occur in some grains and vegetables, may bind nutrients and prevent their absorption. For example, oxalic acid, naturally present in spinach, decreases the absorption of calcium and zinc from this vegetable.

Availability also has to do with the form of the nutrient. Vitamin A in carrots is present, not as the preformed vitamin, but as its precursor, carotene. In order for carotene to have vitamin value in the body, it must be converted to vitamin A before it is absorbed. It takes about twice as much carotene as it does vitamin A to give the equivalent vitamin value.

The assessment of nutritive value also has to consider the presence of other substances which may be highly desirable, though not essential for life. An example is dietary fiber, primary sources of which are whole grains, fruits and vegetables. Dietary fiber contributes to healthy intestinal function and the control of blood lipids. Fiber may also affect susceptibility to some forms of cancer.

Sometimes there are substances in food which relate negatively to health and well-being when present in substantial quantities. Mercury in fish is an example. High levels of nutrients in foods can be harmful or even toxic if excessive amounts of the food are consumed. Vitamin A in liver and fish liver oils is an example: frequently consuming large amounts could be dangerous. Cholesterol, while not a nutrient, is present in certain foods of animal origin and can contribute to high serum cholesterol levels in some people. A high blood cholesterol level increases the risk of heart disease. The presence of saturated fat along with cholesterol promotes an even greater increase in blood cholesterol level (10).

Occasionally the presence of minimal amounts of a nutrient is highly desirable. A low level of sodium is considered by most health professionals to be a positive attribute of a food. Most of us consume too much sodium which contributes to high blood pressure in many people.

Nutritive value also considers how much and how often we usually eat a food. Generally, foods consumed in small amounts or infrequently do not make important conributions to our health, no matter how packed with nutrients they may be. For example, parsley is an excellent source of vitamins A and C, but it makes relatively little contribution to most people's nutritional welfare because it is consumed infrequently and in minuscule amounts.

Evaluating the amount of a nutrient present in a food depends on how much of the food is considered to be a serving. To meet nutritional needs, recommended serving sizes for meats, fish and poultry are 3 ounces of cooked food. Actual serving sizes are frequently larger. In order to make comparisons between different foods, we usually select a serving size of 3 or 3½ ounces. The convenience of using 3½ ounces is that it is the same as 100 grams, and most nutrient tables express nutrient content in amount per 100 grams. The selection of serving size is arbitrary, but if it is known that the usual consumption of a food is more or less than the figures being quoted, the appropriate adjustments in numbers must be made.

In describing serving size, it should be clear whether or not the nutrient content is based on a cooked or raw portion. Most of the time we eat seafood cooked, whereas most nutrient data are expressed on a raw basis. Calculations for estimating the nutrient content in cooked seafood are discussed in Chapter Five. It takes about 4 ounces of raw fish fillet to yield about 3 ounces cooked owing to the loss of moisture. Yield estimates also depend on the method of cooking so this rule of thumb is only approximate. Also, some nutrients may be lost during preparation and cooking.

The nutritional quality of food is affected by processing, handling, storage, and cooking. Uncoated iron cooking pots can enrich foods with iron. The content of some vitamins diminishes with long term storage. Heat destroys certain vitamins; acid and alkali destroy others. Overcooking will diminish most vitamins. Deep-fat frying is an example of how to undermine the nutritive value of a food, not so much because nutrients are destroyed (most are well retained) but because frying greatly increases the fat content of the product, thereby increasing total calories consumed. Deep-fat frying is not always "bad", but as a habit it can contribute to the erosion of good health. The effects of cooking on nutrient retention are discussed in greater detail in Chapter Five.

How we integrate all the above information into a meaningful yet fairly simple nutritive evaluation is discussed in the next section. There is no generally agreed upon assessment tool and every proposal has its supporters and detractors. One of the advantages of nutrition labeling is that it presents nutrition information in a systematic way, even if it stops short of giving a relative appraisal of nutritional merit.

Nutritive value is an assessment of the nutritional merit of a food based on its content of nutrients in the context of its usual serving size. Nutritive value may be considered high when a food contains a large proportion of one or more nutrients we need in addition to energy. Other conditions such as the form of the nutrient, presence of inhibiting or facilitating factors, availability, level of less desirable substances like cholesterol or saturated fat, recommended intake, frequency of consumption and method of storing, handling and preparation will affect how we assess the nutritive value of any one food.

## Assessing Nutritive Value

### Objective Measures

It should be emphasized that it is more appropriate to assess total food intake or food habits as "nutritious" rather than to characterize individual foods as more or less nutritious. That is because good nutrition is derived from our whole food intake, not just from certain foods. Nevertheless, there is a need for assessing and describing the nutritional attributes of individual foods. A nutritious food might be considered as one providing "more than just energy" (11). An excellent discussion of other appropriate criteria for assessing nutritive value is given by Helen Guthrie in (11).

There are both subjective and objective measures of nutritive value. The most common subjective terms we hear are "high" or "low" in one or more nutrients, "rich" in something or an "excellent source of" a nutrient, or simply "nutritious". These terms imply a certain nutritional value, but it is seldom clear what that value is. The most careful use of these familiar terms will be based on an objective measure or established criterion by which a food is described. That is what nutrition labeling tries to do: put an objective basis to statements about a product's nutritive merit.

To assess nutrition information objectively, we need to know the portion of food being considered. Is it a volume measure like half a cup, or an arbitrary unit of weight like 100 grams? We also need to compare the amount present in a serving to the amount recommended for us to consume. Judgements about low or high content can be made later.

Serving size is an arbitrary decision. In order to compare different foods, serving size needs to be expressed in terms of weight, usually grams or ounces. For convenience, the weight of a serving is usually described in household units as well, like one cup or one tablespoon. Household units permit us to visualize an amount on amount on the plate and they relate more clearly to familiar units of measure. Many people are uncertain what 100 grams – or 3½ ounces – would look like on a plate.

Nutrition scientists compare foods on the basis of equal weight. The most common basis of comparison, because it is simple, is 100 grams which is approximately 3 ½ ounces. It is easy to overlook the fact that absolute amounts of nutrients, like number of calories or grams of fat need to be calculated on the basis of usual serving size, as few of us eat servings of 100 grams. Look out for this problem when you read tables of nutrient values. Most of the time you will see figures given for 3 or 3½ ounces or 100 grams of an item whereas the amount we customarily eat may be quite different. As examples, 3½ ounces of caviar would be far too much; while the same amount of steak would appear lonely on most American dinner plates.

It is not easy to decide what a customary seafood serving size is. According to United States Department of Agriculture (USDA) recommen-dations, a serving from the meat group of foods is 2-3 ounces of cooked meat or its equivalent. To meet our daily nutrient needs, USDA recommends that adults eat at least two such servings (12). An entree of fish fillet may weigh between 4 and 9 ounces or even more. An appetizer or soup with shrimp may contain only two ounces of shrimp or less. The decision about serving size should take into account customary food habits and recommended amounts.

The usual basis for gauging how much of a nutrient most healthy individuals and groups of people need is the figures published by the National Academy of Sciences. These figures, known as the Recommended Dietary Allowances (RDAs), are deliberately set above the minimum needs of most people to provide a safety factor for everyone (7). Until recently they were intended to be used as guidelines in planning the nutrition of **groups** of healthy people, not for **individual** dietary assessment. The 1985 revision of the RDAs is expected to be appropriate for individual dietary assessment.

While there is often debate about the actual levels of nutrients suggested in the RDAs, a more serious difficulty is the fact that there are no recommended levels for many nutrients known to be essential. We simply do not have enough information about human requirements to make even sensible guesses.

RDAs have been established for different age groups and for men and women. But having several sets of numbers is too complicated to use in nutrition labeling; one set of figures is needed. The result of this need to compromise is the U.S. RDA, set out in Title 21 of the Code of Federal Regulations (13). These numbers apply to all persons over 4 years old and are based on the most generous estimates of recommended nutrient intakes in the RDAs. It should be emphasized that the U.S. RDAs tend to overestimate the amounts of nutrients we need, but they have the advantage of being safe and permitting product comparisons based on nutrient content. They should not be used as targets for nutrient intake. Moreover, there are no U.S. RDAs for several nutrients like calories and fat.

So we have a dilemma. On one hand there are the RDAs which are not appropriate to use for individuals, and on the other there are the U.S. RDAs, which overestimate the nutrients most of us need. Using a generous "standard" makes it appear that a product is lower in nutrient content than it might really be. For example, if most people need 12 milligrams of a nutrient and the standard is set at 15 milligrams to be on the safe side, the amount of nutrient in a product expressed as a percent of 15 rather than 12 will be smaller. This practice may seem unfair from a manufacturer's standpoint, but is a safer measure for consumers. It is better that a product be likely to contain a higher percentage of vitamins than the amount shown. The disadvantage is that foods making important contributions to the diet do not appear as "nutritious" as they really are on the basis of the numbers found on the nutrition label. Iron is a good example: the U.S. RDA is very high (18 mg) and the amount in iron-rich foods seldom more than 1-3 mg.

In fact, when nutrition labels are devised, manufacturers round their data to the nearest 2, 5 or 10 percent as appropriate. To be on the safe side, the rounding is usually downwards so that the nutrient content of the product is likely to be more than the amount shown on the label. This practice is designed to avoid misbranding of products and to eliminate nutritionally meaningless small differences in nutrient content among products.

In spite of its imperfect nature, the most familiar standard for expressing nutritive value is based on the U.S. RDAs. This system is the backbone of nutrition labeling and the mandatory one for nutrition labels on packages. Use of this system in seafood is discussed in Chapter Six.

As an example of how to evaluate the nutritional qualities of a serving of fish, assume a serving of 4 ounces of baked flounder, which to many Americans would be a small portion. Baked flounder has on the average 30 percent protein (3). The U.S. RDA for protein from animal sources is 45 grams (8). To assess the serving of flounder in terms of its protein content:

1. Convert ounces to grams:
   (1 oz. = 28.4 gm)   4 oz. × 28.4          = 113.6 grams flounder

2. Calculate grams of protein:
   (30% protein)   113.6 × .3               = 34.1 grams protein

3. Express grams of protein as a
   percent of the U.S. RDA for protein
   $\dfrac{34.1 \times 100\%}{45}$           = 75.7% of the U.S. RDA

4. Round answer to the nearest 5
   grams:                                    = 75% of the U.S. RDA

These calculations show that a single, modest serving of baked flounder provides three quarters of the recommended daily protein intake for an adult. Putting this calculation into the perspective of a whole day's food, it means that by this serving alone one can nearly fulfill the day's entire recommended protein intake. Then, consider what the contribution of other parts of the meal and other meals of the day might be to the total protein intake. Clearly, Americans consume abundant protein!

This procedure can be repeated for other nutrients present in flounder to obtain a profile of major nutrients. Condensing the profile into a meaningful general statement about the nutritional value of flounder is the final task and not an easy one. Consideration of characteristics like low levels of less desirable nutrients or substances like cholesterol and sodium needs to be included. Finally, the cooking method must be specified, for it too affects the nutritive properties, especially fat and sodium levels.

Similar calculations can be made using the RDAs as a standard for comparison. This is the standard most frequently used by nutritionists in assessing both individual foods and diets. Less refined estimates have to be used for nutrients where no RDAs exist.

Another way of expressing the nutritive value of a food uses the concept of nutrient density. This approach attempts to relate the amount of one or more nutrients to a common base, usually the energy value of a serving of the food. One example is the Index of Nutritional Quality (INQ) developed by Sorenson and others (14). This is an expression of two ratios which relate nutrient requirements to energy requirements. Other writers have criticized the INQ and proposed different assessment measures (15, 16).

Nutrients such as protein, fat and carbohydrate, which can be converted to energy in the body, can be expressed in terms of calories. Therefore it is possible to compare them on the basis of their respective calorie equivalents.

Nutrients like vitamins and minerals that do not have a calorie value need a different basis for comparison and this requirement has led to another use of nutrient density. Nutrient density may be expressed as the amount in weight of the nutrient per total calories in a serving, or per 100 calories. The differences in units among different measures of nutrient density are confusing and the resulting number difficult to interpret. Calculations of nutrient density are generally not used in consumer information publications.

Expressing fat as a percentage of calories, instead of amount in grams, may have some advantage in communicating the caloric importance of fat, since consumers are unfamiliar with grams. It is unclear whether replacing gram numbers with percent numbers actually helps much in practice. There is an urgent need for simple ways to teach consumers to appraise the amount of fat in foods. Nutrition labels give fat in grams and a simple system of low, moderate and high values or symbols would be very useful. Another difficulty with nutrient density is how to consider all the nutrients present. What does one do with a series of nutrient density figures for each of the nutrients present? One answer is simply to take an average of all the nutrient densities calculated. This would give a single estimate of nutrient density. The problem with averages, of course, is that they are distorted by extreme values. A food with a very high content of one or two nutrients would yield a misleadingly high average value. In the long run, this might not be so bad, since foods with high levels of one or two nutrients tend to be considered nutritious by less rigorous methods of assessment anyway. But this assumption does not always hold (17). An example is oranges, which have large amounts of vitamin C and potassium and very little else. Distorted values do make comparisons between different foods more difficult.

Nutritionists have struggled with the problem of obtaining a single satisfactory numerical rating of nutritive value. A variety of indexes have been proposed and criticized (11, 15). Recently, Russo and colleagues devised a nutrition quotient to estimate the nutritive value of several different kinds of foods (18). This estimate used calories and eight major nutrients as its basis. From the nutrition quotient the authors derived a four star rating scale which could be applied to individual products.

Russo et al. tested their nutrition quotient and rating scale among consumers and found improved attitudes and knowledge. Other formats tested also resulted in improvements. The importance of this particular study is that, in spite of the oversimplification of nutritive value that a numerical index implies, such an index can be helpful to consumers. Perhaps we ought not abandon the challenge of devising objectively based rating scales, in spite of their shortcomings.

We are still left with the problem of missing values for nutrients and what to do about negative attributes of a product, like high sodium or cholesterol level. There are ways of handling these problems but the options become increasingly subjective, even though they may be represented eventually by a single number or illustration. It is important to remember the presence of negative nutrient factors if a realistic assessment of nutritive value is to be communicated and misleading advertising messages avoided.

## Subjective Measures

Subjective measures of nutritive value are opinions. An educated appraisal can be better than nothing in the absence of objective criteria.

Subjective measures of nutritive value purport to give a "rough cut" of how good a source of nutrients a particular food may be. It is helpful to know if a food is high in a nutrient we need or low in something we are trying to avoid. Most of us would rather just be told that something has low, moderate or high nutritional merit. The main problem is that everyone has a different idea about what constitutes low or high, about the relative hazards and benefits of certain substances, about the importance of any single food and about the desirable goals for nutrient intake.

A well publicized example of a subjective standard or goal is the recommendation by the American Heart Association and other professional groups that Americans consume no more than 300 milligrams of cholesterol per day (19, 20). This goal or guideline was derived from the evaluation of numerical data, clinical experience and the opinions of experts in heart disease. Indirectly it has an objective basis, but it is primarily the weight of collected opinion.

Even though a cholesterol intake of no more than 300 milligrams per day is a subjective goal, it can be used as a standard for assessing nutritive value in the following way: compare the cholesterol content of a serving of food with 300 and express the result as a percent of the recommended (maximum) intake. In this way, the contribution of a single food can be put into the perspective of a person's total daily cholesterol intake. Taking this approach with shrimp, which has a reasonable amount of cholesterol, it is clear that with a moderate serving size, e.g., 3 ounces, and the avoidance of other cholesterol-rich foods that day, you can enjoy a shrimp entree and still keep within the recommended cholesterol intake for the day.

The advantage of subjective measures is that they are relatively easy to understand, largely because they are expressed in simple terms. They distinguish between the extremes of low and high nutrient content or merit and they save us the bother of coping with numbers.

The problem is that there is seldom any standard or basis for describing a food's nutritional properties in simple terms. One person may think that 20 percent of the recommended intake of a vitamin contained in a serving of a food makes that food a rich source of the vitamin, while another may rate 20 percent as only fair. The Code of Federal Regulations requires that a "significant" source of a nutrient be at least 10 percent of the U.S. RDA for that nutrient (21).

Where nutrients are scarce, poorly available and generally consumed in inadequate amounts, as is the case for iron, a food source of 5 or 10 percent may make an important contribution to a person's total daily intake, especially if one consumes many foods which have small amounts. The total from the entire day's food becomes more important than any one food source. With a nutrient like vitamin C, which is widespread among fruits and vegetables, some foods may have 5 or 10 percent of the recommended amount and others over 100 percent. If the foods having close to 100 percent of the recommendation are widely consumed, then those having small amounts contribute little to the overall intake of vitamin C. Thus, the 5-10 percent level of vitamin C in foods would be much less important than the similar level is for iron.

A problem subjective measures share with objective measures is that they frequently tell only part of the story. Swordfish is an excellent source of protein but it may also have undesirably high levels of mercury. Tuna, if packed in water rather than oil, has fewer calories and very little fat but is its sodium content out of sight? These are the sorts of issues both consumers and the seafood industry face, but sometimes from different perspectives.

Subjective measures allow considerable freedom to assess negative nutrients and substances like sodium, cholesterol and fat. They permit a clearer interpretation of a numerical value, but only when backed by a sound rationale, objective measures or substantial professional agreement. The reader's instinctive reaction to the descriptive virtues of a food's nutritive value must be the question "On what basis do you say that?" When there is no clear answer, be skeptical.

In the end, the nutritive value of a food does not stand alone. We consume many other foods over the course of a day, week and lifetime. This book attempts to present a perspective on the nutritional merits of different kinds of seafood by looking at the content of various nutrients, and then appraising the ways seafood can contribute to healthful habits. And for healthful living, seafood has a lot going for it!

*Chapter Two*

# Nutrients and Substances in Fresh Seafood

---

## Calories and Protein

### Calories

To the physicist and the body, the calorie is a measure of energy. It is the amount of heat required to raise one kilogram of water one degree Celsius. As you might guess, one calorie* is not much heat or energy.

We can measure the number of calories in a food by completely burning a sample of it in a special heat measuring device called a bomb calorimeter. The amount of heat produced is a measure of the total energy value of the food. The body processes food in a somewhat similar fashion by breaking it down or oxidizing it to release energy. The body is not quite 100 percent efficient, however, and the energy it obtains from foods is somewhat less than that obtained by complete combustion in a calorimeter. Hence the physiologic energy values for food are slightly less than the true chemical values.

We do not usually determine the calorie value of a food by direct measurement. Instead, we calculate by adding the energy value of its components. In most tables of food composition, the energy values have been derived by this type of calculation.

The components of food which yield energy when digested, absorbed and metabolized by the body are carbohydrate (sugars and starch), fat and protein.

*The calorie described above is really a kilocalorie (kcal), or Calorie with a capital "C." It refers to the energy applied to one kilogram of water. The calorie with a small "c" is too small a unit to be useful. Common usage has dropped the kilo from kilocalorie, which means that we measure in kilocalories but talk in calories (22). Calorie in this book refers to kilocalorie.

Each of these has its own physiologic energy or fuel value:

Carbohydrate:   4 calories per gram
Fat:            9 calories per gram
Protein:        4 calories per gram
Alcohol:        7 calories per gram

The calorie value of any food is determined as shown in the example in table 2.1.

---

**Table 2.1.   Sample Calculation to Determine the Calorie Value of 100 grams of Atlantic Cod Fillet.**

| Energy source | Amount in Grams* | Conversion Factor for Calories | Calories |
|---|---|---|---|
| Protein: | 16.4 | 4 | 65.6 |
| Fat: | 0.6 | 9 | 5.4 |
| Carbohydrate: | 0 | 4 | 0 |
| **Total Calories:** | | | 71.0 |

*Data from Table 9.1, Chapter 9.

---

It should be noted that some tables of food composition use slightly different values from those given above. Differences may be particularly noticeable for foods high in protein, like seafood, where values of 5 or greater may be employed as the energy equivalent of protein (23). When it is not stated otherwise, assume that calorie values in this book have been calculated using the

---

**Table 2.2   Finfish Species with more than 2 percent Carbohydrate**

| Species | Grams of carbohydrate per 100 grams |
|---|---|
| European anchovy, raw, whole | 2.1 |
| Silver butterfish | 2.3 |
| Carp | 2.1 |
| Catfish, freshwater, several species | 2.6 |
| Silver hake *(Merluccius bilinearis)* | 7.2 |
| Herring | 6.4 |
| Mackerel, Atlantic | 8.2 |
| Mackerel, king | 2.6 |
| Sardine *(Sardina ocellata)* | 3.9 |
| Tuna, big-eye, dark meat | 2.5 |

Source: Sidwell (3)

---

above conversion factors. In the tables in Chapter Nine where calorie values have been calculated, the Atwater energy values from USDA Handbook No. 8 have been used. They are: protein 4.27 cal/gm, fat 9.02 cal/gm, and 4.0 cal/gm for carbohydrate.

Seafoods have some unusual composition features that do not apply to many other foods. The first is that most fish do not have appreciable carbohydrate. Many species have less than one half of one percent. A few species with more than 2 percent carbohydrate are listed in table 2.2. For all practical purposes, the calorie values of seafood are based only on the fat and protein content. Shellfish may have 5 percent carbohydrate or more and this amount is usually included when calculating the caloric value of shellfish.

The second unusual feature is that a few species have their fat predominantly in the form of wax esters instead of triglyceride. These wax esters are believed to be indigestible by humans, so that the "fat" content would not contribute to the calorie content of the fish. Two examples are orange roughy and black oreo from New Zealand.

Finally, it should be emphasized that all calorie values of foods are approximate. In giving calorie values in recipes, charts, point-of-purchase materials and so on, the values should be rounded to the nearest 5 or 10 calories. It is misleading to imply that the calorie value of food is known to a level of accuracy unwarranted by analytical methods. It is a good habit to quote calorie values as "about 200 calories" or "approximately 200 calories" rather than as exact figures.

Although most seafood has virtually no carbohydrate, it is mentioned here briefly because it is important in breadings and batters used in many popular seafood products. Carbohydrates consist of sugars and starches. Sugars may be composed of one or two simple sugar units. Examples of simple sugars or one sugar units are glucose (dextrose), fructose (found in honey) and galactose. Examples of two sugar units or disaccharides are sucrose (table sugar), lactose (milk sugar) and maltose (corn syrup).

Simple sugars are metabolized quickly by the body to yield energy. Sugars have no nutritional function other than as a source of energy. Because they are sweet, however, they do make many foods more enjoyable. Consuming too many sugar-rich foods contributes to weight gain and tooth decay and displaces more nutritionally worthwhile foods from the diet.

Complex carbohydrates are called starches and they are found only in plants. Starch is composed chemically of repeating units of glucose. Starches are used in breadings, batters and sauces. Small amounts of animal starch (glycogen) are found in some seafoods.

Starch and glycogen are broken down into glucose during digestion. Like sugar, starch is a source of energy. The main reason starches are preferable to sugars is that they can contribute dietary fiber. While processed starch as in pasta does not contain appreciable fiber, the starch found in cereals, grains, fruits and vegetables can make a useful contribution to good health. Because starch takes longer to digest than sugar, it also helps to make you feel full.

The other form of carbohydrate found in foods is a modified form of starch called dextrin. When starch is partially broken down during digestion or processing, smaller units of glucose chains are formed. Called dextrins, these contribute only energy or calories to the body, like sugars and starches.

The most important feature of carbohydrates is that they contribute energy to the body. Sugars, starches and dextrins all have a fuel value of about 4 calories per gram.

## Protein

The cardinal virtue of all seafood is its high quality protein. Seafood supplies not only abundant amounts of protein but also the kinds of protein most efficiently used by the body. Protein supplies amino acids from which the body makes new proteins. To make these new proteins, about nine amino acids are "essential"; that is, they cannot be manufactured by the body (24). Other amino acids used to make proteins can be made in the body and are thus called "nonessential" amino acids. What makes a food protein "complete" or "high quality" is the presence of all the essential amino acids. With few exceptions, most proteins from animal products are complete. All seafood provides complete protein so that less of it is required by the body to meet its daily protein needs.

Another feature of seafood protein is that it is highly digestible. This means that it is readily broken down by the body and easily absorbed. People of all ages, from children over a year to seniors, can enjoy seafood because its protein is highly digestible.

---

# Fat, Omega-3 Fatty Acids and Cholesterol

## Fat

In recent years, the word "fat" has taken on a rather nasty connotation since we have been frequently reminded that many of us possess too much of it, that we should lose some of it and that we eat too much of it. The kinds and amounts of fats in foods have been linked to the development of heart disease. Much advice has been given about how much and what kind of dietary fats we should be eating. It is likely that the advice we hear about the kinds of fat we should eat will be changing. The rapid developments in our understanding of the unique properties of fish oils suggest that the kinds of fat in fish may be especially beneficial for heart health. In order to understand these developments, it may be helpful to refer to the glossary of terms relating to fat in the box on the next page.

Fats belong to a class of substances called lipids. The term lipid refers to any substance that dissolves in an organic solvent like nail polish remover or ether. Lipids include triglycerides or fats, phospholipids, waxes, sterols and others. When we use the term fat we are usually referring to what the biochemist calls a triglyceride. Triglycerides are found in our bodies, in plant and

## Summary of Terms Relating to Fat

**Lipid:**  a general term for all substances that are soluble in organic solvents like ether or nail polish remover. Lipids include triglycerides, phospholipids, waxes and steroids.

**Triglyceride:**  the most common form of "fat" in food and the body. Triglycerides are composed of a 3-carbon chain to which are attached 3 fatty acids as shown below:

*Fig. 2.1   Shorthand Structure of a Fat or Triglyceride:*

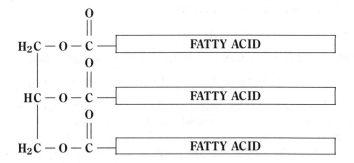

**Oil:**  a fat that is liquid at room temperature; it contains unsaturated fatty acids.

**Fatty Acid:**  a molecule consisting of a chain of carbon atoms to which many hydrogen atoms and two oxygen atoms are attached. The structure of fatty acids may be written in shorthand with the number of carbon atoms before the colon and the number of double bonds after. Palmitic acid, a saturated fatty acid with no double bonds, would be written 16:0

**Saturated Fat:**  these fats are comprised mainly of fatty acids that cannot take on more hydrogens in their structure and thus are "saturated." Saturated fats are solid at room temperature and are found mainly in foods of animal origin as well as in coconuts, avocados, margarine, shortening and palm oil.

**Unsaturated Fat:**  a general term referring to fats that contain fatty acids which can take on additional hydrogen atoms in their structure. These fats are soft at room temperature.

**Monounsaturated Fat:**  these fats contain fatty acids that can take on two hydrogen atoms in their molecular chain. These fats are usually soft at room temperature.

**Polyunsaturated Fat:**  these fats contain fatty acids that can accept four or more hydrogen atoms in their chain. Highly polyunsaturated fats like those in fish oils can take on many hydrogen atoms. Polyunsaturated fats are liquid at room temperature and are found in vegetables, grains, nuts and seafood. Examples are corn oil and cod liver oil.

**Phospholipid:**  like triglycerides, phospholipids are derivatives of glycerol with a 3-carbon chain backbone. They have two fatty acid chains plus a phosphate-containing group attached to the glycerol. The phosphate may have attached to it a variety of molecules or "groups" which define each particular phospholipid. For example, lecithin is a phospholipid where choline is attached to the phosphate group.

animal foods and in seafoods. Triglycerides differ from one another by the kinds of fatty acids they contain. Those containing polyunsaturated fatty acids are liquid at room temperature and are called oils. Corn and safflower oil are familiar examples. Those containing a large proportion of saturated fatty acids are solid at room temperature. Examples of these are beef fat, lard, vegetable shortening and butter.

Fats from foods serve us in several important ways.

- First, they furnish the essential fatty acid, linoleic acid.

- Second, they supply abundant energy for physical acitivity, the body's chemical processes and heat.

- Third, fats often provide fat-soluble vitamins.

- Fourth, food fats are a relatively inexpensive form of calories.

- Fifth, fats add both palatability and pleasure to the foods we eat.

We need a small amount of fat in our food. Fats, especially vegetable oils, contain an essential fatty acid called linoleic acid that the body cannot make for itself. The amount of linoleic acid required is small and is easily obtained from the foods we commonly eat, especially vegetables and seafood. It also appears that linolenic acid, a second fatty acid, is probably essential in humans. The evidence for its essentiality comes from studies with non-human primates and clinical conditions in people (25, 26). It may also be that the omega-3 fatty acids in fish oils are necessary for optimum health, but definitive evidence for this is still lacking (27, 28).

It is easier to criticize fat than to admire it, but we can certainly respect it for its engineering. Fat was designed as a lightweight energy source to provide fuel between meals. Long ago, when humans were hunters and gatherers, time between meals was often lengthy. By being able to store more than twice as much energy per unit of weight in the form of fat, rather than as less efficient fuel sources like carbohydrates and proteins, man avoided the need to develop a massive frame to carry his energy needs with him.

Nowadays, we still carry our energy reserves with us as fat, but we tend to use it less often between meals. For many of us, this results in a gradual weight gain over time.

It is wise to heed the health warnings about eating too much fat. Most of us consume 40 percent or more of our daily energy or calories as fat. It appears that this is too much, from the stand-point of heart health, body weight and obesity, diabetes and some forms of cancer. We would be better off at a level of about 30 percent or less. The bottom line for good health is "eat less total fat". This is just what the Dietary Guidelines, published by the USDA and the Department of Health and Human Services, advise us to do (29, 30).

The other aspect of dietary fats is the type or composition of the fat. While all fats have the same energy or calorie value of about 9 calories per gram, which is about 40 calories per teaspoon, fats differ in their composition. Fats are made of different kinds of fatty acids, that in turn differ in the amount and arrangement of the carbon and hydrogen atoms they contain. The body handles these fatty acids in different ways which have implications for health. We still have a great deal to learn about how the body processes different fatty acids, but it seems clear that some fatty acids are more beneficial for health than others.

In particular, fatty acids which are polyunsaturated, that is, those having a chemical structure that can take on more hydrogen atoms, have been shown to be more favorable for healthy blood lipid (fat) levels than saturated fats. In many

### Table 2.3  Fat Content of Selected Finfish [a] (figures are percentages)

**5% or less fat**

| | | | | | |
|---|---|---|---|---|---|
| Orange roughy | <1 | Striped bass | 2.2 | Spanish mackerel | 5.9 |
| Red hake | <1 | Crevalle jack | 2.2 | Spot | 6.1 |
| Cod, Atlantic and Pacific | <1 | Atlantic whiting | 2.2 | Bluefin tuna | 6.1 |
| Haddock | <1 | Pacific halibut | 2.2 | Cisco | 6.4 |
| Cusk | <1 | Yellowfin tuna | 2.5 | Coho salmon | 6.6 |
| Lingcod | <1 | Brook trout | 2.5 | Sardine | 6.8 |
| Northern pike | <1 | Skipjack tuna | 2.7 | Amberjack | 7.0 |
| Pollock, Atlantic & Pacific | <1 | Ocean perch | 2.8 | Albacore tuna | 7.2 |
| Blue shark | <1 | Wolffish | 2.9 | Arctic chart | 7.9 |
| Mahi-mahi | <1 | Bluefish | 2.9 | Sockeye salmon | 7.9 |
| Red drum | 1.0 | Barracuda | 3.1 | Atlantic herring | 8.0 |
| Red grouper | 1.0 | Scup | 3.2 | Carp | 8.5 |
| Yellow perch | 1.0 | Atlantic sturgeon | 3.2 | Whitefish | 9.0 |
| Rockfish | 1.0 | Tullibee | 3.3 | California pilchard | 9.4 |
| Snapper | 1.1 | Weakfish | 3.5 | Lake trout | 9.4 |
| Tilefish | 1.2 | Atlantic halibut | 3.6 | Pompano | 9.5 |
| Flounder | 1.2 | Sea catfish | 3.6 | Pacific herring | 9.8 |
| Jewfish | 1.3 | Striped mullet | 3.7 | | |
| Walleye | 1.4 | Chum salmon | 4.2 | | |
| Black drum | 1.5 | Swordfish | 4.4 | **More than 10% fat** | |
| Monkfish | 1.5 | Channel catfish | 4.4 | Atlantic mackerel | 10.7 |
| Bigeye tuna | 1.6 | Spanish sardine | 4.6 | Lake sturgeon | 10.8 |
| Pacific whiting | 1.6 | Pacific mackerel | 4.8 | Butterfish | 11.2 |
| Atlantic croaker | 1.7 | Anchovy | 4.8 | King salmon | 11.4 |
| Jack mackerel | 1.8 | Pink salmon | 5.0 | Spiny dogfish | 11.4 |
| Black sea bass | 1.9 | | | Inconnu | 11.8 |
| Blue runner | 1.9 | **5.1% – 10.0% fat** | | Shad | 12.5 |
| Spotted sea trout | 1.9 | Bonito | 5.5 | Sablefish | 14.2 |
| Pacific pompano | 2.0 | Atlantic salmon | 5.6 | American eel | 15.8 |
| Smelt | 2.1 | Rainbow trout | 5.8 | Buffalo | 16.6 |

Source: Table 9.1, Chapter 9.

[a] Fat content shown is the average value for each species; fat content varies with season, sex, geographical location, etc. These values are approximate and should be used only as a guide.

people, achieving a better blood lipid pattern can lower the chances of heart attack or stroke (10). The best ways to achieve a healthy blood lipid pattern are to eat less fat in total, to limit the amount of saturated fats consumed and to keep cholesterol intake below 300 mg per day (31).

Most seafood is relatively low in total fat and relatively high in its proportion of polyunsaturated fatty acids. These features give seafood a clear health advantage, as research is beginning to demonstrate.

Let's take a closer look at fats in seafood. Seafood can be divided into different categories on the basis of fat content. Low fat varieties might arbitrarily be considered as those having no more than 5 percent fat in the muscle on a raw basis. Moderate fat content would be between 5 percent and 10 percent fat and levels above 10 percent fat could be viewed as "high". These divisions are somewhat arbitrary, since there are no agreed upon or government standards for what constitutes low, moderate and high fat. The levels given here are consistent with those recommended by professional nutritionists and health professionals and have been used by others (32).

It turns out that most varieties of finfish and all shellfish contain less than 5 percent fat in the raw muscle. There are only a few species containing on average more than 10 percent fat. Thus a simple categorization of low fat/ high fat species has been suggested (33). The argument for retaining three categories is that other foods having between 5 and 10 percent fat have been described as

### Table 2.4   Fat Content of Shellfish

| Molluscs | % Fat |
|---|---|
| Abalone | 0.5 |
| Surf clam | 0.5 |
| Squid, long fin | 0.7 |
| Scallops | 0.6 – 0.8 |
| Octopus | 0.8 |
| Quahog (cherrystone) | 1.0 |
| Soft-shell clams | 1.2 |
| Squid, California | 1.4 |
| Squid, short fin | 1.8 |
| Mussels | 2.2 |
| **Crustaceans** | |
| Gulf shrimp, mixed | 0.4 - 0.8 |
| Crayfish, freshwater | 0.5 |
| Crabs, mixed species | 0.8 – 1.9 |
| Northern shrimp | 1.0 |
| Spiny lobster | 1.2 |
| Lobster | 1.5 |

Source: Table 9.2, Chapter 9.
For more comprehensive and detailed figures, see table 9.2.

moderate, not high, by others and that three categories is consistent with an easy-to-remember low/moderate/high approach to nutrient quantities (32). For purposes of consumer education, simple memory devices have much to recommend them.

The fat content of the major species of fish is shown in Table 2.3 and of shellfish in Table 2.4.

Fat content of fish is not a straightforward matter. It varies widely with the species (34), within individuals in a species (35), with season (33), physiological status and spawning (36), location in the muscle or body (36, 37), between wild or cultivated sources (38), diet of the fish (37) and geographic location (35, 39, 37).

Oil content may vary from a high of 30 percent during intense feeding to a low of 1-2 percent following spawning (36). The oil content of some species may reach as high as 75 percent (36)! The range for most species is unknown.

An example of the seasonal variation in fat content of spot is shown in Table 2.5.

---

*Table 2.5   Seasonal Variation in the Fat Content of Spot*
*(Leiostomus xanthurus)*

| Date | Average % fat in fillet |
|------|-------------------------|
| May 1979 | 6.73 |
| July 1979 | 8.69 |
| October 1979 | 6.51 |
| November 1979 | 3.84 |
| February 1980 | 0.60 |

Data from Reference 40

---

Most of the data collected on the total fat, fatty acid and sterol content of fish and shellfish are based on very limited samplings and incomplete descriptions of the source of the samples. We know there is great variability, but we have no information to quantify or to correct statistically the values available. This situation is a potentially serious limitation of the seafood nutrient data we have, as emphasized by Stansby (35). Of course, these limitations apply not only to fat, but to protein and to water content as well.

The amount and nature of the fat obtained from different parts of the fish varies enormously. In most species, relatively little fat is found in the muscle, and much of that present is in the form of phospholipid as part of cell membranes (33, 37). Deposits of fat may be found just below the skin, often along the lateral line, and around the belly wall. Since the skin is frequently not eaten, consumption of fish fat may be less than is implied from certain data in nutrient composition tables.

Within the flesh, the oil content is highest in cross-sectional slices closest to the head and least in those near the tail (36). Fat content is also higher in dark flesh than in light (37).

A few species like orange roughy and black oreo from New Zealand have as the predominant fat wax esters instead of triglyceride. For the most part, these wax esters are not digested (33, 41, 42). The fats from these species are sometimes used comercially as liquid waxes.

Fish liver oils differ in fatty acid composition from the oil in the flesh. They usually contain very high levels of fat soluble vitamins as well, whereas the flesh is low in these vitamins. The distribution of fatty acids from the liver, compared with that from the body, generally reveals a lower proportion of the most highly saturated fatty acids. Since the liver contains a great deal of fat, however, the liver becomes an important source of polyunsaturated fatty acids. Thus, consuming whole fish, such as herring or sardines, can greatly increase the amount of polyunsaturated fat from fish.

The fat content of fish varies enormously with how the fish is prepared. Sushi bars notwithstanding, most fish is consumed cooked. High fat fish can have less fat after cooking if methods that allow the escape of fat are used. Such methods as broiling, barbecuing, poaching or steaming on a rack will help remove fat. Trimming away the skin before eating will also remove much of the fat. Conversely, any fish that is fried or has butter added during cooking, or is served with a rich sauce, will have a very high fat content by the time it reaches the dinner plate. The fat content of fish as eaten depends partly on how much fat is present to begin with and partly on how much fat is added or removed during its preparation.

There are two outstanding features about the fat in seafood: the total amount is very low in most varieties and the fat is rich in polyunsaturated fatty acids. The amount of fat eaten with seafood is more likely to come from fat added in preparation and serving than from the fish itself. Polyunsaturated fatty acids help to reduce blood lipids, thereby helping to protect against heart disease.

Seafood oils also have unique properties which render them particularly valuable in healthful diets. These attributes are discussed in the following section.

## Omega-3 Fatty Acids

Fish oils possess at least two unique properties not shared by any other foods. The first is the presence of a relatively large amount of odd carbon chain fatty acids. These are fatty acids with 15, 17 or 19 carbon atoms. The significance of these fatty acids is unknown. The second property is the presence of a high proportion of highly polyunsaturated fatty acids – those having more than four double bonds. While vegetable oils also have a preponderance of polyunsaturated fatty acids, their fatty acids have two or three double bonds. Fish oils have a large proportion of omega-3 fatty acids, having either five or six double bonds. Furthermore, the location of the double bonds in vegetable oils and fish oils is different. The differences in location of the double bonds give rise to differences in the names of the oils from each source.

The vegetable oils contain mainly the omega-6 series of fatty acids while fish oils contain primarily the omega-3 series of fatty acids, although soybean oil contains some omega-3 fatty acid (linolenic acid).

It will be recalled that polyunsaturated fatty acids can take on hydrogen atoms in their carbon chain. The positions where they can do so are known as double bonds and these are created by the removal of hydrogen from the oil molecule. The presence of double bonds, or points of unsaturation, confers several properties on the oil. One of these is a change in the shape or conformation of the fatty acid chains. Changes in the conformation of a molecule often affect its biological activity.

The level of unsaturation renders polyunsaturated fatty acids highly susceptible to oxidation. Fish high in oil content become rancid very quickly if not properly chilled to low temperatures.

The predominant polyunsaturated fatty acids in fish oils are the omega-3 fatty acids. The name comes from the location of the first double bond in the fatty acid chain. Counting from the methyl end of the fatty acid, which is also the last or omega carbon atom in the fatty acid chain, the first double bond is located at the third carbon atom; hence the name omega-3 fatty acids. Omega-3 fatty acids are sometimes called n-3 fatty acids. The terms omega-3 and n-3 are synonymous.

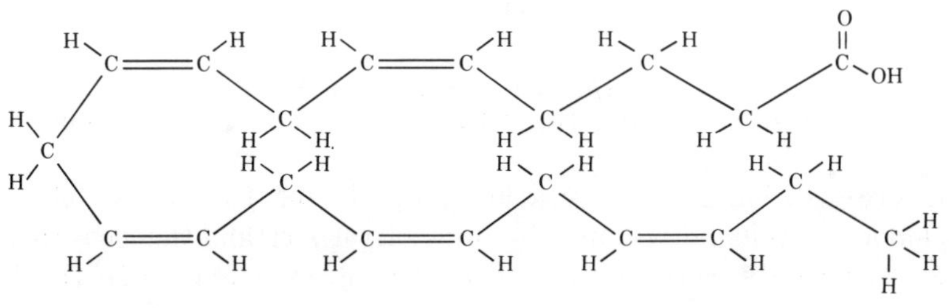

*Figure 2.2    Chemical Structure of EPA (Eicosapentaenoic Acid)*

There are about seven omega-3 fatty acids in fish oil of which two predominate (43). These two are called eicosapentaenoic acid and docosahexaenoic acid – EPA and DHA for short. EPA is a fatty acid with 20 carbons in its chain and five double bonds. DHA has 22 carbon atoms and six double bonds. Diagrams of both detailed and simple structures of the two major omega-3 fatty acids in fish oil are shown in Figures 2.2 through 2.5.

The omega-3 fatty acids in fish derive from the phytoplankton in the food chain that fish eat. Fish, and animals consuming fish, are the primary food sources of these fatty acids, although plant leaves contain small amounts of a similar omega-3 fatty acid (44). Omega-3 fatty acids, like other polyunsaturated fatty acids, remain liquid at cold temperatures, thereby allowing fish cellular membranes to remain fluid in icy waters (45).

Omega-3 fatty acids are distributed in several human tissues including nerve cells, retina, brain and spermatozoa, but to what extent they are essential

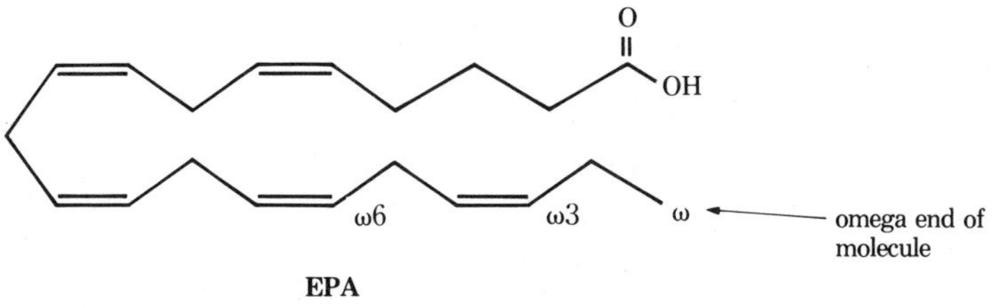

34

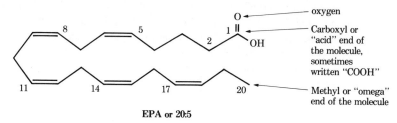

O
‖
OH

ω6    ω3    ω    ← omega end of
                   molecule

EPA

**Figure 2.3    Shorthand version of the Chemical Structure of**
**Eicosapentaenoic Acid (EPA).**

for the proper functioning of these tissues is unknown (45). It is becoming clearer, however, that they are involved in several biochemical pathways (45, 46) and so may influence health.

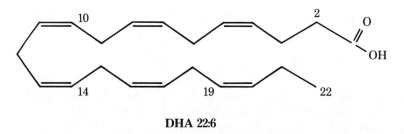

**Figure 2.4    An Alternative Numbering System for EPA**
**Starting from the Methyl or Omega (ω) End of the Carbon Chain.**

Interest in omega-3 fatty acids grew during the 1970s, following the studies among Greenland Eskimos by Bang, Dyerberg and their co-workers (47-51). These scientists were among the first to draw attention to the fact that

DHA 22:6

**Figure 2.5    Shorthand version of Docosahexaenoic Acid (DHA)**

Greenland Eskimos have a much lower incidence of heart disease and other medical conditions compared with Danes and Americans. They associated the low rates of heart disease with several observations: lower levels of plasma cholesterol, lipoprotein and triglycerides; prolonged bleeding times; and altered platelet fatty acid composition. These findings, in turn, were related to the fact that the diet of Eskimos is rich in EPA and DHA, (as well as fat, protein and cholesterol) and that the fatty acids EPA and DHA came from eating marine animals and fish.

Oddly enough, it had been known in 1956 from the work of Ahrens and co-workers (52) that fish oils lower plasma lipids and some workers, notably Stansby, had speculated on the desirable nutritional properties of fish oils (37, 53). An early clinical study, begun in 1952, gave one of the first demonstrations in America of the benefits of a high seafood diet on mortality from heart disease (54). Nevertheless, emphasis was put on lowering plasma cholesterol by consuming vegetable sources of polyunsaturated fatty acids, and the unique properties of fish oils went largely unappreciated. Also, fish oils contain cholesterol, whereas vegetable oils do not. In fact, the cholesterol content of the diets used in earlier studies complicated the interpretation of the results.

Another observation helped focus attention on fish oils. Dramatic reductions in plasma trigyclerides occurred following the intake of omega-3 fatty acids in both healthy subjects and those with abnormally high levels of triglycerides (52, 55-57). Much smaller effects on plasma triglycerides were observed with vegetable oil compared with the fish oil.

Investigators also began studying the reasons for the prolonged bleeding times or slowness of blood clot formation among Eskimos. Several changes in blood platelets were observed, and now the effects of omega-3 fatty acids on a number of biochemical reactions in blood vessel cells, platelets and other blood cells is being studied. Progress is being made rapidly. The research is very exciting and promises a much better understanding of the biochemistry of disease processes and health.

These studies have generated enthusiasm for the potential metabolic and health advantages of dietary fish oils. There remains much to be discovered and such basic questions as how much fish oil is needed to obtain some level of health benefit cannot be answered. The following section summarizes our information to date about omega-3 fatty acids and health. No doubt in the next five years our understanding of the mechanisms of omega-3 fatty acid action will be more sophisticated. We will have a better idea of whether or not everyone can benefit from fish oils and how much seafood we need to consume to enjoy these benefits.

## General Effects on People

The implication from the observations among Greenland Eskimos is that fish oils are protective against heart disease, stroke and possibly diabetes and other diseases as well (45, 58). The Japanese, who eat much more fish than Americans, also have lower death rates from coronary heart disease and where fish consumption is highest in Japan, death rates from heart disease are lowest (59, 60). Finally, a recent study among the Dutch reported lower twenty year mortality rates from heart disease among men who consumed fish than among those who did not (61). The Dutch epidemiologists concluded that "as little as one or two fish dishes per week may be of preventive value in relation to coronary heart disease". While additional data are needed to support this optimistic conclusion, the evidence from these studies definitely points in that direction.

## Effects on Plasma Lipids

**Cholesterol**  In 1959 it was observed that feeding fish oil was more effective than vegetable oil in reducing plasma cholesterol levels (52). A more recent study, in 1983, compared the effects on plasma lipids of feeding salmon oil or mixed vegetable oil (corn and safflower oils) to 12 healthy subjects (62). The effects on plasma cholesterol were similar for the two oils: a modest 11 percent reduction. Other studies have reported reductions in plasma cholesterol but the results are variable (45, 48, 63). The studies are difficult to compare because of differences in study design, levels of fat and cholesterol fed and subjects used. It appears, though, that fish oils are at least as effective as vegetable oils, and may be more so, in lowering plasma cholesterol levels in healthy people (45). By contrast, in people with certain types of blood lipid disorders plasma cholesterol has dropped as much as 45 percent with fish oil enriched diets (57), but there has been no change in patients with other types of lipid abnormalities (64).

**Triglyceride**  The most striking effect of feeding fish oils is a dramatic decrease in the level of plasma triglyceride – a drop of 33 percent in those fed salmon oil compared with no change in those consuming the vegetable oil diet (62). This decrease in plasma triglycerides has been observed by others (55, 63, 65, 66). The implications of this observation in healthy people are unclear, partly because the function of triglycerides in the heart disease process is poorly understood.

The use of fish oils in treating people with disorders of triglyceride metabolism has been remarkable. Decreases in triglyceride from 28 to 70 percent have been reported, depending on the type of disorder (57, 64). Such results are equivalent to what one might expect with pharmacologic doses of drugs. There appears to be enormous potential for the use of fish oil to help people with some forms of high blood lipids.

**Lipoproteins**  Lipoproteins are particles in the blood that transport different lipids, mainly triglyceride and cholesterol. As the name implies, they are composed of lipids and various proteins. Lipoproteins are distinguished from each other by their composition, size and density. They are usually described by their shorthand names of chylomicrons, very low density lipoproteins (VLDL), low density lipoproteins (LDL) and high density lipoproteins (HDL). Those of low density have relatively more lipid than protein – about 80 percent and 20 percent respectively. Those of high density have about equal amounts of protein and lipid.

Chylomicrons and VLDL transport mainly triglyceride, while LDL and HDL carry mainly cholesterol. In the core of lipoproteins, cholesterol is present mostly in its esterified form as cholesteryl ester, but it is most commonly referred to simply as cholesterol.

Fish oil diets have profound effects on plasma lipoproteins and we are only now beginning to understand what some of these changes mean. Healthy subjects fed salmon oil or other fish oils have lower levels of VLDL (very low density lipoproteins) than either the comparison group fed a mixed fat diet or that fed vegetable oil (55, 62, 63). This observation goes along with the finding of lower triglyceride levels, since VLDL is a major carrier of triglyceride in the blood.

In liver, the oxidation or "using up" of fatty acids is apparently greater in animals fed fish oil than in those fed vegetable oil (67). Also, the synthesis or production of fatty acids is reduced, thereby decreasing the need for triglyceride synthesis (67, 68). These observations further support the interpretation that fish oil diets suppress VLDL production in the liver.

How omega-3 fatty acids contribute to the lowering of plasma triglyceride is not known. Goodnight and coworkers have speculated that perhaps VLDL production is diminished or that VLDL removal from blood is enhanced (45). The changes could also arise from alterations in the flux of fatty acids through the liver. Either fewer fatty acids are being brought to the liver from adipose tissue or fewer triglycerides are synthesized from free fatty acids in the liver (45).

Reduced VLDL production by the liver also has consequences for LDL levels in the blood. LDLs are the major carriers of cholesterol and are believed to arise from the metabolism of VLDL particles (69). If there is less VLDL, less LDL would be expected as well. Reduced LDL levels would be beneficial to most people, since a high LDL level is a risk factor for heart disease.

The third major category of lipoproteins is high density lipoproteins or HDL. These particles have gained a favorable reputation for their positive association with lower risk of heart disease (70, 71). In healthy people consuming fish oil diets, HDL levels appear to be no different from those in people fed other dietary fats (55, 62). On the other hand, Nestel observed slightly lower HDL levels in his study of fish oil diets and others have reported increased HDL levels (55, 63, 65). It looks as though the jury is still out on this one.

**Platelets:**  Platelets are the cells in blood responsible for blood clotting. Their composition and function are sensitive to dietary lipids and they become enriched with omega-3 fatty acids when fish or fish oil diets are consumed (50, 65, 72). Changes in platelet composition and function have been suggested to explain some of the clinical findings associated with fish oil diets.

Eskimos have prolonged bleeding times or a greatly increased time required for blood clot formation (50, 73). Since heart attacks result from the formation of one or more clots in heart vessels, clearly factors which discourage clot formation might be protective against heart attack and stroke. Studies have also shown that in Eskimos and others fed fish oils, platelets are much less likely to stick together or aggregate – a measure reflecting clotting (72, 74-76). Pursuit of explanations for these findings has opened an entirely new field in the biochemisty of platelets and ultimately in our understanding of heart disease.

Another effect of fish oil diets is a reduction in the number of platelets (50, 72). This finding could also help explain the reduced blood clotting.

Platelet function can be affected by omega-3 fatty acids. Platelets not only clot blood, they interact with blood vessel walls where fatty plaques accumulate and they produce chemical products such as thromboxanes that affect blood clotting. One scheme to account for the ways in which omega-3 fatty acids might be exerting their effects through platelet and cell membrane metabolism is

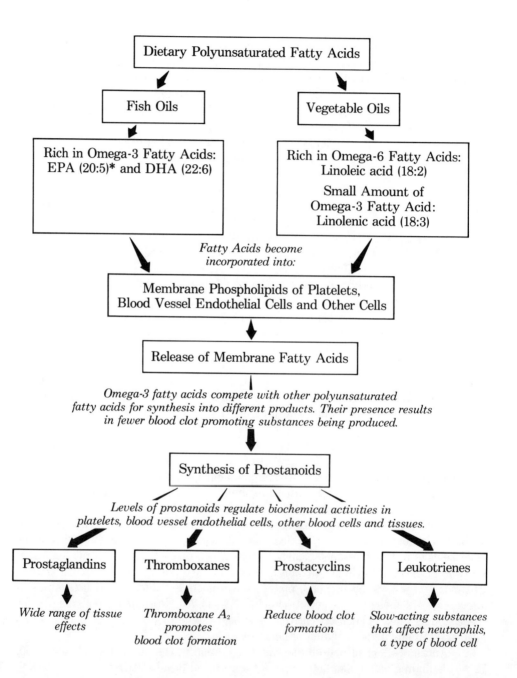

**Figure 2.6  Greatly simplified scheme showing how omega-3 fatty acids might interact with platelets and cells in the blood vessel wall to influence tissue functions and blood clotting.**

*The number before the colon is the number of carbon atoms; the number after the colon is the number of double bonds.

outlined in Figure 2.6. The diagram is greatly simplified, but serves to illustrate how dietary polyunsaturated fatty acids from fish and vegetable oils may be influencing both platelet and blood vessel wall function. The scheme is hypothetical but consistent with evidence accumulated to date.

When omega-3 fatty acids become incorporated into cell membranes, they become available for the synthesis of a group of potent substances known collectively as prostanoids. In Figure 2.6 examples of these substances are given as prostaglandins, thromboxanes, prostacyclins and leukotrienes. Prostaglandins affect a "bewildering" number of body functions and it has been stated that "there is hardly a single organ or function in the body that is not influenced one way or another by prostaglandins" (77). Some of these effects are general such as the contraction of smooth muscle; others are specific, such as the aggregation of platelets. Prostaglandins affect the reproductive system and are potent abortion agents. They affect kidney function, gastrointestinal tract secretions, the respiratory system, especially in asthma, and they lower blood pressure by dilating blood vessels.

One way omega-3 fatty acids might operate is by competing with another polyunsaturated fatty acid, arachidonic acid, for the formation of certain prostanoid compounds. When omega-3 fatty acids are abundant, less of the platelet aggregating substances like thromboxane $A_2$ are produced. When omega-3 fatty acids are absent, different prostanoids predominate. The relative amounts of the different prostanoids are thought to influence metabolic activities in many tissues. Effects of omega-3 fatty acids in the diet have been associated with such diverse clinical conditions as bronchial asthma, psoriasis, inflammatory reactions, immune disorders, epilepsy, arthritis, multiple sclerosis, and malignancies (78, 79). Research in these areas is in the early stages but we can be cautiously optimistic about the outcomes.

There is a growing demand for recommendations about how much fish or fish oil people should consume in order to derive health benefits from omega-3 fatty acids. This question is difficult to answer because we have no information about how little fish might be useful. We know that Eskimos and others who eat fish or other marine foods containing omega-3 fatty acids nearly every day appear to be the healthier for it. We do not know if most Americans would respond the same way, even if we could convince them to eat fish several times a week, but there is no reason to think not.

An important consideration is the interaction in the body between fish oils and other dietary fats. Many of us have become used to considering the amount of saturated fat and unsaturated fat in the diet with the idea that less saturated fat and more unsaturated fat is better. With fish oils as an important source of polyunsaturated fatty acids, perhaps we need to ask the question how much polyunsaturated fat from each source, that is from vegetables and fish, we should be consuming.

If we assume that it is still desirable to keep down the intake of total fat, then fish oils may be an important substitute for other dietary fats – those from animal and vegetable foods. That means substituting fish for fatter cuts of meat and for dairy products. We also consume much of our fat from vegetable sources

### Table 2.6  Omega-3 Fatty Acid Content of Finfish*

| 0.5 grams and under | | | | | |
|---|---|---|---|---|---|
| Sole | 0.1 | Pacific whiting | 0.5 | Pacific mackerel | 1.1 |
| Northern pike | 0.1 | Weakfish | 0.5 | Atlantic herring | 1.2 |
| Pacific cod | 0.1 | Skipjack tuna | 0.5 | Pacific herring | 1.2 |
| Atlantic cod | 0.2 | **0.6 to 1.0 grams** | | Sardine | 1.2 |
| Walleye | 0.2 | Channel catfish | 0.6 | American eel | 1.2 |
| Yellow perch | 0.2 | Red snapper | 0.6 | Atlantic halibut | 1.3 |
| Haddock | 0.2 | Yellowfin tuna | 0.6 | Sablefish | 1.3 |
| Yellowtail | 0.2 | Turbot | 0.6 | Atlantic salmon | 1.4 |
| Sturgeon | 0.2 | Thread herring | 0.6 | Lake trout | 1.4 |
| Rockfish | 0.3 | Chum salmon | 0.6 | Anchovy | 1.4 |
| Brook trout | 0.3 | Striped bass | 0.7 | Coho salmon | 1.5 |
| Silver hake | 0.4 | Wolffish | 0.7 | Pink salmon | 1.5 |
| Striped mullet | 0.4 | Spot | 0.8 | Bluefin tuna | 1.5 |
| Atlantic pollock | 0.4 | Swordfish | 0.9 | Atlantic mackerel | 1.9 |
| Ocean perch | 0.4 | **More than 1.0 gram** | | King salmon | 1.9 |
| Carp | 0.5 | Rainbow trout | 1.1 | Spiny dogfish | 1.9 |
| Pacific halibut | 0.5 | Cisco | 1.1 | Albacore tuna | 2.1 |
| | | | | Sockeye salmon | 2.7 |

* Data based on 100 grams of raw fillet. Figures have been rounded to the nearest 100 mg. Data represent the sum of eicosapentaenoic acid (EPA) and docosahexaenoic acid (DHA). Source: Table 9.1.

as grains and processed foods. It may turn out that a more healthful balance of fat is not necessarily based on the amount of saturated fat compared with unsaturated fat, but rather how much of the unsaturated fat from all foods comes from fish oil. In other words, if we keep the saturated fat down, how much omega-3 fatty acid should we eat? As Lands has expressed it, is the ratio of omega-3 to omega-6 fatty acids in vegetable fats the key (79)? Quite simply, what should be the ratio of fish oils to vegetable oils? It will take more feeding studies in people to answer that question.

The fish with the greatest amounts of omega-3 fatty acids are those with the highest fat content. Sockeye salmon is a particularly rich source of these fatty acids. The amounts of omega-3 fatty acids in fish are given in table 2.6. Although the amounts in lean fish are lower than in fattier species and the omega-3 content of shellfish is generally low, small amounts of omega-3 fatty acids may be quite useful and lean fish and shellfish should not be discounted.

It should also be pointed out that canned fish are a good source of omega-3 fatty acids, but fish packed in oil do not have more of these acids. The oil used in canned fish is vegetable oil, not fish oil.

Omega-3 fatty acids can also be obtained from fish oil supplements. Such non-food sources are rich in these fatty acids. They are also very expensive. Most fish oil preparations are made from fish livers which may contain high levels of fat-soluble vitamins and possibly other undesirable organic substances. The labels of these preparations seldom indicate how well purified the oil is. Capsules and liquid preparations also make it easier to consume excessive amounts which might then interfere adversely with blood clotting. It is safer, cheaper and more palatable to obtain omega-3 fatty acids from fish.

Several cautions about fish oils should be observed:

- Fish oils contain high levels of vitamins A and D which could be toxic if consumed as dietary supplements. Unless these vitamins have been "stripped" or greatly reduced, fish oil concentrates should be avoided.

- We have no idea about the kinds of doses or amounts that are safe or effective for healthy people. Currently, the safest way to get your omega-3 fatty acids is by consuming fish, not fish oil supplements.

- Increases in certain disorders such as apoplexy have been observed among populations consuming large amounts of fish (22). Other undesirable consequences may be as yet unrecognized.

- Fish oil preparations may contain high levels of cholesterol which may be hazardous to people with certain types of lipid disorders; the fish flesh itself is low in cholesterol.

- Large amounts of omega-3 fatty acids might be expected to increase vitamin E requirements.

Recommendations need to be applicable to the general population, to be safe as well as useful and to have good data behind them. We are obtaining the data now but are still quite far from having a data base to help us determine the quantity of omega-3 fatty acids that can be distinctly useful in health. On the other hand it is very clear from the Dutch study and from clinical studies among patients with heart disease that increasing the amount and frequency of seafood in the diet is beneficial in several ways:

- it can reduce the total amount of fat we eat;

- it can reduce our intake of saturated fat;

- it can lower our intake of cholesterol;

- it can provide omega-3 fatty acids.

We can take immediate advantage of these benefits by eating fish at least once a week, especially if it substitutes for a fatter entree. Whether we need to eat fish as often as two or three times a week or more to obtain markedly improved heart health is not known. It certainly would not hurt.

**Advice: Eat fish at least once a week.**

42

## Cholesterol

The word cholesterol is terrifying to many people. The fear derives from the association between cholesterol in foods and the build up of cholesterol-rich material in arteries and blood vessels, which is in turn related to heart attacks and stroke. Many of us have the idea that to consume foods with cholesterol is to invite heart disease; but things are not quite that simple. There are many factors besides food cholesterol which contribute to the build-up of deposits in the blood vessels. Genetic background, amounts of exercise, age and other factors all influence the nearly inevitable accumulation of "plaque" (fatty deposits) in our blood vessels.

Our bodies make cholesterol for use in cell membranes and hormones. The more cholesterol we take in from foods, the less our body makes, but this regulatory system is only partly effective in controlling blood cholesterol levels. High blood cholesterol levels can result from: our genetic make-up; consuming too much cholesterol in foods; excessive cholesterol production in the liver; or failing to excrete the extra amounts. Just how important the dietary source of the body's cholesterol may be appears to be different for different people. Some people are more susceptible than others to the build up of extra cholesterol in their blood. Others can handle the excess without developing high levels of blood cholesterol. This means that for susceptible people, dietary cholesterol is much more critical than for less susceptible people. Only a physician can determine if a person is more than usually susceptible.

Most people are probably not greatly affected by dietary cholesterol, so long as their cholesterol intake is within a moderate level, no more than about 300

### Table 2.7 Approximate Cholesterol Content of Finfish

| | Approximate cholesterol content (mg/100 gm raw muscle) |
|---|---|
| Skipjack, albacore, mullet | less than 30 |
| Hake, whiting, butterfish, spiny dogfish, jack mackerel, red snapper, pollock, Atlantic herring, Atlantic halibut, haddock, channel catfish, sole, flounder, cod, Atlantic salmon, swordfish | 31 – 60 |
| Chum salmon, carp, Atlantic mackerel, big-eye tuna. northern pike, canned chunk light-meat tuna | 61 – 90 |
| Anchovy, canned Atlantic sardine | more than 91 |

**Note:** Reliable data on the cholesterol content of seafood are scant. Cholesterol content varies appreciably with the the method of analysis, sampling, species, etc. and may be viewed as approximate plus or minus 20 percent (109).

Data from References 3, 80-83.

mg a day. People consuming cholesterol in amounts above 500 mg appear to be at greater risk of accumulating the extra cholesterol in their blood. Also, people who are known to be susceptible to heart disease because of their genetic background are urged to consume no more than 300 mg cholesterol a day.

Seafood is not a major dietary source of cholesterol. There are a few exceptions to this general observation, and they are squid, fish roe, black abalone and perhaps blue crab. None of these species is consumed in large amounts by Americans. White shrimp, rock shrimp and spiny lobster have moderate amounts of cholesterol while American lobster meat is not particularly high in cholesterol.

*Table 2.8   Approximate Cholesterol Content of Shellfish*[a,b]

| Approximate Cholesterol Content | Raw | Cooked[c] |
|---|---|---|
| **Molluscs:** | | |
| Abalone | 111 | 160 |
| Soft shell clams | 25[d] | 40 |
| Hard shell clams | 40[d] | 65 |
| Razor clams | 107 | 172[d] |
| Surf clams | 31 – 41[d] | 50 – 66 |
| Mussels | 63 | 60 |
| Octopus | 122 | –[e] |
| Oysters, all species | 50 | 78[d] |
| Scallops, all species | 36 – 43 | 72 – 86[f] |
| Squid | 250[g] | – |
| **Crustaceans:** | | |
| Deep sea red crab | – | 60 – 78 |
| Blue crab | 102 | 120 |
| Jonah crab | – | 78 |
| Rock crab | – | 60 – 71 |
| King crab | 60 | – |
| Lobster | 70 | 85 |
| Spiny lobster | 95[f] | 106 |
| White shrimp | 66[f] | 90 |

[a] Cholesterol content varies appreciably with the method of analysis, sampling species, season, etc. and should be read as plus or minus 20 percent (109).

[b] Data from references 82-86.

[c] Values for cooked seafood are often higher than for the same item raw because of moisture losses during cooking. Cholesterol is well retained by most cooking methods (see Chapter 5).

[d] Estimated from yield data in Chapter 5, assuming 95 percent retention.

[e] Dashes denote lack of yield data from which to estimate values.

[f] Estimated from yield data in Chapter 5, assuming 100 percent retention.

[g] Range is 150 - 400 (5).

But if you are fond of eating the tomale or liver of lobster, you will be consuming a substantial amount of cholesterol. Tables 2.7 and 2.8 present summaries of the cholesterol content of seafood.

Some shellfish have additional sterols besides cholesterol. It is not known whether these have any major effect on human blood lipid levels (4). These other sterols, which are usually plant sterols from the phytoplankton a shellfish consumes, are thought to compete with cholesterol for uptake from the intestine, thus reducing the amount of cholesterol that is absorbed (87).

Finally, most people in America do not eat fish and shellfish often enough or in sufficiently great quantity for the amount of cholesterol present to make much difference. With the findings that most shellfish are low to moderate in cholesterol content, it can be safely assumed that nearly all seafood can be included in both normal and low cholesterol diets (4). With a few exceptions, noted above, cholesterol is not a primary concern with seafood.

## Vitamins and Minerals

### Vitamins

Today in America frank vitamin deficiency is rare. We are more likely to suffer from excess vitamin intake than from too little. This does not mean that everyone is consuming all the right amounts of necessary vitamins, but that the once common deficiency diseases like pellagra are apt to occur only in very unusual circumstances. Some groups of people, like the elderly, pregnant women, teens and children regularly consume smaller amounts of certain vitamins than recommended.

The amounts of several vitamins in seafood have not been adequately investigated. Among the reasons for this are the lack of reliable analytical methods (e.g. for vitamin E), the immense task of analyzing thousands of samples, and the many sources of variation in nutrient content in foods. We also have much to learn about the effects of processing and cooking on vitamin content and availability.

The U.S. Department of Agriculture has undertaken a systematic reanalysis of the composition of foods for nutrients for which reliable laboratory methodologies exist. For other nutrients, we await progress in science and technology. Data from the U.S.D.A., from the National Marine Fisheries Service and from research publications form the basis for the nutrient tables and discussion in this book.

### Fat-Soluble Vitamins: A,D,E and K

**Vitamin A.** Recently, there has been renewed interest in vitamin A because of the suggestion that some forms of the vitamin may be protective against certain cancers. There is not enough evidence at this time to indicate how vitamin A may be involved and it appears that other dietary factors, perhaps selenium, may also be important (88). Vitamin A is toxic in large amounts and convincing evidence for beneficial effects in cancer remains to be shown.

We do know, however, that vitamin A is indispensable for proper vision, especially at night. Insufficient vitamin A leads to night blindness and eventually total blindness. Although the condition is rare in this country, it is widespread in many poor countries. Vitamin A also functions in bone and tooth growth, and tissue integrity (89).

Vitamin A is found in its active form in many animal foods. Because it is fat soluble, it is associated with the fat portion of foods. It is highly concentrated in fish liver oils, but only small amounts are found in fish muscle or fillets. Not surprisingly, high fat fish have more vitamin A than lean fish. Fish are not a major source of this vitamin for most people.

Other food sources of vitamin A are eggs, liver and vitamin A-fortified milk products.

Vitamin A is also found in a "precursor" or inactive form in many plants, particularly yellow and dark green vegetables. This precursor form, carotene, is converted to the active forms of the vitamin upon absorption by the body. Owing to inefficiencies in both absorption and conversion of carotene to vitamin A in the body, only about one sixth of the carotene in foods as eaten becomes available for use in the body as vitamin A. This inefficiency, along with the low consumption of vegetables by many people, contributes to rather low vitamin A nutriture in many groups of the population, especially children. On the other hand, the vitamin A which is consumed is stored in the liver, providing a carry-over for times of dietary shortfalls.

There is another concern with vitamin A. Precisely because it is stored in the body, the potential for vitamin A toxicity is real. Taking vitamin supplements, especially megadoses, or treating acne with vitamin A preparations quickly results in very large vitamin A intakes. Cases of toxicity in both children and adults have been reported with intakes ten times above the Recommended Dietary Allowance (7). Vitamin supplements can be a source of disease, not protection.

**Summary:**

- Modest amounts of vitamin A are present in high fat fish

- Commercial fish oils and liver are a concentrated and "natural" source of vitamin A, but are not commonly consumed

- Lean fish have very little vitamin A

- Fish oil supplements pose a risk of vitamin A toxicity unless the preparations have been "stripped" of their fat-soluble vitamins

**Best Food Sources:**   Liver, vitamin A-fortified milk products, fish oils, carrots, butternut and hubbard squash, spinach, sweet potatoes (yellow) and dandelion greens.

### Table 2.9   Vitamin A Content of Some Fish Liver Oils

| Species, fish liver oil | Approximate Vitamin A Content | |
|---|---|---|
| | RE per gm[a] | I.U. per gm[b] |
| *1980 RDA for adult men* | *1000*[b] | *5,000* |
| *US RDA* | *1500* | *5,000* |
| Cod[c] | 120 – 1,200 | 400 – 4,000 |
| Shark[c] | 135 – 1,800 | 450 – 6,000 |
| Atlantic pollock[d] | 240 – 750 | 800 – 2,500 |
| Petrale sole[e] | 1,200 – 52,500 | 4,000 – 175,000 |
| Spiny dogfish[e] | 3,300 | 11,000 |
| Rockfish[e] | 4,200 – 90,100 | 14,000 – 300,000 |
| Great blue shark[e] | 6,000 | 20,000 |
| Halibut[c] | 6,000 – 108,000 | 20,000 – 360,000 |
| Albacore tuna[e] | 7,500 | 25,000 |
| Bonito[e] | 10,500 | 35,000 |
| Skipjack tuna[e] | 12,000 | 40,000 |
| Yellowfin tuna[e] | 15,000 | 50,000 |
| Halibut[e] | 19,000 | 63,500 |
| Bluefin tuna[e] | 22,500 | 75,000 |
| Soupfin shark[e] | 22,800 | 76,000 |
| Sablefish[e] | 27,000 | 90,000 |
| Swordfish[e] | 75,000 | 250,000 |
| Lingcod[e] | 52,500 | 175,000 |
| Black sea bass[e] | 90,100 | 300,000 |
| **Species, whole fish body** | | |
| Pacific herring[e] | 27 | 90 |
| Pilchard[e] | 30 | 100 |
| Menhaden[e] | 150 | 500[f] |

[a] RE = retinol equivalents = 1 microgram retinol
= 3.33 International Units (I.U.) retinol
= 10 I.U. beta-carotene
1 I.U. vitamin A = 0.3 micrograms retinol
1 teaspoon oil is approximately 4.7 grams

[b] RDAs express vitamin A consumption in retinol equivalents to include both preformed and precursor (carotene) forms of vitamin A in foods. The terminology of I.U. is widespread and has been retained in the US RDAs and on nutrition labels. Most of the vitamin A in liver is preformed.

[c] Data from Reference 90; species not given.

[d] Data from Reference 91 (1949)

[e] Data from Reference 92; average value of all samples.

[f] Range of values given.

**Vitamin D**   Many readers will remember distastefully the days of taking a spoonful of cod liver oil before setting out for school. This was a common practice before dairy products became fortified with vitamin D and dates back to 1842, when Scheutte recommended cod liver oil for the treatment of rickets, a disease characterized by bone deformities (93). It was well known that children developed rickets over the winter and lack of exposure to sunshine was recognized to be part of the problem. In the 1840s, cod liver oil was also being used in the treatment of tuberculosis, although its efficacy was dubious.

In the 1920s, it was shown that rickets could be produced by inadequate diet, but not in animals exposed to sunshine. Eventually it was discovered that the active substance in cod liver oil was also produced in the skin through the irradiating action of sunlight. Since this was the fourth unidentified nutrient to be discovered, it was called vitamin D. It turns out that vitamin $D_3$, as it is now called, is made in the skin from a molecule closely resembling cholesterol.

Vitamin D has several active forms with vitamin $D_3$ coming from animal sources and vitamin $D_2$ from plants. Chemically modified forms of these vitamins are active in different body tissues.

Vitamin D is more properly considered a hormone than a vitamin, although its function in the body is closely tied to other nutrients, especially calcium.

---

*Table 2.10   Vitamin D Content in Several Fish Liver Oils*

RDA for children[a] = 400 I.U. or 10 μg cholecalciferol
RDA for adults over 23 yrs = 200 I.U. or 5 μg cholecalciferol
U.S. RDA = 400 I.U.

| Species | Vitamin D I.U. per gram[b] |
|---|---|
| Fat fish, e.g. herring, salmon, pilchard, sardine, fresh or canned[c] | 2-18 |
| Dogfish[d] | 10-30 |
| Shark[c] | 13-50 |
| Haddock[d] | 50-100 |
| Pollock[d] | 80-100 |
| Cod[c] | 80-300 |
| Ling[d] | 100-200 |
| Halibut[c] | 200-4,000 |
| Swordfish[c] | 2,000-25,000 |
| Yellowfin tuna[e] | 10,000-45,000 |
| Bluefin tuna[e] | 20,000-70,000 |
| Albacore tuna[e] | 20,000-250,000 |
| Skipjack tuna[e] | 25,000-250,000 |
| Bonito[e] | 50,000 |

[a] RDA for children is greater than for adults to meet the needs of bone growth.
[b] I.U. International Units = 0.025μg cholecalciferol (vitamin $D_3$).
[c] Data from Reference 90. Species not given.
[d] Data from Reference 91 (1949). Species not given.
[e] Data from Reference 92.

Vitamin D is converted to its metabolically active forms first in the liver and finally in the kidney. Thereafter it acts in three major sites: the gastrointestinal tract, bones and the kidney.

In the gut, the active form of vitamin D appears to promote the synthesis of proteins which transport calcium across the intestinal wall. Vitamin D is essential for the uptake of calcium by the body.

In bone, another metabolite of vitamin D is active in promoting bone growth. Bone cells are continually renewing bone structure and vitamin D acts to foster the deposition of minerals in bone. It also interacts with other hormones to affect bone metabolism. Vitamin D is required for proper calcium deposition in the treatment of bone disease (osteoporosis) in the elderly.

In the kidney, vitamin D affects the movement of calcium and phosphorus. It also affects the activity of certain kidney enzymes.

Vitamin D does not occur in appreciable amounts in the foods we usually eat. We rely upon exposure of our skin to sunshine and fortification of dairy foods to furnish what we need. The vitamin is concentrated in fish liver oils, but these are not widely consumed in America. Indeed, the concentration of vitamins A and D is so high in some fish oils as to pose risks of toxicity.

The fattier species of fish such as herring, mackerel, lake trout and salmon have some vitamin D. Because these fish are not regularly consumed by most groups, except native populations in the far North, this dietary source does not make an important contribution to the vitamin D welfare of most Americans.

The vitamin D we obtain from sunshine is tightly controlled by the body. The amount varies with the intensity of the sun, the darkness of the skin, and how long the skin is exposed. Fortunately, vitamin D production via skin irradiation is very slow and long periods of "sun bathing" result in the production of compounds other than the vitamin, thus preventing vitamin D toxicity (94). Incidentally, formation of the vitamin is not achieved behind a sunny window – the glass screens out most of the ultraviolet rays necessary for vitamin D production. Fog, smog and foul weather have the same effect. The vitamin is stored in the liver, so a little goes a long way.

## Summary:

- Moderate amounts of Vitamin D are found in fish with a high fat content, but these do not contribute importantly to the nutrition of most Americans

- Fish oils may contain large, potentially toxic, amounts of vitamin D, but these are not widely consumed; they are one of the few "natural" sources of vitamin D

- Vitamin D is obtained mainly from exposure to sunshine and from the fortification of dairy products

- Vitamin D intake is not a major health problem in the USA and is of concern mainly in certain endocrine and bone disorders; it is important, however, in the treatment of osteoporosis in the elderly

• For people who do not consume vitamin fortified milk, and are not regularly exposed to outdoor sunshine, cod liver oil is an appropriate source of vitamin D

**Best Food Sources:**    fish liver oil, high fat fish, eggs, vitamin D-fortified milk and milk products.

**Best Source of all:**    sunshine on a clear day – a fine reason to go fishing!

**Vitamin E**    Another fat-soluble vitamin, known to exist since the 1920s, came to be called vitamin E because it was the fifth vitamin to be discovered (93). This vitamin, found in vegetable oils, was rapidly destroyed by cod liver oil and rancid fats. Only by feeding very large amounts of the vitamin to animals given cod liver oil could the damage from the fish oil be prevented.

The puzzle was solved when it was learned that vitamin E functions as an antioxidant to prevent fats from going rancid. Cod liver oil, because of its large quantity of highly unsaturated fatty acids, required large amounts of the antioxidant vitamin to keep it from going rancid or being oxidized. Similarly, diets containing large amounts of polyunsaturated fatty acids, as are found in most vegetable oils, require increased amounts of vitamin E in order to prevent the oxidation of the fats. The requirement holds for food not only on the shelf or refrigerator but also when consumed. Fortunately, vitamin E is found in most of the same foods as unsaturated fatty acids, so the sources tend to be together.

Current assays are generally regarded as being insufficiently reliable to give firm quantitative estimates of vitamin E in foods (95). The data we do have indicate that seafood is only a modest source of vitamin E. High fat fish have greater quantities than lean varieties and shellfish have very little vitamin E (96). Fish oils are highly susceptible to oxidation or rancidity because of their polyunsaturated fatty acids. It is not known to what extent vitamin E is present in sufficient amounts or is effective in deterring fat oxidation in seafood. Antioxidants may be less effective in fish oils than in other fats (37).

Vitamin E intakes do not appear to be a problem among Americans.

**Best Food Sources:**    vegetable oils, especially soybean, corn, sunflower, and cottonseed; margarine made from these oils; mayonnaise, wheat germ and walnuts.

**Vitamin K**    This is the vitamin involved in blood clotting. It is found mainly in plants, especially green leafy vegetables, broccoli and cauliflower. There are only small amounts in most fish. Most of our supplies are produced "in house" by the bacteria in the intestine, so that supply is not a problem. Only the newborn infant needs vitamin K until its intestinal flora become established a few days after birth.

**Best Food Sources:**    green leafy vegetables, broccoli, cauliflower, liver.

## Water-Soluble Vitamins

**Vitamin C or Ascorbic Acid**   The association of this vitamin with citrus fruits is usually traced to the days of scurvy aboard British sailing vessels in the 18th century. Although the antiscorbutic effects of citrus fruits had been known for at least two hundred years before, it was not until the work of James Lind in 1747 that citrus juice and limes became a regular ration in the Royal Navy. This practice earned the British sailors the nickname 'limeys' and also abolished the dreaded scurvy.

Today, most people are aware of Linus Pauling's efforts to link vitamin C intake with the common cold. Fewer people are aware that this vitamin appears to do nothing to reduce the likelihood of catching a cold, but may slightly decrease the length of the illness. It has become fashionable to take very large amounts of ascorbic acid, thereby increasing risks of kidney stone formations, disorders in the intestine, and subsequent dependency on large amounts of the vitamin (97). It is especially inadvisable for pregnant women: it can lead to scurvy in the mother if intake is suddenly reduced and to unusually high requirements for the vitamin in the newborn.

Vitamin C has important functions in the body. It is necessary for proper wound healing, and for the formation of collagen, a structural part of arteries, veins, gums, cartilage and bone (89). Ascorbic acid participates in a variety of chemical reactions in the body involving hormones and amino acids. It also increases the absorption of other nutrients, especially iron and folic acid.

Ascorbic acid is widespread among fruits and vegetables, especially citrus fruits. Other fruits like strawberries, kiwifruit, mangoes, cantaloupe and vitaminized apple juice provide good sources. Broccoli, red and green peppers, kale, brussel sprouts, collards and turnip greens are excellent vegetable sources. Potatoes can be a good source as well. Seafood, meats, poultry and dairy products are not particularly good sources of vitamin C.

Ascorbic acid is easily destroyed by heat and much may be lost in cooking. (Stability of this and other vitamins is discussed in Chapters Four and Five).

**Best Food Sources:**   citrus fruits, red and green peppers, strawberries, broccoli, greens, potatoes.

## The B Complex Vitamins

**Thiamin**   The notion that foods contain components which are remedies for disease goes back at least to Hippocrates, who advocated liver for the treatment of night blindness. In the late 1890s, a Dutch military doctor in the East Indies observed that chickens fed highly polished rice developed polyneuritis, a disease of the nerves (90). Those fed rice still in the husk thrived. At first it was thought that the polished rice contained a nerve poison and that the rice husk contained a substance which neutralized the poison. Shortly after, the correct interpretation was given: rice husks contained an essential nutrient which could prevent the nerve disease. Soon the feeding of whole rice instead of polished rice to prisoners eradicated the disease beriberi from prisons.

The early work with thiamin supported the concept of "vitamines" which were thought to be organic substances (amines) essential for life (vita). Just how important thiamin turned out to be was shown in the late 1930s when it was discovered that thiamin was essential for the conversion of carbohydrate toenergy. Because of its importance in energy metabolism, the recommended intake of the vitamin is expressed in relation to total energy intake.

Thiamin works in the body as a "coenzyme" – a necessary participant for enzyme activity. It is involved in amino acid metabolism, in the transfer of carbon dioxide groups from one substance to another and in the metabolism of sugars containing 5 carbon atoms. These metabolic activities affect the body's cardiovascular, nervous and muscle systems.

Thiamin is widespread among foods but is seldom found in large amounts in any single food. Most fish and seafood have small amounts of thiamin. Pork is exceptionally high in thiamin. Wheat germ, liver, cooked dried peas and beans, enriched bread and whole grain cereals are the richest sources.

Thiamin is very sensitive to heat and oxygen and as much as 70 percent may be lost in canning and cooking.

**Best Food Sources:**    Pork, wheat germ, liver, cooked dried peas and beans and enriched bread and cereals.

**Riboflavin**    In the early investigations of individual nutrients, much confusion arose over the existence of several "factors" in the water soluble fractions of plant extracts. It was not simple to demonstrate the presence of more than one factor and the crude diets used in feeding experiments were often deficient in more than one nutrient. Nevertheless, astute observers reasoned that more than one nutrient existed in certain vegetables and grains and that nutrients other than thiamin were responsible for the growth-promoting properties of certain vegetables. Distinguishing between thiamin and riboflavin, largely because riboflavin is heat stable and thiamin is not, led to the demonstration of a nutritive yellow substance, then called vitamin $B_2$ (90, 93).

We now know that riboflavin is crucially involved in the conversion of energy from one chemical form to another in every cell. It is used in converting the energy from the fats and carbohydrates in foods to the energy used in muscles and other tissues. Like thiamin, it works as a coenzyme in chemical transfer reactions. It is also necessary for healthy eyes and skin and for growth.

Seafood is a modest source of riboflavin. The dark flesh of some species like pilchard and mackerel are good sources. Fish consumed whole, like smelt, sardines and canned herring are also good sources of riboflavin.

**Best Food Sources:**    liver, milk, meats, dark-fleshed fish, mushrooms, broccoli, turnip and collard greens, okra, winter squash, asparagus.

**Niacin**    Niacin, another of the B vitamins, has a rather famous history, owing to the pioneering work of Dr. Goldberger and his colleagues among the inmates of State institutions in the South. In 1915, Dr. Goldberger demonstrated that the disease pellagra, which was widespread among inmates, could be eradicated by dietary supplements of yeast, meat or milk (93). However, it took another twenty years before the definitive link between pellagra and nicotinic acid, a form of niacin, was demonstrated.

Pellagra, the disease resulting from inadequate amounts of niacin and protein in human diets, had long been associated with diets high in corn. In Mexico, on the other hand, where maize or corn is the staple food, pellagra was almost never seen. Why was this so? It happens that the niacin in corn exists in a "bound" form which is not available for metabolism. In Mexico, maize is prepared by first boiling it with mineral lime. This alkaline process releases the bound niacin and the vitamin becomes available for metabolism.

In humans, niacin can be made from the amino acid tryptophan. Therefore, diets which are low in niacin but abundant in protein will protect against pellagra. For this reason, the dietary requirements for niacin are expressed as niacin equivalents to take into account the conversion of tryptophan to niacin.

Niacin metabolism is antagonized by the amino acid leucine. High dietary levels of leucine can lead to niacin deficiency symptoms. This is not a problem in the U.S., but occurs in some parts of South Africa, Egypt and India (89).

Seafood is a moderately good source of niacin, but there is considerable variation in amount depending on the variety of fish. Some varieties are rich in this vitamin, particularly mackerel, salmon, sardines, swordfish, and tuna. Lean white fish and shellfish tend to have lesser amounts.

Niacin is important in the body in the release of energy from carbohydrates. It is needed for the synthesis of fats and cholesterol and is required for the "respiration" of every cell. It exists in two chemical forms: nicotinamide and nicotinic acid.

- intakes are sometimes expressed as niacin equivalents to take into account the conversion of tryptophan to niacin; 1 niacin equivalent = 1 mg niacin or 60 mg tryptophan.

- more precise recommended intakes are expressed in terms of total caloric intake to reflect the fact that the need for this vitamin is linked to energy metabolism; thus the RDA recommends 6.6 niacin equivalents per 1000 calories, and not fewer than 13 niacin equivalents for intakes less than 2000 calories.

**Best Food Sources:** fish, meat, poultry, eggs, enriched cereals and breads, dried peas and beans.

**Pyridoxine (Vitamin B$_6$)** It was not until the 1930s that a group of similar compounds including pyridoxine was isolated and shown to cure rats of a nutritional deficiency once thought to be pellagra. It was later still that pyridoxine was shown to be essential for humans. Pyridoxine has three active chemical forms that are involved in many reactions in amino acid metabolism. It permits the formation of new amino acids, assists in the breakdown of surplus amino acids and helps in the synthesis of many other substances like hemoglobin, antibodies and niacin. It is a part of more than 50 enzymes. The need for this vitamin increases with the amount of protein consumed. Because American diets are relatively high in protein, the recommended intake for pyridoxine is also relatively high, about 2 milligrams. Need for pyridoxine is increased among pregnant and lactating women and among alcoholics. Taking oral contraceptives also increases the need for pyridoxine.

Fish and shellfish are among the best sources of pyridoxine. Tuna and salmon are especially rich in the vitamin. Pyridoxine is widespread in fish, meat and poultry, and, to a lesser extent, in vegetables such as avocados, peas, potatoes, spinach and tomatoes.

**Best Food Sources:**   poultry, meat, fish especially tuna and salmon, dark green vegetables, some fortified cereals.

**Folacin**   Another vitamin with several active forms is folacin. The active form in tissues is folic acid. Before its identity was known, its presence in yeast and its effectiveness in treating megaloblastic anemia had been shown by Dr. Lucy Wills in India (90). It was first isolated from spinach in 1941 and given the name folic acid.

Folic acid is essential for the production of red blood cells in bone marrow and for the synthesis of nucleic acids in cells. It is also involved in the metabolism of certain amino acids. Special attention to folic acid is important for pregnant women in order to avoid anemia. Dietary supplements are frequently recommended to ensure adequate intake of this vitamin. Taking oral contraceptive pills increases the need for folacin.

Folacin is widespread among foods. It is particularly abundant in dark green leafy vegetables, liver, dried peas and beans, and peanuts. Fish, whole grains, oranges and many vegetables are moderately good sources.

**Best Food Sources:**   dark green leafy vegetables, liver, roasted peanuts, romaine lettuce, beets, raw cabbage, whole wheat, oatmeal, avocado, orange juice and eggs.

**Vitamin B$_{12}$**   Another vitamin important for healthy blood cells is B$_{12}$. It took over twenty years to identify and isolate this compound whose discovery was the result of a search for a growth factor for bacteria (90). It was quickly shown to be effective in the treatment of Addison's or pernicious anemia, a fatal disease.

There are several curious features unique to this vitamin. The first is that it contains cobalt as part of its structure. For this reason it is called cyanocobalamin. The second is that it requires normal stomach function in order to be absorbed. The stomach secretes an "intrinsic factor", a special protein which permits the vitamin to be absorbed in the intestine. Without this protein, the vitamin is not absorbed.

Another feature of this vitamin is that it is found exclusively in animal foods. It is not present in plant foods unless they are contaminated with insects or have been treated with certain molds as in tempeh, a soy product. Fish and shellfish are rich sources of vitamin $B_{12}$, with anchovies, herring, sardines, pilchards, oysters and clams at the top of the list.

Vitamin $B_{12}$ is one of the few water-soluble vitamins which are stored in the body. Most adults will have a two to five year supply stored in the liver.

**Best Food Sources:**   fish, especially anchovies, herring, sardines, pilchards, oysters and clams; liver; liverwurst; meats and milk.

**Biotin and Pantothenic Acid**   These two lesser known vitamins are involved in different aspects of energy metabolism and both are vital to cell metabolism. Both are involved in antibody production. Biotin functions in the breakdown of amino acids and pantothenic acid is involved in making fats and substances which transmit nerve impulses.

Both vitamins are fairly widely distributed in foods, although refined cereals and grains have only small quantities. Organ meats and eggs have both vitamins. Egg yolk is a rich source of biotin. Our intestinal bacteria also manufacture biotin, and this source is available for absorption. Fish and shellfish are believed to be good sources of biotin.

Pantothenic acid is abundant in animal foods, whole grains and legumes (dried peas and beans). Smaller amounts are found in milk, vegetables and fruits. Seafood is a good source of this vitamin.

## Summary of Water Soluble Vitamins

Ascorbic acid or vitamin C is important for its participation in wound healing, the absorption of iron and the metabolism of other nutrients. There is very little of the vitamin in seafood and it is readily destroyed by heat. The B vitamins on the other hand, are relatively abundant in seafood with niacin, vitamin $B_{12}$ and pyridoxine (vitamin $B_6$) present in good amounts. In general, the B vitamins are critical for biochemical processes in energy metabolism, lipid and protein metabolism and the activity of certain enzymes. Thiamin is present in seafood in fair amounts but is rather easily destroyed by heat, especially in canning. Because these vitamins are water soluble, they are readily leached into washing, cooking and canning liquids so that care during preparation and cooking is important to conserve them.

# Minerals

The study of the importance of minerals to the health of animals developed, in part, from the study of plants. It also followed the work of early scientists studying individual tissues like bone and from chemists studying the "ash" components of semi-purified diets. The attraction of both domestic and wild animals to salt licks led to the study of sodium and potassium in animals, while the study of bone fostered an understanding of calcium and phosphorus. Within the last thirty years efforts have been devoted to the trace minerals – those needed in minuscule amounts – with the discovery of the essentiality of such minerals as selenium, chromium, manganese and others.

There has been renewed public interest in calcium in conjunction with osteoporosis, a type of bone disease. Fluoride continues to be debated, in spite of the clear benefits it confers to teeth. Doubtless, the spotlight will shine on other minerals as our knowledge of disease and its prevention progresses.

Seafood is an important food source of several minerals and has the advantage of being low in those widely consumed in excess (sodium for example). The way seafood is processed and cooked also affects its mineral content. This aspect is discussed in Chapter Four.

**Calcium**   Although this mineral is best known as the major constitutent of bones and teeth, calcium has several vital functions in other body tissues. It is needed for blood clotting, for muscle contraction and for the transmission of nerve impulses. Once thought to be a rather static component of bone, calcium is now known to be in a dynamic state of flux. Regular dietary intake of calcium is required to maintain bone strength.

Other nutrients affect calcium absorption and metabolism. Vitamin D is needed for calcium absorption. The amount of calcium absorbed is greater when the need for calcium is increased, as in pregnancy and growth, when the amount of vitamin D present is increased and when the usual intake of calcium has been low. Lactose, the sugar in milk, also increases the absorption of calcium.

There are also conditions which lower calcium absorption. One of these is the presence in foods of substances which interfere with calcium uptake. The best known of such substances are phytates and oxalates. Phytates are present in whole grains and some types of fiber, and oxalates are present in some dark green leafy vegetables like spinach, chard and beet greens. Oddly enough, turnip, mustard and collard greens are low in oxalates. These compounds bind calcium tightly and prevent its being absorbed in the intestine. Other conditions which interfere with nutrient absorption also affect the uptake of calcium and other minerals.

The presence of other minerals, especially phosphorus, affects calcium absorption. High levels of phosphorus may interfere with calcium uptake and may be of concern in some conditions. Because phosphorus is widely present in the food supply, especially in highly processed foods, people concerned about obtaining adequate amounts of calcium need also be alert to possible excessive phosphorus intake.

Since vitamin D is also required for calcium absorption, conditions which limit the availability of this vitamin would also diminish calcium absorption. For most people, this is unlikely to be a problem.

There is considerable debate over how much calcium we should be consuming. The need for calcium is greater when protein and phosphorus intakes are high, as is the case for the usual American diet. Growing children, adolescents and pregnant women need large amounts of calcium. It also appears that post-menopausal women need more calcium than most are getting, in order to offset the calcium loss from their bones which leads to osteoporosis. People with habitually low intakes of calcium seldom show any problems until old age.

Because of our usual diet and the need for calcium as we age, the National

Academy of Sciences recommends a fairly high level of calcium for everyone. For nutrition labeling purposes, the amount used is 1000 milligrams or 1 gram. Seafood, milk products and some vegetables are the most important sources of calcium. The soft bones of several small fish and of canned varieties are especially valuable dietary sources of calcium.

**Best Food Sources:**   soft bones of small fish like sardines, smelts and those in canned salmon; milk and milk products; dark green leafy vegetables; dried peas and beans.

**Phosphorus**   This mineral is involved in bone structure and in important metabolic reactions in cells. Phosphorus forms a special chemical bond to store energy for cells and works with the B vitamins in energy transfers. It also helps maintain the proper level of acidity in tissue fluids. Phosphorus is widely distributed in foods. It is high in protein-rich foods like seafood, meat and dairy products, and in many processed foods as an additive. It is recommended that we consume about the same amount of phosphorus as calcium, but in practice most diets contain more phosphorus. Taking large amounts of antacids containing aluminum hydroxide will prevent the absorption of phosphorus and other minerals and may lead to depletion.

**Best Food Sources:**   seafood, meat, milk products, grains.

**Magnesium**   Magnesium is important in bone structure, nerve transmission, protein metabolism, energy release in cells and many enzyme reactions. It is widely distributed in foods, especially vegetables, and deficiencies are rare. Its absorption from foods is related to the presence of other minerals, especially calcium and phosphorus, to the level of magnesium present and to other dietary components like fat, sugar and alcohol. High levels of magnesium have a cathartic effect.

**Best Food Sources:**   anchovies, periwinkles and snails, freshwater catfish, tuna canned in oil, milk products, cereals, wheat germ, dried peas and beans, green leafy vegetables.

**Iron**   Iron is best known for its contribution to healthy blood. It is a component of hemoglobin, the protein which carries oxygen to tissues and removes carbon dioxide from them. When there is not enough iron available, the red blood cells respond by having smaller amounts of hemoglobin and this, in turn, limits the oxygen exchange in tissues. In this way, iron deficiency results in anemia and a feeling of low energy.

Iron is also a component of myoglobin in muscle, where it functions like hemoglobin in blood, i.e., to exchange oxygen and carbon dioxide. Some enzymes in the body also have iron in their structures.

In general, iron is rather poorly absorbed from foods. Once absorbed, however, very little leaves the body, except in cases of blood loss. As with calcium,

## Table 2.11  Iron Content of Selected Seafoods

| Finfish | mg/100 gms | | mg/100 gms |
|---|---|---|---|
| Anchovy | 1.5 | Salmon, silver | 1.3 |
| Barracuda | 0.8 | Salmon, sockeye | 0.9 |
| Bass, striped | 2.8 | Shad | 0.8 |
| Bonito, Atlantic | 5.9 | Swordfish | 0.8 |
| Bonito, Pacific | 6.0 | Trout, rainbow | 1.5 |
| Carp | 1.0 | Trout, brook | 1.4 |
| Catfish, channel | 1.0 | Tuna, albacore | 1.3 |
| Catfish, ocean | 0.9 | Tuna, bigeye | 1.5 |
| Cod, Atlantic | 0.4 | Tuna, bluefin | 1.2 |
| Cod, Pacific | 0.2 | Tuna, skipjack | 1.9 |
| Croaker | 0.8 | Tuna, yellowfin | 1.7 |
| Flounder and sole | 0.6 | Turbot, greenland | 1.0 |
| Haddock | 0.8 | Whitefish | 0.3 |
| Herring, Atlantic | 1.0 | Whiting | 0.4 |
| Herring, Pacific | 1.4 | | |
| Mackerel, Atlantic | 1.1 | | |
| Mackerel, Pacific | 2.0 | **Shellfish** | |
| Mackerel, Spanish | 1.0 | Abalone | 2.6 |
| Mahimahi | 1.7 | Clam, quahog | 2.8 |
| Monkfish | 1.5 | Clam, razor | 11.0 |
| Mullet, striped | 1.2 | Mussel | 7.3 |
| Perch, lake | 0.6 | Octopus | 4.8 |
| Perch, ocean | 0.8 | Oyster, Pacific | 6.5 |
| Pike, Northern | 0.4 | Oyster, Eastern | 7.1 |
| Pike, walleye | 0.8 | Oyster, European | 3.5 |
| Pompano, Atlantic | 0.6 | Crab, blue | 0.6 |
| Pompano, Pacific | 2.7 | Crab, king | 2.0 |
| Rockfish | 0.3 | Crayfish | 1.8 |
| Salmon, Atlantic | 1.0 | Spiny lobster | 2.3 |
| Salmon, king | 1.1 | Shrimp, brown | 1.8 |
| Salmon, chum | 0.5 | Shrimp, pink | 0.2 |
| Salmon, pink | 0.9 | Shrimp, Northern | 0.4 |

Source: Tables 9.1 and 9.2

iron absorption increases with the body's need for iron. Iron is more readily absorbed from some foods than from others. Iron present in organic or "heme" form, such as that found in seafood and meat, is much more readily absorbed than that present in inorganic form, such as is found in plants. The conditions present in the intestine at the time of absorption greatly influence the amount of iron absorbed.

Uptake is increased by the presence of vitamin C, citric acid and certain unknown factors in some foods like cauliflower and sauerkraut. The presence of organic iron at the same time as inorganic iron increases the uptake of the inorganic iron. That means that mixing a little meat with grains or legumes will increase the iron available from the vegetables.

As with calcium, several substances will reduce the amount of iron absorbed from foods. One of these is tannic acid in tea. Just one cup of tea taken with a meal will reduce the absorption of non-heme iron by about half. Antacids taken with or shortly after meals reduce iron absorption, as do calcium and phosphate salts found in some medications. The food additive EDTA binds iron to make it unavailable and unknown substances in certain foods like spinach, soybeans and bran also decrease iron absorption.

Iron needs are most difficult to meet:

1. in infants whose milk based diet is usually low in iron;

2. in children and adolescents who are growing rapidly;

3. in women during the child-bearing years, because of menstrual losses; and

4. in pregnancy, because of the increased demands of the fetus, placenta and maternal blood supply.

Surveys of the American population have repeatedly indicated shortfalls in iron nutriture, especially among children and adolescents. Greater consumption of seafood, especially of certain underutilized species like herring, sardines and mackerel, could make an important contribution to the iron intakes of millions of Americans, helping to combat the major public health problem of anemia.

The best sources of iron in foods are red meats, especially organ meats, shellfish, dark fleshed fish, poultry, dried peas and beans, dark green leafy vegetables, enriched grains and cereals, prune juice, watermelon and seeds.

Seafoods, especially shellfish and the darker fleshed fish, are some of the least often recommended sources of iron but may be equal to or better than the well known red meat sources. In addition, much of the iron in seafood is present in the organic form most available to the body. Sardines, smelts, bluefish, herring, mackerel, mussels, clams, oysters and scallops are especially rich in iron. Iron content of selected seafoods is shown in Table 2.11.

**Best Food Sources:**   organ meats; red meats, dark fish and many shellfish; poultry; dried peas and beans; dark green leafy vegetables; enriched grains and cereals; prune juice; seeds.

**Best Seafood Sources:**   mussels, oysters, clams, herring, sardines, bluefish, shrimp, mackerel, smelts, scallops, light meat tuna.

**Zinc**   The importance of zinc to good health has gained considerable attention in the past few years. Zinc is found in more than 100 enzymes whose activities are vital in synthesizing our cellular genetic material (nucleic acids), as well as in healing wounds, in vitamin A metabolism, in sexual development, in growth, in fighting infections and in maintaining healthy skin.

Zinc deficiency in man has been observed in the Middle East where diets are extremely low in zinc. Low levels of dietary and tissue zinc have been documented in the United States and marginal zinc deficiency has been observed in children. As a result, much more attention is being given to the zinc content of usual diets and to defining our needs. Current estimates suggest that usual diets fall below the RDA of 15 milligrams for zinc. Zinc may be of concern to vegetarians because of the low availability of zinc from vegetables and grains. It is likely that rich food sources of this mineral will become increasingly important.

As with iron, zinc is more readily absorbed from animal foods than from plants. Absorption of zinc is higher than for iron, with the average believed to be about 40 percent. Again as with iron, absorption of zinc is increased in the presence of protein, particularly animal protein. Unlike iron, however, zinc absorption is not improved in the presence of vitamin C. Dietary fiber, phytate, oxalate and other minerals such as iron and lead all decrease the absorption of zinc from foods. As with many other minerals, the interactions among dietary components present at the time of digestion all exert an effect on the amount of nutrient absorbed. It is complicated!

As a rich food source, seafood scores again. Oysters have become famous as an extraordinarily concentrated source of zinc. Just three ounces of oyster meats may contain up to 75 milligrams of zinc – 5 times the U.S. RDA! Other molluscs like mussels, scallops and clams are also rich in zinc. Crustaceans like crab, lobster and shrimp are good sources and pilchard also seems to be high in zinc.

**Best Food Sources:** oysters, other molluscs, crustaceans, some fish, liver, red meats, poultry, milk products, eggs, seeds and legumes.

**Copper** Copper, like iron, is involved in healthy red blood cells. It is a component of several proteins and enzymes and is involved in iron metabolism. Copper deficiency in man has been observed in severely malnourished children and with excessive antacid consumption; otherwise, it is rare. Copper is fairly widely distributed in foods and its absorption is related to other components of the meal. Acid promotes copper absorption, as does starch compared with sugar. By contrast, high levels of zinc interfere with copper uptake.

The distribution of copper in foods has not been widely studied. Known food sources are organ meats, shellfish – especially oysters, crab and lobster – nuts, corn oil margarine and legumes.

**Best Food Sources:** liver, kidney, oysters, nuts, crab, lobster, legumes, corn oil margarine.

**Iodine** Iodine was discovered in 1811 by Courtois, who was working to keep Napoleon supplied with gunpowder. He was using dried kelp as a source of lye to make the niter for gunpowder and discovered the iodine in it. Shortly thereafter, a

Swiss physician successfully treated goitrous patients with iodine, but overdoses resulted in toxicities and the treatment fell into disrepute. In the 1920s, American school children were successfully treated for goiter with small amounts of iodine. Soon the thyroid hormone thyroxine was discovered to contain iodine and the link between iodine and the enlarged thyroid or goiter was firmly established.

In spite of our understanding of the most common cause of goiter, the condition remains endemic in many parts of the world. Iodine content in foods is related to the amount of iodine in the soil, the availability of foods from the sea and the types of food processing. In some third-world countries goiter remains a problem where soil iodine levels are low, food supplementation is not feasible and most food is produced and consumed locally.

In the United States, the problem of goiter was largely overcome by adding iodine to table salt. In addition, much of our food supply comes from different parts of the country so that most regions are not dependent only on their local harvest. However, some foods, like milk, have large regional differences in iodine content.

More recently, iodine intake has increased because of the use of iodine-containing additives in food processing and animal feeds. Major sources of iodine are dairy foods, grain and cereal products, meat, fish, poultry and sugars. The last source is thought to derive from the use of iodine-containing red food colors. Iodine is also available from medications, the air, water and other beverages. As a result of its widespread distribution in the U.S. food supply we no longer rely on iodized salt as the major source of iodine.

Seafood has long been a reliable, natural source of iodine. Many varieties of finfish, molluscs and crustaceans have substantial iodine levels. Iodine is also found in edible sea plants.

**Best Food Sources:**   milk and dairy products; grains and cereals; seafood, especially hake, striped mullet, squid, haddock, herring, mackerel and clams.

**Fluorine**   This element is present in small amounts in soil, water, plants and animals. Very little is present in the food supply and the main dietary source is drinking water. Small amounts of fluorine or the ion fluoride, as it is found in water, become incorporated in teeth and bones. Teeth with fluoride are much more resistant to decay. Bones with fluoride are stronger and perhaps less prone to osteoporosis. The easiest way to obtain fluoride is through the addition of the element to the public drinking water. In some communities this public health measure has been resisted, largely owing to the spread of misinformation and fear.

Data on the amount of fluorine in foods are scarce. The information we have about seafood indicates that cod and haddock have a moderate amount of fluorine. Salmon and herring have somewhat more than cod, while shrimp, oysters and crab have very little. Blue mussels, on the other hand, are rich in fluorine. Three ounces of steamed mussels contain about 3 milligrams of fluorine, which is the upper range of the recommended dietary intake for this element. Canned sardines are also rich in fluorine.

**Best Food Sources:**   fluoridated drinking water, mussels, sardines, salmon

**Best Food Sources:**   fluoridated drinking water, mussels, sardines, salmon and herring.

**Sodium**   There has probably been more publicity about this element in the past few years than virtually any other nutrient. This is largely because sodium is strongly linked to high blood pressure, or hypertension, a stealthy disease you do not feel which leads to stroke and heart attack. Most Americans consume too much sodium in foods and many efforts have been directed toward lowering people's intake of sodium. Thus, the desirable emphasis with sodium is on how little sodium is present, rather than how much.

Sodium's job is to regulate water balance and maintain proper fluid volume in the liquid surrounding the cells. Sodium acts like a sponge to hold water. When too much sodium is present excess water may be retained and this leads to high blood pressure. The insidious part of high blood pressure is that we feel no symptoms of it, often until too late. Furthermore, it has been estimated that over sixty million Americans have some degree of high blood pressure, so that this condition is a major health problem.

Controlling the amount of sodium we consume can be helpful in lowering high blood pressure or in discouraging it from developing. This means using mainly foods naturally low in sodium, like seafood, fresh poultry and meats, fresh fruits, vegetables and unprocessed whole grains. It also means throwing out the salt shaker and limiting the use of salty foods, like canned and dried soups, pickles, olives, deli items, frozen dinners and many cheeses. People with severe hypertension may need more drastic restrictions.

Other ways to control blood pressure are: achieving desirable body weight for your age, sex and body frame; following your doctor's recommendations for taking medications; and getting regular exercise.

Sodium and salt are often confused. Salt is made of sodium and chlorine and contains about 40 percent sodium. Salt is also the major source of sodium in foods, so salty foods are the highest in sodium. Sea salt is the same as table salt and has no nutritional benefits.

Fresh seafood is one of the best choices for curbing sodium intake since all varieties are low in sodium. On the other hand, smoked and cured fish, most canned and some frozen fish have sodium containing additives and/or salt added to them. These additives may not be listed on the label so the consumer and retailer may be unaware of them. A good example is the sodium tripolyphosphate added to frozen fish fillets (see Chapter Three). Canned tuna and salmon also contain high levels of salt.

Most fresh fish range from about 60 to about 100 mg sodium per 3½ ounces (100 grams) of raw muscle. This is considered "low sodium" by the FDA labeling regulations. Most shellfish and crustaceans, on the other hand, have more sodium, usually in the range of 200 – 400 mg per 3½ ounces. Squid and scallops fall in between at about 160 mg.

Sometimes, fish canned in water, bouillon or tomato sauce have more sodium than the same variety canned in oil. This situation often puts the consumer in a "no win" situation. The water pack has much less fat and fewer

62

calories, but has a much higher sodium content. The solution is to drain and rinse the water packed product in fresh water before using. This will get rid of much of the excess sodium. Alternatively, diet pack canned fish packed in water without added salt is available.

Since most people consume too much sodium, the recommended range of intake for good health is 1100-3300 milligrams per day. By contrast, many people consume from 2300-6900 mg or more per day.

**Foods Lowest in Sodium:**   fresh seafood, meat and poultry; no-salt canned fish; fresh, plain-frozen or no-salt added canned vegetables and fruits; unprocessed whole grains like oatmeal, rice, bulgur wheat, barley; unsalted nuts and seeds; pasta; dried peas and beans; low salt or sodium reduced cheese.

**Potassium**   This mineral acts in the opposite way to sodium, in terms of balancing electrical charges inside and outside the cell. Sodium is found primarily outside the cell, while potassium is found mainly on the inside. The concentration of both minerals is regulated by the kidney.

Most people consume enough potassium. Those taking diuretics for the control of high blood pressure or other conditions may lose too much potassium from the body. By contrast, overuse of salt substitutes made from potassium can lead to excessive potassium intake.

Seafood is a relatively rich source of potassium. Many finfish have between 300-400 mg potassium per 3½ ounces and nearly all is retained during cooking. Shellfish and crustaceans tend to have less potassium, generally in the 200-300 milligram range. Blue mussels are very high in potassium: 3½ ounces of steamed mussels have over 1100 mg potassium! Other rich seafoods are scallops, canned clams, tuna canned in oil, sardines canned in tomato sauce, steamed Atlantic pollock and mackerel.

**Best Food Sources:**   Excellent food sources are those providing 400 mg or more of potassium per serving. Such foods are: mussels, scallops, canned clams, drained tuna canned in oil, sardines canned in tomato sauce, bananas, cantaloupes, orange juice, baked or boiled potatoes, nectarines, butternut squash.

**Selenium**   Selenium was not discovered to be an essential nutrient until the late 1950s when it was shown to be required by chickens and sheep. Re-evaluation of the need for this trace mineral in man soon followed, and it is now known that selenium is an essential component of at least one enzyme in red blood cells, glutathione peroxidase (98). This enzyme destroys hydrogen peroxide which can be a dangerous product of fatty acid metabolism.

The metabolism of selenium is inter-related with that of vitamin E and the amino acid methionine. In foods it is most commonly found bound to methionine. The selenium content of foods is directly related to the level of selenium in the soil (89). Selenium is present in seafood in important amounts with shellfish having somewhat greater amounts than finfish.

Selenium is of current interest for two reasons. One is that it appears to be protective against the deleterious effects of methylmercury and inorganic mercury which is sometimes found in seafood (see Chapter Three). The other is that it may exert a controlling effect in the development of some forms of cancer (89). The activity of certain carcinogens may be enhanced by selenium while the toxicity of others diminished (89, 99).

**Best Food Sources:**   seafoods, kidney, liver, grains, legumes and nuts.

**Chromium**   The importance of chromium for the health of laboratory animals was observed in the 1950s and its association with an improved ability to handle glucose was reported in 1959 (100, 101). Although a definitive demonstration of its essentiality in man has not been shown, it is generally believed to be required in small amounts. Chromium has been associated with better efficiency of insulin in the handling of blood glucose and with changes in blood lipoprotein levels, but unequivocal evidence is lacking (89).

**Best Food Sources:**   meat, liver, brewer's yeast, whole grains, nuts and cheese; seafood is not a particulary good source of this mineral.

**Manganese**   Manganese has been shown to be an essential nutrient for animals and, because it participates in a number of biochemical pathways in people, it is assumed to be required. Manganese is found as part of several enzymes which function in carbohydrate synthesis and lipid metabolism (89). It has also been associated with cholesterol metabolism: subjects who are deficient in manganese also have low cholesterol levels.

Manganese is involved in brain metabolism and can affect brain function by either its deficiency or its excess (102, 103). It is thought to be involved in the successful treatment of Parkinson's disease with a drug called L-dopa. Low manganese levels in blood have been associated with epileptic seizures in people but the significance of this association is not known (104).

There is concern about manganese exposure among workers in manganese mines who inhale the dust from the ores. Toxicity has been reported. Excessive dietary intakes are not believed to be a problem. Manganese is not abundant in seafood.

**Best Food Sources:**   tea is exceptionally high in manganese; plants are richer in this mineral than animal foods

### Miscellaneous Trace Elements

**Cobalt**   is an essential nutrient because it is a constituent of vitamin $B_{12}$, to which it conferred its name, cyanocobalamin. A requirement independent of the vitamin has not been shown. The best dietary source of cobalt is green leafy vegetables.

**Molybdenum**   is an essential constituent of several enzymes involved in energy metabolism. It has been associated with several clinical conditions. The main food sources are meat, grains and legumes. Molybdenum is present in seafood. There is more in shellfish than finfish.

**Silicon**   Silicon was recognized as an essential nutrient for the chick in 1972, but there is no proof of its essentiality in man (105, 106). Silicon appears to be important in bone mineralization and in the formation of cartilage and connective tissue in bone joints. It also interacts with molybdenum.

**Arsenic and Cadmium**   Both minerals are known for their toxicity rather than their essentiality. Arsenic has been suggested to be important in zinc and/or arginine metabolism, but it is not known if this is of any practical significance (89). Both minerals are present in seafood.

Seafood has more arsenic than other foods. Estimates of the amounts vary greatly; one source reports that shellfish, especially crustaceans, have more than finfish, while a report from FDA's Bureau of Foods listed finfish as having more than twice the level of shrimp (107, 108). The FDA report combines arsenic analyses from a wide variety of finfish and states that their analyses do not permit them to ". . . draw conclusions about the species likely to have higher arsenic contents" (107). Nevertheless, seafood is a major source of this element. Arsenic is thought to be poorly absorbed and is readily excreted by the body, suggesting that its presence in foods at the levels observed is not a health problem.

*Chapter Three*

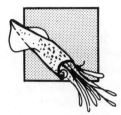
# Additives in Seafood

The term "additive" has taken on a pejorative meaning largely because of its use as a catch-all for substances of questionable safety, added deliberately to foods by manufacturers or processors. It suggests something added to food that is not food (110). But most people realize that not all additives are harmful – sugar, anyone? – and that manufacturers are generally concerned with improving their products, not poisoning their patrons. The food industry may have fanciful ideas of product quality or shelf life. Excesses have occurred and harmful substances been used but malicious intent is not proven. We need a dispassionate look at the subject.

Additives include substances in food added either intentionally, as in vitamin enrichment, or unintentionally, as in trace metals from mixing equipment. Their honest use is to foster improved safety, quality, quantity or availability of food. Additives can also adulterate food, creating a false impression of quality. Pure water is one of the most notorious of such additives. Whether a substance is helpful or harmful depends not only on its safety, but also on how it is used. Each substance needs to be considered on a case by case basis.

A suitable definition of the term additive has challenged governments throughout the world. It is not clear what distinguishes an ingredient from a food or even what a food is. It is just as difficult to define a contaminant. Since foods are shipped all over the world, a common system of nomenclature would greatly assist countries in developing reasonable food trade policies.

Under the auspices of the United Nations Food and Agriculture Organization and the World Health Organization, over 100 countries have worked to establish a set of food standards to govern international trade. The body charged with this difficult mission is the Codex Alimentarius Commission. Codex has defined food additive* and has set forth general principles for their use. This

---

*'Food additive' means any substance not normally consumed as a food by itself and not normally used as a typical ingredient of the food, whether or not it has nutritive value, the intentional addition of which to food for a technological (including organoleptic) purpose in the manufacture, processing, preparation, treatment, packing, packaging, transport or holding of such food results, or may be reasonably expected to result, (directly or indirectly) in it or its by-products becoming a component of or otherwise affecting the characteristics of such foods. The term does not include 'contaminants' or substances added to food for maintaining or improving nutritional qualities (128).

definition has not yet been adopted for use in international trade, but in the way of governments, slow progress has been made toward that goal (110).

In the United States, food additive is defined in a stricter way than the proposed international definition and takes into account the presence of radiation processing and of substances generally recognized as safe. The US definition excludes the following: pesticide chemicals in or on raw agricultural commodities, color additives, prior sanctioned substances and new animal drugs (110). The complete definition of food additives as stated in the Federal Food Drug and Cosmetic Act 1958 amendment is presented in Appendix 3. For a superbly readable discussion of the meaning of the U.S. definition of food additives and why certain substances are categorized the way they are see Wodicka's review in reference (110). The article is both entertaining and informative.

The U.S. Food and Drug Administration (FDA) has the responsibility for determining whether or not a particular substance may be safely added to foods or food packaging. Its authority comes from the 1958 Food Additives Amendment and the 1960 Color Additive Amendment to the Federal Food, Drug and Cosmetic Act. These changes increased FDA's jurisdiction to include a larger number of substances and established a narrower definition of safety (111).

Defining the term "safe" was an attempt to improve on the ambiguity of the term "harmful" that had prevailed. "Safe" is "reasonable certainty of no harm" but, according to Congressional intent, it "does not, and cannot, require proof beyond any possible doubt that no harm will result under any conceivable circumstances" (112).

The legal changes to the 1938 Food and Drug Act meant that the burden of proving the safety of an additive was placed on the manufacturer, and pre-market safety data were required. FDA procedures require a manufacturer to file a petition seeking approval for using the substance, to provide test results that prove the substance is safe in at least two animal species and to give practical methods for detecting and measuring the additive in foods.

The regulatory options available to FDA include doing nothing, requiring labeling, limiting the use of the substance, or banning the substance (111). If approval is turned down, the petitioner has the option of providing more data and applying again for approval. The decisions of regulators involve not only their own interests, but those of scientists, lawyers on behalf of their clients, and policy makers who represent the public interest. Regulators need to consider their decisions in the light of consumer reaction, enforcement procedures and requirements, and the impact on future decisions. Present procedures are deemed inadequate by nearly all parties (58).

Since all substances are potentially toxic, even pure water, some restriction must be imposed on the amounts added to food. These restrictions are known as "tolerance levels". They are set "not to exceed the smallest amount needed, even though a higher tolerance may be safe" (1). Animal studies are employed to determine the maximum amount of a substance that does not produce any undesirable effects. Usually 1/100th of that amount will be set as the tolerance level in order to ensure a wide margin of safety.

Curiously, very few naturally occurring constituents in foods enjoy such a generous margin of safety. Amounts of trace minerals like selenium, goitrogenic substances and aflatoxin undoubtedly have a margin of safety less than 10 fold. The margin for salt is probably less than 5, and among people with high blood pressure is less than 1 (113). Safety margins for the fat soluble vitamins A and D may be about 25-40 in adults and less than 10 for infants. These observations suggest that nature worries less about the hazards of certain food substances than do the FDA and consumers. It also implies the need for a wide variety of foods in the diet, a not very exciting but certainly sound bit of advice (29).

Food safety is further ensured under a legal provision known as the "Delaney clause". This states that no potentially carcinogenic substance may be added to food. Thus, substances which have been shown to cause cancer in animals may not be added to foods. Levels of naturally occurring carcinogens, however, are regulated by establishing tolerance levels. Exceptions to the carcinogen ban can be created through Acts of Congress. That is what has happened to permit saccharin in the marketplace. Extensions of the saccharin approval appear to circumvent the usual rules. Products containing saccharin are required to carry a health warning and a notice that it causes cancer in laboratory animals.

FDA takes the position that a substance must be proven safe before it may be added. Given the kinds of chemicals on trial, this is not a bad premise. But neither is it a perfect one. It is extremely difficult to prove safety because the object is to demonstrate lack of an effect, and you cannot always know what to look for. It is also difficult to know how long to continue looking for results, since the long term effects of the consumption of minute amounts of a substance may take decades to detect. Then there are the difficulties of establishing cause and effect with any certainty. An additional problem is synergy: the effect of two substances together being greater than that of either one by itself. There are other problems too, but these are the fundamental ones.

On the other hand, hasty approval of substances for human consumption poses risks which are difficult to foresee. Take aspartame for example. First approved for use in 1981, the safety of aspartame has been questioned by consumer groups, the American Medical Association, the American Academy of Pediatrics, the Center for Disease Control, the American Diabetic Association and numerous physicians, researchers and consumers. Then, in 1985, FDA suggested privately that pregnant women use aspartame in moderation (114). What about the rest of us? FDA is reviewing the data on aspartame safety, levels of consumption and reports of side effects. Whether there will be changes in the regulations governing the use of aspartame is not known, but the experience will at least serve to make everyone more cautious about food additives.

There are two groups of substances which are exempt from the usual testing and approval procedures of FDA. These are "prior sanctioned substances" and those "generally recognized as safe", or GRAS. Prior sanctioned substances are those which were approved in writing by the FDA before the passage of the 1958 Food Additives Amendment. It is difficult to know which substances are covered under the "prior sanctioned" provision because few of these approvals are published. As Wodicka has pointed out, many are based on laws of 1906 and 1907 before there was a Code of Federal Regulations and many are contained in letters to processors which may be irretrievable (110). GRAS substances are ingredients such as spices and flavorings which historical usage suggests are not harmful. The original GRAS lists were compiled by FDA in response to the most frequent inquiries about specific food components. They were intended as a convenience, not as a definitive list. In fact, from the legal point of view, most of the food supply and the utensils used to process foods are GRAS.

The Food Additives Amendment of 1958 established a legal and procedural watershed. Those substances already on the GRAS list at the time were considered legal; those added thereafter were subject to review, according to the procedures already described. The review process would then establish whether the substance or process would be GRAS or a food additive. The irony is that what may be "defined as a food additive, i.e. an ingredient added in small quantities to affect the properties of the food, may be either a food additive or a GRAS substance under U.S. law" (110). There are obvious advantages to having a substance classified as GRAS rather than as an additive.

Nowadays, because of our more sophisticated analytical technology, we can detect vanishingly small quantities of substances we might not otherwise wish to find. The major question then turns on the issue of risk. To what and how much risk are we exposed by virtue of minute quantities of certain substances? To what extent can we control those risks? As Middlekauff has pointed out,

> "The term risk implies a lack of control. To the public in general, it appears that there are conditions in the environment over which they have no control and which will cause their early demise. The public tends to fear more those matters over which they have no control than those matters over which they do have control. A complicating factor is that if a hazard is found naturally, it may be acceptable, whereas an equivalent or even less significant hazard caused by man is unacceptable." (111).

Concepts of risk assessment are being widely debated as we come to grips with a basic dilemma: virtually everything carries an inherent risk; what level of protection or safety should we rightly expect from our government and its regulations? What risks are we, as consumers, willing to assume, in order to maintain a safe, abundant and economical food supply? How much are we willing to pay for how much less risk?

The resolution of such questions is no easy matter. It involves, at least, three main disciplines: science, for the provision of data and technology; law, for interpreting, applying and sometimes creating laws and regulations; and politics, for generating legislation and expressing the will of the people. As Middlekauf expressed it when discussing carcinogens in foods, "the scientific determination of carcinogenicity confronts the legal issue of the applicability of the Delaney clause... and the policy issue of whether the substance should be permitted in the food supply." (111).

There are no easy answers. The need to protect people from undue risk is clear; the best ways of achieving consumer protection without stifling progress in science and technology are less so. Industry, consumers, government and academics have begun to work together to devise a workable system (115, 116). Dialogue has begun, thanks largely to the need for regulating carcinogens in food. The Interagency Risk Management Council (IRMC) was formed in 1983 by FDA, USDA, the Environmental Protection Agency (EPA), the Consumer Product Safety Commission and the Occupational Safety and Health Administration (OSHA). IRMC has been charged with the task of developing common principles of risk assessment, with FDA as the lead agency for the group (111, 116). To what extent IRMC can achieve its goals remains to be seen. Readers interested in the issues and problems posed in risk assessment are encouraged to consult references (111, 117-122).

One can argue that the most compelling aspect of food additives, intentional or otherwise, is food safety. Issues surrounding food safety are ancient, but the study of food safety as such is relatively new. It encompasses chemistry, microbiology and nutrition as well as many related disciplines like food science, toxicology and epidemiology (123). As our knowledge increases, and the realization grows that all foods can be viewed as a mixture of chemicals, the way we view the relative risks from the food supply is changing.

Slowly we are moving away from the view that a substance, *per se*, is either safe or harmful towards the notion that a substance at certain levels is harmless to most people, yet in greater amounts may be dangerous. In this perspective, the critical problem is 'what is a safe level?' Linked to this question is the larger one, 'what level of risk is an individual or society willing to accept?'

If you feed substances to laboratory animals, are there any nasty side effects as a result? The concept of **toxicity** includes the concept of dose, or amount fed. How much does it take to produce an effect? The **hazard** of a substance is its capacity to produce injury under the circumstances of exposure (113). This means, how likely are people to incur side effects within the range of amounts most might receive? Many toxic substances are present in food, but few are hazardous. For example, oxalate is toxic, but its presence in spinach is not a hazard. Shellfish contain lead, mercury and fluoride, but shellfish are not toxic.

There are enormous numbers of naturally-occurring toxicants in foods, yet the usual "diet consumed by normal, healthy individuals" presents relatively little hazard (113). The reasons why this is so are:

1. the concentration of each toxic substance is very low and only exaggerated consumption of a limited number of foods with such substances will be be a problem;

2. toxicities of thousands of different chemicals in our diet each day are not cumulative; and,

3. the toxicity of one element may be offset by the presence of another (113).

Foods containing toxic substances may be hazardous under abnormal or unusual circumstances. These will occur when the concentration of the toxic substance is abnormally high; when excessive amounts of a food are consumed over a long period of time; when a person has an "abnormal" susceptibility to a food component; or when a toxin is present inconsistently.

## Indirect Food Additives

These are substances found in food as a consequence of the natural environment where the food originated, or as a result of handling or processing. They have not been added deliberately, but neither were they part of the original composition of the food substance. Some examples are soil contamination of grains, bacterial toxins such as those associated with "red tide" in shellfish and the presence of parasites such as nematodes in fish.

Chemical residues might be considered unintentional additives by virtue of their nearly universal distribution over the earth and the imperfect mechanisms living things have of dealing with them. In some cases, the liver of the animal, fish or shellfish will concentrate the chemical in an attempt to detoxify it, to prepare it for excretion, or as a means of excluding it from the rest of the body. In other cases, heavy metals such as lead, mercury and cadmium can accumulate in systemic tissues and bones. Still others like arsenic may be taken up by the body and mostly excreted. It is not always clear how much of an environmental contaminant enters the food supply, nor how much remains in the body.

### Food Safety Issues Related to Seafood

The USDA has attempted to establish a priority listing of the most pressing issues of food safety, in part so that reasonable budget allocations can be made (124). It turns out that nearly all of the ten priorities relate to unintentional additives. Potentially harmful food additives rank eighth on the priority listing, suggesting that many other hazards associated with foods are more urgent.

A similar listing of the actual hazards associated with foods was developed by FDA in 1978. In this listing, food additives ranked sixth behind toxigenic and pathogenic microorganisms, malnutrition, environmental contaminants, toxic natural constituents of food and pesticide residues.

Let us take a look at the USDA list, in order of priority, especially as it relates to seafood:

**Mycotoxins.**   These are the toxic products of mold. By far the most potent of these are aflatoxins, carcinogenic compounds that may contaminate peanuts and peanut butter, nuts, grains and animal products if the animals have consumed contaminated grain. Because aflatoxins can be produced while a plant is growing, it may be impossible to eliminate them completely from the food supply. FDA has set very low tolerance levels for aflatoxin: no more than 15 parts per billion in foods destined for interstate commerce (125). Aflatoxins are not associated with seafood.

**Bacterial toxins.**   The most notorious of these poisons is produced by the bacterium, *Clostridium botulinum*. Frequently fatal, botulism is contracted by eating foods contaminated with the botulinus toxin. The bacteria thrive in an environment deprived of oxygen, low in acid and at least 38°F. The bacteria themselves are readily killed by heat and usual processing methods but the bacterial spores are not. Hence, under improper processing conditions the spores may generate active bacteria which produce the deadly toxin. The toxin is destroyed by boiling so that canned items that have been cooked after opening are harmless (1). Home canned low acid foods such as vegetables, and vacuum packed smoked seafoods are the most vulnerable.

Botulism is a major concern to seafood processors who use canning, vacuum packaging and modified atmospheres as methods of preservation. Because each of these methods has the potential for creating a hospitable environment for *Clostridium botulinum*, strict procedures and low temperatures are required to ensure freedom from botulinum growth. These processing conditions are well known and specified (126). In outbreaks of bacterial contamination involving canned seafood, the problem has invariably been traced to defective equipment, not faulty processing (126). Seafood processors can never relax their vigilance against this threat.

**Bacterial infections from food.**    Thousands of cases of food poisoning can be attributed to the consumption of foods contaminated with harmful bacteria. Usually the presence of these bacteria can be traced to poor food handling in the home or food service operation. Only rarely is food poisoning attributable to errors in commercial processing (127).

By far the most common form of foodborne illness is caused by the organism *Salmonella*. This bacterium thrives in a wide variety of foods, especially when time and temperature permit its growth. It is a hazard because of poor food handling. Seafood is not exempt as a host, particularly when processing is carried out where sanitation is poor.

A type of bacterial poisoning, called scombroid poisoning, can occur with the bacterial degradation of fish like tuna, skipjack, bonito, and mackerel. The poison produced is believed to be a histamine-like substance, and while the affliction is not usually fatal, it can be. Such poisonings can most often be traced to high temperature storage.

**Chemical residues**    The phrase chemical residues is a catch-all term for a wide variety of organic and inorganic compounds found throughout the environment. It includes insecticides, herbicides, industrial chlorinated compounds, petroleum compounds, various nitrogenous compounds, chemotherapeutic agents and industrial chemicals and by-products. Many substances in these categories are toxic to sea life, laboratory animals and humans, but the conditions that make them hazardous to man are not well known. A recent summary of the literature on the toxicity to aquatic life of various chemicals in these categories was published in 1982 (129). Myers and Hendricks give an excellent summary of chemicals that have been tested for carcinogenicity and of the range of substances warranting concern. It is surely not exhaustive. Pollution of water resources comes from many sources:

- transport from land applications downstream to estuaries and the sea;

- the application of pesticides to marshes and shorelines;

- flow of surface waters to lakes and streams;

- deposits in silt;

- chemicals and contaminated dust carried by the wind;

- industrial and municipal dumping into waterways.

Current FDA action levels for poisonous or deleterious substances in seafood are shown in Table 3.1.

*Table 3.1  FDA Action Levels for Certain Chemical Substances in Seafoods*

| Substance | Products | Action level (Parts per million) |
|---|---|---|
| Aldrin | fish & shellfish | 0.3 |
| Dieldrin | fish & shellfish | 0.3 |
| Benzene hexachloride | frog legs | 0.5 |
| Chlordane | fish | 0.3 |
| DDT, DDE, TDE | fish | 5.0 |
| Endrin | fish & shellfish | 0.3 |
| Heptachlor | fish & shellfish | 0.3 |
| Heptachlor epoxide | fish & shellfish | 0.3 |
| Kepone | crabmeat | 0.4 |
| N-methyl mercury | fish, shellfish, & crustaceans | 1.0 |
| Mirex | fish | 0.1 |
| PCB | fish | 2.0 |
| Toxaphene | fish | 5.0 |

Source: FDA

There are several reasons why chemical residues, especially pesticides, are worrisome. The first is that they are long lived; that is, they resist chemical and bacterial degradation so that their continued use results in accumulation of the substance in the environment. Another reason is that they are incorporated into phytoplankton, the first link in the food chain, and become concentrated through the food chain. One example of such magnification: mullet feeding on plankton with residues of 50 parts per billion, themselves contained residues in the range of 1 - 15 parts per million (roughly a 100 fold increase). Porpoises feeding on the mullet had residues of 800 parts per million for another 100 fold increase in concentration (130).

Some chemical residues like the polychlors (cyclic organic molecules with several chlorine atoms attached) can penetrate the skin and gills of fish so that residues may be acquired other than by feeding.

Many chemical residues can be absorbed by animals but are not easily excreted so that they accumulate in body tissues. Most organic compounds are distributed in fat tissues, liver and other organs that are usually not consumed so that even contaminated fish may have negligible levels of toxic chemicals in the edible flesh. The caution is raised about fish oil supplements that may contain high levels of noxious substances because these supplements may be derived from fish livers and waste tissues.

The extent of pollution is a function of the chemical stability of the contaminants and the rates at which they are added to and removed from the environment. The moisture level and temperature of the environment also affect their activity.

Pollution of estuaries is a particularly serious problem because they are the nurseries that support the microscopic plants and animals that sustain both young and mature fish. Their destruction undermines local and distant populations because the young are eliminated.

There is room for cautious optimism, however, because progress in cleaning major waterways has been made in several states, including New York, Connecticut and Massachusetts. Salmon are returning to some East Coast rivers. Legislation has been enacted controlling some of the most devastating chemicals, like the banning of DDT and PCBs. Controls on many other chemicals are under review. The review and legislative process is time-consuming, controversial and political as is obvious in the case of acid rain. Much damage accumulates while arguments continue. Short term solutions usually prevail over long term ones and these are seldom in the best interests of the environment or aquatic life.

Our record in preserving wildlife species and fragile environments is dismal. Astonishing achievements have been made but by and large they are exceptional. Painstaking documentation of man's failure to husband the resources of the sea was recently published in a sobering volume by Farley Mowat called *Sea of Slaughter* (131).

**Heavy Metal Contamination**   The metals of primary concern as contaminants of seafood are mercury, lead, cadmium and arsenic. Of these, mercury has been the most important and received the greatest attention. The toxicity of mercury in man has been well documented in studies of Minamata disease in Japan and Canada. Mercury enters the food chain first in phytoplankton and then becomes concentrated in the flesh of certain species of fish. It is present in fish mainly in the form of methylmercury. The species most widely associated with high mercury are swordfish, Pacific halibut, tuna, shark, king mackerel and tilefish (132). Large, long-lived fish usually have the highest levels, although the size/concentration relationship was reported to be weak for some species (133). Freshwater fish in rivers and lakes where mercury wastes are disposed may also have high mercury levels.

Methylmercury is completely absorbed from food and is nearly completely retained. There is some indication that selenium may be protective against the harmful effects of mercury but the evidence is so far inconclusive. The current FDA activity level for mercury in fish is 1 part per million based on methylmercury content (134). A 1978 study assessing the likelihood of consumers exceeding a safe level of mercury from eating seafood concluded that "Mercury in seafood poses little hazard to the overall seafood eating public" (132). Even among those groups consuming varieties with the most mercury and those who might be most susceptible to adverse effects (women of child-bearing age and children) the risk of consuming such seafoods was not found to constitute a hazard. Presently, FDA regularly monitors mercury in swordfish and certain other species. It appears that the action level of 1 ppm methylmercury is adequate protection against health risk from mercury to American seafood consumers.

Arsenic has entered the food supply through its use in pesticides and animal feed additives (107). The use of arsenic-containing pesticides on food crops has decreased since the late 1960s, accounting for the decrease in arsenic levels in all food groups. Seafood is the leading source of dietary arsenic with smaller amounts present in meat and poultry. Arsenic, however, unlike mercury, is readily excreted from the body. Table 3.2 presents levels of arsenic observed in six species of seafood from the recent National Food Processors Association study. The figures are much higher for shrimp and flounder than those reported by Jelinek and Corneliussen in 1977, but lower for salmon and whiting (107).

**Table 3.2   Levels of Arsenic in Six Species of Seafood from the National Food Processors Association Study**[a]

| Species | Raw | Baked | Broiled | Microwaved | Breaded and fried |
|---|---|---|---|---|---|
| | | | *Parts per million* | | |
| Flounder | 4.9 | 6.0 | 5.8 | 6.0 | – |
| Sockeye salmon | 0.3 | 0.4 | 0.4 | 0.4 | – |
| Atlantic mackerel | 1.3 | 1.7 | 1.5 | 1.5 | – |
| Shrimp[c] | 15.4 | 13.4 | 13.4 | 3.7[b] | – |
| Alaska pollock | 1.2 | 1.4 | 1.7 | 1.3[b] | 1.4[b] |
| Pacific whiting | 0.5 | 0.8 | 0.8 | 0.8[b] | 0.6[b] |

[a] Data are for means of 11 samples
[b] Data are means of 5 or 6 samples
[c] Data varied from 2.24-27.20 ppm

**PCBs**   PCBs or polychlorinated biphenyls are synthetic compounds formerly used industrially as insulating fluids and now banned from production. PCBs are extremely resistant to destruction and degradation and high temperatures are required to detoxify them. They are also highly toxic and believed to be carcinogenic (135-139).

PCBs are widespread in the environment and are especially concentrated in river and marine sediments as well as the fatty tissues of fish and animals consuming fish. They are poorly excreted and accumulate in fatty tissues. Some species of fish are more likely than others to have high levels of PCBs because of their feeding habits, geographical location or exposure and their relatively high fat content. PCB levels also vary with the size of the fish and the season. Data for bluefish and striped bass show greater amounts of PCBs in larger fish compared with smaller ones and for striped bass caught in summer compared with those caught in winter (135, 138).

Once contamination occurs there is little that can be done to remove the PCBs from the water or the fish. The only way to avoid PCBs in fish is to remove the contaminated fish from the marketplace if it contains PCBs above the FDA action level of 2 ppm - or to avoid consuming fish known to contain PCBs. PCBs have been detected in a large number of freshwater and marine fish in widely varying amounts. In fact, one of the difficulties in assessing exposure to PCBs is the wide variability in the amounts of PCBs in fish. There may not be many fish with very high levels, but it is extremely desirable to detect and avoid those that do have significant contamination. New York, New Jersey and Massachusetts are three of a number of states that have been monitoring PCB levels in a variety of fish caught in their waters. When levels above the legal tolerance of 2 ppm are found, strict fishing limits are imposed.

According to a State report, the species most usually affected in New Jersey are striped bass, American eel, bluefish, white perch and white catfish. FDA has identified other species with high PCB residues: mackerel, drum, porgy (scup) and sea trout. In general, freshwater species are higher in PCBs than estuarine and marine ones; shellfish have less than finfish (135).

Because PCBs are most concentrated in the fat, it is possible to avoid eating the parts of the fish most likely to be highest in PCBs. By trimming the fatty portions – the belly flap, skin, lateral line and dark meat – and by broiling or baking instead of frying, the consumer can minimize the risk of eating appreciable amounts of PCBs.

People who eat a wide variety of seafoods are obviously less at risk than those who eat mainly the varieties known to have significant PCB levels. Several sport fish from the Great Lakes are heavily consumed by some people; other people eat predominantly contaminated species from Eastern coastal waters. Such population groups need to be especially aware of the risks of PCBs. Women of child-bearing age, especially pregnant and nursing women, need to be alerted to the risks of consuming PCB-contaminated fish. Among the adverse effects of PCBs are reproductive disorders and possible risk to nursing infants.

FDA has urged state and local health officials to evaluate their local circumstances and alert people as appropriate. FDA does not have the authority to close waters to fishing or to prohibit harvesting or possession of fish but it can impound or prohibit fish from interstate commerce.

Monitoring seafood supplies for PCBs (and other contaminants) requires a thorough, well designed surveillance system that will detect changes in substance levels, give an accurate range of the amounts present and identify all affected species. Analytical data need to be related to edible portions of fish as consumed so that reasonable estimates of human exposure can be derived. Information from monitoring activities can form a data bank from which trends can be determined and risk assessments made. To achieve this, comparable sampling and survey methods are required. Few surveys are comparable and some are poorly designed (135, 139), making reliable estimates difficult to make. Nevertheless, the FDA action level of 2 ppm appears to provide adequate protection from PCBs in seafood.

To minimize exposure to PCBs in seafoods:

- avoid species known to have PCBs, such as striped bass, bluefish, eel, white perch, white catfish, mackerel, drum, scup and certain Great Lakes sport fish;

- eat lean fish in preference to fattier species;

- broil or bake instead of fry;

- remove the skin, fatty portions and red muscle to reduce the consumption of the fattest parts of the fish;

- eat a variety of species rather than one or two.

**Naturally occurring toxicants and allergens**   The distinction between an allergen and a toxicant has to do with the kind of adverse reaction the substance elicits. An allergen is a substance in a food which results in an immunologic reaction when the food is eaten – that means that it triggers the production of an antibody. A toxic substance or poison acts directly upon a person without the involvement of the immune system. An example of a seafood allergen is histamine, whereas the substance called saxitoxin is the toxin responsible for paralytic shellfish poisoning.

Much as we prefer to think otherwise, nature is not always benign. Nasty substances occur naturally in a wide variety of foods, and many people are particularly susceptible to their effects. Especially with allergies, susceptibility varies with the individual, being strongly associated in families. Allergies to seafood are discussed in Chapter Seven.

Many marine animals produce toxic substances, but fortunately only a small number are related to food poisoning in people living in America. Poisoning from seafood is still a major problem in Japan, China and other countries. An excellent summary of seafood toxicants is provided in reference 140. The three major sources of toxicants in seafood are those produced by algae or plankton, those produced inherently in certain species of fish and those produced by bacterial contamination of fish. The last was discussed above in the section on bacterial toxins.

One of the best known forms of seafood poisoning, paralytic shellfish poisoning, is that which afflicts humans eating shellfish which have themselves ingested certain microscopic plankton. The dinoflagellate plankton do not affect the shellfish, but the associated toxin is accumulated by the animal and is toxic to humans when consumed. The shellfish are harmful only during times of intense plankton concentration, when the amount may be so great as to change the color of the water. Hence the term "red tide". Once the plankton quantities subside, the shellfish rid themselves of the organisms and are no longer toxic. Most mussels, clams and cockles cleanse themselves of the organisms fairly quickly, but the Alaska butter clam accumulates the poison in its siphon and may retain it for several months.

The resulting disease is called paralytic shellfish poisoning (PSP). It is characterized by numbness, muscular uncoordination, respiratory distress and possibly death. If the dose ingested is not excessive, the victim recovers with no long-lasting effects. Shellfish harvesting is controlled by the States under a Federal Program called the National Shellfish Sanitation Program. Under this arrangement, shellfish waters are continuously monitored for pollution and other contaminants. Areas found contaminated are closed to shellfishing. State Departments of Public Health will sample the beds during the prime red tide season and post notices when shellfish become excessively contaminated. FDA has set the maximum level for sagitoxin in fresh, frozen or canned shellfish at no more than 80 micrograms per 100 grams of shellfish meat (140).

A major difficulty with shellfish poisons is that they are stable to heat and processing. That means raw, cooked or canned shellfish may be poisonous if the concentration of toxin is high enough. The poisons also resist enzymatic digestion in the gut, making avoidance the only safe preventive measure.

Other types of poisons linked to plankton and blue-green algae have been identified and associated with oysters such as asari poisoning in Japan and Florida. Oddly enough, some shellfish poisons that are toxic in the laboratory have not been associated with shellfish poisoning.

There is at least one shellfish, the red whelk *Neptunea antiqua*, that produces its own toxin. Poisoning results from consuming the creature either raw or cooked. The Japanese ivory shell, *Babylonia japonica* is also poisonous. The only defense is knowledge and recognition of the species.

Another important public health problem involving seafood poisons is ciguatera poisoning. It occurs mainly in hot climates and is usually confined to the consumption of reef fishes such as snappers, barracudas, surgeon fishes, jacks, groupers, sea basses, sharks, trigger fishes, wrasses, parrot fishes and eels (140). Outbreaks of the disease are becoming more numerous as people travel more and tropical fish reach northern fish markets. The toxic substance involved comes from algae or plankton and reaches the larger species of fish through the food chain. The toxin accumulates primarily in the fish liver and viscera and to a small extent in the flesh. Outbreaks of the poisoning are sporadic, and the toxin is seldom fatal, but its effects can linger for months. There appears to be no way to detect the toxicity in the fish prior to consumption. The toxin is not destroyed by cooking.

Yet another manner in which fish may be poisonous is by virtue of their own domestically produced poison. Such is the case with the pufferfish (sometimes called blowfish or fugu), which produces the deadly substance tetrodotoxin. The fish is considered a delicacy in Japan and China, but pufferfish poisoning is a public health problem in Japan and accounts for at least 100 deaths annually (140). The Japanese government trains and licenses chefs in species recognition and in the safe removal of the puffer viscera, so that eating the flesh in a reputable establishment is less risky. Very small quantities of puffer may be imported into the U.S. from Asia. A variety caught in the Atlantic is not comparable in terms of toxicity. Historically marketed as "sea squab" because it is said to taste like chicken, there have been no documented cases of toxicity. However, it is definitely inadvisable to eat the liver or roe.

**Process-induced toxicants**   The technologies of freezing, canning, drying, smoking, pickling etc. carry with them a certain potential for adverse consequences. Reactions between the contents of a tin and its metal lining are well known, especially for acid foods. Most canned seafood is low in acid, but sardines in tomato sauce is an example of a high-acid seafood product. Harmful quantities of metal can be acquired by a product when a chemical reaction starts between the acidic food and the lining or the lead-soldered seam of the can. Many seafood processors are using cans specially lined with C-enamel to avoid this problem.

There are products of the smoking process which may contain harmful substances, depending upon the materials and procedures used. Smoked food may contain polycyclic aromatic hydrocarbons (PAH) residues and other products from wood smoke. Some of these are precursors to potentially carcinogenic compounds; others are mutagenic. This is an area where very little information exists, but suspicions have been raised.

**Viral infections**   Shellfish have been associated with viral diseases, especially hepatitis type A (infectious hepatitis). Contamination of shellfish with this virus is usually due to fecal contamination of the water where the shellfish were raised (141). Hepatitis can be severe, and there is no treatment for it except rest and the body's own healing mechanisms (1).

Shellfish from sewage polluted water can also transmit a variety of other viruses which result in severe gastrointestinal disease. The most common viruses are enteroviruses, rotaviruses, and paroviruses.

**Potentially harmful food additives**   See discussion of direct food additives, in this Chapter, below.

**Development of toxicants in the body**   This is a relatively new area of study that achieved much attention with the recognition that gastrointestinal flora, our own native and presumably friendly bacteria, produce nitrosamines, which at high levels are carcinogenic in animals.

We know very little about the achievements of our gut bacteria. Changes in the kind of bacteria in the intestinal tract can have major effects on digestion, and the extent to which diet influences these changes is an area of active research. Studies on colon cancer, the effects of dietary fiber on gut bacterial activity, the production of nitrosamines and other digestive system processes indicate that the body's usual routine may not be as innocent as we thought.

The body's production of toxicants has been most widely investigated in conjunction with specific food additives. Some examples of the ways food additives result in potential biological hazards are discussed in the food additives section, below. It is well to keep in mind that a substance may be toxic yet not hazardous, simply because our exposure may be very low, our body's defense mechanisms capable of dispatching the agent or our susceptibility inadequate.

**Parasitic infections**    Animal flesh is susceptible to parasitic infection, but parasites are a relatively minor health problem. The best known food parasite in the U.S. is *Trichenella spiralis*, or trichina, the organism sometimes found in pork (and certain wild meats like bear and walrus) that is responsible for trichinosis. Like all parasites, trichina are destroyed by heat. Thorough cooking to an internal temperature of 170°F. will destroy the worm.

There are three main types of helminth or worm parasites transmitted to man from fish (142). These are tapeworms (Cestodes), flukes (Trematodes) and roundworms (Nematodes). Parasites are only a problem when fish (and meat) are consumed raw as in sushi, sashimi and ceviche, fish roe and steak tartare, and "green" herring, or when infested products are undercooked, as sometimes occurs with pork and sausage. With the rapidly growing popularity of raw seafood such as sushi, the possiblities of parasitic infection are increased.

It has been estimated that 100,000 cases of tapeworm occur in the U.S. every year, from all sources (143). The most commonly affected fish species come from fresh water: walleye pike, perch and burbot. On the West Coast infected salmon is a source. Control can be achieved by freezing at -4°F. (-20°C). for 24-48 hours or by consuming only cooked fish.

Tapeworm infection causes pernicious anemia that results from a deficiency of vitamin $B_{12}$. The tapeworm preferentially takes up the vitamin (and other nutrients) from the gut, leaving the host an inadequate supply. In countries where diets are marginal, parasitic infection seriously undermines health, particularly in children.

Flukes are most common outside North America, mainly in China and throughout Asia, where rates of infection surpass 40 percent in some areas (142). The use of human feces as fertilizer and of fecally contaminated water ensure that the parasite thrives. The cultural habit of consuming raw fish is so widely entrenched that attempts to disrupt the life cycle of the parasite by encouraging cooking are almost futile. Imports of live or fresh shellfish that might carry the fluke are prohibited. Shellfish imports may come only from waters that are inspected and approved by the FDA under the Shellfish Sanitation Program.

Roundworms or nematodes appear from time to time in fish available at the retail level. Although they are harmless, "worms" are repelling and discourage consumers from buying and using fish, especially fresh fish. As has been pointed out previously, nematode infections are transitory among different species of fish, their occurrence being related to the available food supply and health of the species (17). Candling the fish before sale permits removal of the parasites.

Although nematode infections occur in many species they are strongly associated with cod harvested from certain areas. Popularly known as "codworms" they have been found in bottom or near bottom dwelling fishes from continental shelf waters, usually where there are large populations of seals, which are the host animal (145). The prevalence and level of infection increases with the size and age of the fish. Actual infections of codworm in man, although not unknown, are extremely rare (145).

One serious nematode health risk associated with the ingestion of raw fish is anisakiasis. This disease, caused by the nematode *Anisakis simplex*, first appeared in humans in the Netherlands and was associated with the consumption of green herring. In Japan, its occurrence is associated with sashimi consumption. In the U.S. *Anisakis* larvae have been found in fish available in markets throughout the country (146, 147). This particular nematode burrows into the gastrointestinal wall causing acute abdominal pain, frequently requiring surgery. The crisis is worth avoiding.

Fish, squid, crabs, crayfish, snails and shellfish can all be hosts to various parasites. The way to avoid infection is to cook seafood before eating it. Freezing to -20°C. is effective as well. There is some indication that codworms, and perhaps other nematode larvae, can survive some conditions of light smoking but definitive conditions are not known (145). Irradiation is potentially useful for the destruction of parasites, but its use in seafood handling is not yet approved in the U.S. It may be expected that with the increasing popularity of raw or marinated raw fish, more outbreaks of parasitic infection will occur.

## Direct Food Additives

It could safely be argued that more attention has been paid to intentional or direct food additives – those substances, other than foodstuffs, that food manufacturers and processors deliberately add to food – than to all other natural hazards in our food supply combined. That intentional food additives are regulated, easy to identify (because they are regulated) and frequently the target of consumer advocates is obvious. What is less evident, is the lack of information that frequently underlies the sinister image of these substances. No one will assert that all additives are perfectly harmless, but neither are we being slowly poisoned by the substances we add knowingly to food.

Unquestionably, intentional food additives have improved the availability, safety, stability, quality and nutritional value of our food supply. Vitamin enrichment and food fortification are two of the best known examples of the desirable use of food additives; cellulose and excessive salt are two of the worst. But it is tedious to talk about the commonplace; sensationalism, whether real or imagined, captures headlines. So it is the problem that gets attention.

When food manufacturing or processing goes awry, enormous media attention is devoted to the event. Sometimes the attention is justified because of food safety, as in the case of product recalls. It is unjustified, however, when speculation substitutes for fact. The latter is more frequently the case, as in the example of the alleged association between hyperactivity in children and salicylates in certain foods.

The result is widespread fear and mistrust of particular foods or ingredients and even of the food industry in general. Large sums of research dollars are spent disproving allegations founded on nonsense or poorly designed studies. The public often does not learn the final conclusions and nurtures the myth long after it has been discredited – as is the case with hyperactivity and food additives.

It is a very large task to dispel those fears, explain complex ideas simply and honestly, and produce the facts necessary to combat misinformation. Frequently the responsibility for banishing consumer misperceptions falls to the producer of the maligned product, whose vested interest in the subject undermines his credibility no matter how earnestly he presents the facts. We need a consortium of consumers, food scientists, nutritionists, government officials, industry representatives and communications specialists to offer an authoritative perspective to the public. No single party, so far, has gained the public's confidence on issues of food and health.

What is the basis for consumer fears? An irrational mistrust of the food supply derives from many sources: partial understanding of the facts, misinformation, ignorance of scientific principles, negative health experiences with food, "frivolous" applications of food technology, occasional outbreaks of industry-based food contamination, anti-science prejudice, increasing distance between the original source of the food and the final product, misleading advertising and health claims, abundance of nutritionally questionable or worthless products, "anti-business" or "anti-institution" bias of vocal groups, media attention to bizarre and exceptional events relating to food and so on.

Scepticism about food goes back a long way. In the Middle Ages, people were concerned about the adulteration of their food by merchants who diluted the milk, added chalk to flour and sold them short weights. It is well to raise questions and demand explanations about product composition. Fortunately there are laws and regulations to protect consumers against product adulteraton and fraud; and advocacy groups to promote awareness and action about questionable products. But we cannot always tell which products are better and which are worse.

Dishonesty in the food system has become more sophisticated. Not long ago, consumers were treated to finely ground wood chips in their bread, and this "additive" has now been reincarnated as a smoke flavoring. Replacement foods, like juice drinks, cheese food and frozen french fries may unfairly represent the original foods they replace (100 percent juice, cheese, potatoes) either because they lack some of the nutrients present in the original (potassium in fruit juices) increase the amount of "negative nutrients" (additional sodium in cheese food) or add substances that were never present in the first place (fat in french fries, food colors and artificial flavors in juice drinks).

The concern that replacement foods, new food products (especially those bearing little resemblence to traditional familiar foods) and modified or highly processed foods might adversely affect our nutritional welfare is well founded. There are plenty of examples to support the following observations in processed foods: missing trace elements; exorbitant amounts of sodium; additions or increases in total fat or saturated fat; removal of dietary fiber; unwarranted addition or increase of sugar; chemical destruction of nutrients; loss of vitamins and so on. Many of these observations can be offset by positive aspects: vitamin and mineral enrichment of flour and some cereals; development of reduced and low sodium foods; and the use of antioxidants which protect fat soluble vitamins. But there remains much to be desired in the nutritional quality of many processed foods.

The seafood industry is not immune from these observations just because it has fewer products on the shelves. In fact, the rapid development of markets for surimi-based products places particular responsibility on seafood processors. (A full discussion of the nutritional aspects of surimi and of processing in general can be read in Chapter Five). The seafood industry is confronted with new technology in handling, product development, processing and packaging which promise ease, convenience, longer shelf life and new products but which pose similar dilemmas when it comes to nutritional quality. Many of these new technologies depend upon food additives at some point in their implementation. Because the manufacturer has most of the responsibility for maintaining the nutritional value of his product, it is important that nutritional quality be considered equally with food safety and product appeal.

The following section describes the food additives most widely used in seafood processing and gives the nutritional consequences, if any, of each. Additives are grouped according to their technical functions within two main divisions: processing additives and final product additives. The categories are based on the data collected from the food industry through surveys conducted by the National Academy of Sciences/National Research Council (148-150). Where a substance performs more than one function, its classification is that used by the NAS/NRC. If the substance has GRAS status, this is mentioned; otherwise, the substance is regulated as a food additive.

## Processing Additives

These substances are used at the industrial level to facilitate the processing, storage, handling, or packaging of foods. In general, they are not functionally active in the final product although they may be present in low concentrations (148).

**Phosphates** Phosphates are salts of phosphoric acid. They may be condensed with either sodium or potassium but the sodium salts are the most common. Although there are several different kinds of phosphate salts, the ones most effective in seafood treatment are sodium polyphosphate (sodium tripolyphosphate) and sodium pyrophosphate. The pyrophosphate contains two phosphorus atoms and the polyphosphate contains three. A third phosphate, sodium hexametaphosphate is used in canned seafood to prevent the formation of struvite crystals.

Polyphosphates do several things: they help prevent the loss of water or drip from cut fish and shellfish which improves yield and physical appearance; and they prevent oxidation and minimize texture changes (151, 152). They are effective during both refrigerated storage and freezing. Too much polyphosphate, however, will extract protein from the flesh and give a slimy, translucent appearance.

Polyphosphates help the flesh to bond and this property improves the appearance and texture of thawed fish. It also means that frozen fillets need to be separated by a plastic film if they are to be easily separated later.

Polyphosphates act primarily on the surface of the fish or shellfish and do not penetrate the flesh. For this reason, flatfish, whose surface area is large relative to their weight, take up more polyphosphate than round fish. It is difficult to assess how much polyphosphate is taken up by fish because of the large variation in natural phosphate content (153). There is no doubt, however, that such dips increase the phosphorus content. Polyphosphate treatment also increases the uptake of water in the flesh. Unscrupulous operators often use excessive phosphate to increase the weight of the product.

The nutritional implications are unclear: the amount of phosphorus, a necessary nutrient, contributed by the phosphate dipping of seafood, is difficult to assess. It is believed to be relatively small. Certainly the amount of phosphates in other kinds of foods like baked products, processed meats and processed cheese contribute greater amounts of phosphorus to the diet than seafood dips (154). Tripolyphosphate binds calcium and magnesium. There has been some concern over total dietary phosphate decreasing calcium deposition, especially in children. This would have a negative effect on nutritive value were it not for the fact that most seafood is not particularly abundant in these minerals.

**Other dips**   Specialty dips have been developed for seafood destined for further processing. These solutions may contain isolated soy protein along with salt, phosphate, sugar and sometimes other ingredients. They claim to increase the water uptake of fish or shrimp by 25-30 percent (155). This water is unbound and is usually lost during cooking. After dipping, fish or shrimp are processed with breading or batter and frozen. These dips are also proposed for use in extending scallops processed as "restructured scallops" using sausage casing. This type of dip suggests adulteration to the author. The addition of water as well as soy protein is supposed to be listed on ingredient labels.

## Washing/Surface Removal Agents

**Chlorine**   Dilute chlorine solutions are very often used for washing fish to assist in removing bacteria. The recommended procedure calls for washing fish from bulk storage with chlorinated sprays containing 2-10 ppm (parts per million) chlorine (156). How much if any chlorine remains in the flesh is unknown. Minute amounts of chlorine may be detectable in the final product. Chlorine is needed in small amounts but the requirement is more than filled by the chloride in table salt (sodium chloride).

## Final Product Additives

These substances remain functionally active in the final food product after processing.

**Sulphites**  This category includes sodium and potassium bisulphite, sodium and potassium metabisulphite, sodium sulphite and sulfur dioxide. The major use of these substances is in fresh produce items; sodium bisulphite is authorized for use, however, in shrimp, because it prevents the development of melanosis, or "black spot." Recent awareness of the sensitivity of certain people, particulary asthmatics, to sulphites has led to review of their usage by the FDA. In fact, shipments of shrimp into the U.S. were impounded because of the suspected excessive levels of sulphite. The FDA is presently reviewing its position on sodium and potassium bisulphite and has recently proposed a ban on the use of five sulphite compounds on fresh vegetables and salads. To date, sulphites remain on the GRAS list. The nutritional implications are minor. While it has been recognized for a long time that sulphite destroys the vitamin thiamin, the amount of thiamin is fairly low in seafood and its destruction is not a major issue. Thiamin is obtained mainly from whole grains and enriched flour. Sulphite does have a protective effect on certain amino acids preventing their involvement in browning (157). It also enhances the retention of vitamin C (ascorbic acid).

**Nitrates, nitrites**  Nitrates are naturally occurring salts of nitrogen, oxygen and usually sodium. They can be converted to nitrite. Nitrite, most commonly in the form of sodium nitrite, is used as a preservative in certain vacuum packed foods such as bacon, hot dogs and sausages to protect against the deadly microorganism, *Clostridium botulinum*. Nitrites are also used to impart a characteristic pink or red color and a distinctive flavor to cured foods.

Much concern has been expressed over the relationship between these substances and the formation of closely related compounds, nitrosamines. Some nitrosamines are carcinogenic to laboratory animals, but neither nitrite nor nitrate are themselves carcinogenic. Large amounts of nitrite are toxic.

Nitrate is widely distributed in plants and under certain "natural" circumstances of storage may be converted to nitrite. Nitrates and nitrites are also synthesized in the body, even in the absence of dietary intake (158). The conversion of nitrate to nitrite occurs naturally through the action of microorganisms in the mouth. What worries people is the conversion of nitrite to nitrosamines in the body and in foods, and the possible risk of cancer from this group of compounds. It has been estimated that the natural synthesis of nitrosamines in the body is the largest source of human exposure to these compounds (159). Several researchers in the field have also concluded that the presence of nitrite in cured meats does not increase natural nitrosamine formation in people (160).

The formation of nitrosamines from nitrite can be inhibited by the presence of other substances, particularly ascorbic acid (vitamin C) (161). Vitamin E also inhibits nitrosamine formation in some systems. Much attention has been given to cooked bacon as a source of nitrosamines. One possible reason cooked bacon retains nitrosamines is that very little water remains at the end of cooking, compared with other cured meats. It has been suggested that lack of water means that fewer of the volatile nitrosamines can be carried off during cooking (162). The use of nitrosamine inhibitors has enabled the use of substantially smaller amounts of nitrite in bacon curing: 40 parts per million (ppm) instead of 120 ppm (163). Presently, bacon is monitored to ensure that the final amount of the major volatile nitrosamine in bacon does not exceed 10 parts per billion (164).

Nitrites and the nitrosamine issue are important to the seafood business. They are used in curing and smoking but very little is known about the formation and retention of nitrosamines in cured and smoked seafood. Nitrites have been considered indispensable in cured meats as a protection against botulism. Presumably, they would be similarly useful in seafood. Whether conditions in seafood favor nitrosamine formation and retention as readily as in bacon or as inconsistently as in other cured meats is unknown.

Nitrites are inhibited from forming potentially harmful nitrosamines by ascorbic acid and vitamin E. Ascorbic acid levels are very low in seafood, so that this interaction is negligible. Vitamin E levels in seafood appear to be relatively low as well. Nitrites can interact with lysine resulting in the loss of this essential amino acid, thereby reducing the biological value of the protein. To what extent this actually happens is not known.

**Potassium Sorbate**   A GRAS substance used in processed fish products to retard the growth of fungi and molds. Recently, sorbate in dip solutions has been shown to retard bacterial growth in fresh seafoods. Commercial preparations incorporating potassium sorbate are now in use.

**Salt**   A GRAS substance and probably the most ubiquitous food additive, salt is used frequently in seafood processing. It may be a component of poly-phosphate mixtures used to dip fish, or it may be the only ingredient in a brine dip. Concentrated brines are used for freezing tuna, crabs and salmon. Seawater may be used as a cooking and cooling medium and also for refrigerated storage at sea.

Salt fulfills various functions depending on the concentration used. At high concentrations it is a preservative; at low concentrations it is a flavor agent. There is no clear separation of these functions except that concentrations above 2 percent may taste excessively salty.

Salt is clearly used as a preservative in salt dried cod and in pickled or marinated seafoods. It is a customary component of seafood canning liquids, except in diet pack fish.

The nutritional implications are important: because most Americans consume excessive amounts of sodium, and sodium contributes to high blood pressure in millions of Americans, the FDA and health professionals have urged the food industry to reduce the customary levels of salt added to products. Salt is not needed as a preservative in fresh, frozen or canned seafood so that amounts presently added to these forms of seafood could safely be lowered. The amounts of salt present in smoked, dried and pickled seafood products is very high, and cannot be effectively removed after purchasing the product. Developing ways of making these processing methods less dependent upon high levels of salt would be a major health and happiness achievement. Seafood processed without salt or brine has distinct health advantages.

## Flavors and Flavor Modifiers

**Vegetable Broth**  This is an optional packing fluid for canned tuna with the following standard of identity: "consists of a minimum of 0.5 percent by weight of vegetable extractives and to be prepared from two or more of the following vegetables: beans, carrots, cabbage, celery, garlic, onions, parsley, peas, potatoes, green bell peppers, red bell peppers, spinach, and tomatoes" (165). The nutritional implications are minor: usually the amount present (no more than 5 percent of the volume of the container) is too small to be able to contribute important amounts of nutrients. Broth is frequently discarded or drained, so that nutrients are lost. Broth does not contribute calories but usually contains large amounts of sodium, either from salt or monosodium glutamate or both.

**Lemon Flavoring**  May be added to canned tuna if it conforms to the following standard of identity: "prepared from lemon oil and citric acid together with safe and suitable carriers for the lemon oil which are present at non-functional and insignificant levels in the finished canned food. . . a safe and suitable dispersing ingredient may be added in a quantity not exceeding 0.005 percent by weight of the finished food" (165).

**Monosodium Glutamate (MSG)**  This substance is widely used as a flavor enhancer in protein rich foods. It is also a well known constituent of Oriental style food. Some people are sensitive to it and develop transitory side effects. MSG is frequently found in surimi based seafood products.

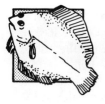

*Chapter Four*

# Nutrition Consequences of Different Processing Methods

## Handling

How the fish is handled and stored after harvesting has a great deal to do with how well and how long it will retain its quality. Temperature is probably the single most important factor, but such features as physical abuse, bruising, density of packing, time before cleaning and gutting, washing, and sanitation procedures all affect how much the fish will have deteriorated before it reaches the next stage in processing. A good summary of the consequences of physical damage to seafood quality is presented in (166). Deterioration in quality, of course, affects the ultimate nutritional value of the product through losses and chemical changes.

There are three categories of concern in the immediate handling of seafood that are linked to the retention of nutritional value. These are:

- fish spoilage, primarily relating to bacterial activity, lipid oxidation and autolysis (self-digestion)

- drip loss from the cut surfaces of fish

- washing procedures

## Causes of Fish Spoilage

Fish is widely known to be one of the most perishable of all food items. Its fragility is related to the composition of the product and the presence of bacteria. Unlike meat, fish muscle is not protected by a layer of fat or connective tissue; the skin, however, is a deterrent to bacterial invasion. Seafood develops off flavors and odors quickly if it is not properly handled after catching and odor alone can discourage a consumer from buying seafood. If odor cannot be checked, it is more difficult to determine the freshness of a seafood item, but biochemical and sensory tests are available (167). A brief and excellent review of the major sources of damage to seafood is given in (166). Tips for handling fish to maintain top quality in processing, packaging and shipping operations are given in (156, 168).

Several different types of spoilage activity are involved in eroding the quality of seafood. There is enzymatic action from enzymes in the fish itself; bacterial spoilage from bacteria in the fish and surrounding environment; and the chemical breakdown of fat or autoxidation. Because the native bacteria and enzymes involved in these processes are adapted to work at cold temperatures, a certain amount of activity will occur after harvesting, even under well-iced conditions. Canning destroys and freezing or icing greatly retards these activities. The rule: COOL, QUICK, CLEAN is aimed at minimizing the effects of spoilage agents (144).

It has long been thought that being able to monitor various spoilage processes over time might be a useful way of determining freshness in seafood. Several biochemical tests have been developed for this purpose but many of them have serious difficulties in implementation and are not suited to all species (167). It is useful to review the major sources of spoilage in fish, because different types of processing affect these activities in different ways. Other types of deterioration are reviewed in (166).

**Temperature**   probably the most critical factor for preserving freshness and quality is cold. Near freezing temperatures, or slightly below 32°F. are ideal for maintaining seafood quality. The higher the temperature, the shorter the keeping time.

**Autolysis**   this term simply means self breakdown. When the fish dies, cells release enzymes which act on the tissue of the animal. There are several breakdown products which result from enzyme activity. The main ones for seafood are amino acids from the breakdown of protein, lactic acid from the breakdown of glycogen in muscle, hypoxanthine from the breakdown of cellular nucleotides, and trimethylamine oxide breakdown to trimethylamine. Measurements of hypoxanthine and trimethylamine have been particularly encouraging for the monitoring of freshness in certain seafood species.

**Bacterial Activity**   Bacteria present in the gut and visceral organs are ready to spring into action on the fish muscle once the animal has died. That is one reason why it is especially important to gut and wash fish as soon after harvest as possible. Bacteria also reside on the flesh as a result of cross contamination – the unintentional transfer of microorganisms from storage sites, fish handlers' equipment and other places to the fish. The use of cleaning solutions, rinses and good sanitation practices will minimize this problem.

The amount of bacterial growth is determined by the numbers of bacteria present to begin with, the temperature and the type of bacteria present. Psychotrophs, or cold-loving bacteria, thrive at freezing temperatures, whereas others are killed or inactivated. Modified atmospheres, like the increase in carbon dioxide and the reduction in oxygen used in certain packaging techniques, favor the growth of gram-positive bacteria over the original population of predominantly gram-negative bacteria (169). Increasing temperature, as mentioned above, gives nearly all bacteria a boost.

The major results of bacterial action are "off" flavors and odors and the production of several chemicals, chiefly trimethylamine (TMA), lactic acid, diamines like putrescine and cadaverine, and histamine (especially in mahimahi) (167, 170).

**Fat Breakdown or rancidity**   Known as autoxidation, this term refers to the chemical breakdown of fat in the presence of oxygen. It is a problem mainly for species of fish having more than 5 percent fat content (See Tables 2.3 and 2.4 in Chapter Two). Autoxidation, which is a major concern to the fish industry is difficult to prevent because the chemical process is self-generating. It is particularly prone to occur in polyunsaturated oils, continues or is enhanced at freezing temperatures, is not particularly deterred by the usual food antioxidants and causes much fish spoilage (171, 172).

Fish oil is especially vulnerable to rancidity because of the large share of polyunsaturated fatty acids with many double bonds. The double bonds are highly susceptible to taking up oxygen, which can result in the formation of ketones, aldehydes, and hydroxy-acids. Fat oxidation results in the development of unpleasant "fishy" odors.

Oxidation is enhanced in the presence of compounds containing iron or copper, so that the red muscle parts of the flesh are much more easily spoiled. This can be a problem for such species as tuna, swordfish, bluefish, mackerel and others. Fish oils also oxidize more quickly when frozen or irradiated rather than when iced and stored (36, 166). Rancidity is retarded in frozen seafoods that are vacuum packaged (166). A more elaborate discussion of oxidation in fish is given by Stansby (171) and Kramer (166).

The main nutritional implication of fat oxidation is that the nutritional value of the fat is decreased because the amount of polyunsaturated fatty acids is reduced. Oxidation also destroys fat soluble vitamins, especially vitamins E and A. Note, though, that the function of vitamin E is to prevent fat oxidation, and in the process it becomes oxidized itself. The need for vitamin E is greater when the diet contains plenty of polyunsaturated fatty acids (7). Also, the vitamin A content of most fish muscle is very low; however, it is extremely concentrated in fish liver oils.

## Drip Loss

Once the fish has been cut, the surface of the flesh loses water. This water loss occurs in both fresh and frozen fish (upon thawing) and can be extensive. Values of 5-10 percent have been reported for salmon, halibut and fresh-water species, with values up to 30 percent being known (173-175). Drip is apparently greater from salt-water fish than from fresh water species (174, 175).

While the loss is primarily water, the drip also contains water soluble proteins, B vitamins and minerals (176). Fish that has been thawed and refrozen exhibits much greater drip loss, fatty acid oxidation and other signs of inferior quality (177, 178). Measures to reduce drip are related directly to the methods of handling and to the use of polyphosphate dips. Polyphosphate dips increase water pickup. They also increase the amount of sodium and phosphorus in the fish while retaining moisture, protein and minerals (152, 174). The use of phosphates in preventing drip loss is further discussed in Chapter Five.

## Washing

Sanitation and handling procedures aboard ship and in the fish processing plant require washing fish sometimes several times before it reaches its final packaged form. In addition to keeping the fish clean, however, washing leaches out protein and minerals, particularly sodium and potassium. It has been estimated that in fish washed by the melt water from icing, about 60 percent of the initial sodium and potassium are lost. In fish washed with seawater or brine, however, potassium is still lost, but sodium uptake increases (179). The loss of protein and potassium and the gain in sodium all diminish the nutritive value of the fish.

The effects of washing in the treatment of minced fish is discussed separately in Chapter Five.

---

# Freezing

Freezing is one of the best ways to prolong shelf life of seafood and if done under exacting conditions, is effective in retaining high quality and flavor. Textural changes are inevitable, but these are not necessarily very noticeable at the consumer level. Freezing of less than top quality product or using slow freezing procedures that are known to damage the fish will reduce the quality of the frozen product. In the past, both practices were common, and have contributed to the negative image of frozen seafood, especially finfish, in the mind of the consumer. Today's practices of freezing as soon as possible after harvest, treating freshly caught fish with great care, using superior packaging materials, and ensuring transport and storage well below 0°C., have resulted in very high quality product. Summaries of the current freezing methods used in fish processing are given in (180) and (181).

The possible adverse consequences of freezing include the following:

- texture loss through breakdown of the physical structure of the muscle;

- denaturation of proteins with the loss of amino acids;

- breakdown of fats with the accumulation of unpleasant by-products and a loss of fatty acids and vitamins;

- chemical interactions between proteins and lipids and proteins and carbohydrates;

- loss of protein, B vitamins and minerals through drip.

These changes occur as a result of chemical processes, enzyme activity and microbial action. There are fewer data on nutrient changes with freezing in seafood than there are for many other food categories.

Overall, freezing results in a high degree of nutrient retention – better than most other seafood preparation methods (182). It slows down enzyme activity (but does not eliminate it completely), it inhibits microbial growth, and retards chemical reactions. Lipid oxidation reactions still occur, however, and in some cases proceed more rapidly in the frozen state than in the chilled (183). Enzyme assisted reactions may also be accelerated during freezing and thawing possibly due to the release of subcellular materials when the cells are damaged during freezing (178). It is not safe to assume that freezing and storage conditions have been ideal throughout the distribution system or that substantial nutrient losses may not have occurred. The most important factors in nutrient retention in frozen seafood are:

- top quality product at the outset

- low bacterial counts

- short time between harvest, cleaning and freezing

- rapid chilling

- very low freezing and storage temperatures (below 0°F. or -18°C.)

- rapid time to reach the frozen state

- fat content of the fish – fattier fish oxidize more readily

- packaging material – resistance to breakage, passage of oxygen and tightness of fit are important

- presence of air (oxygen) – oxygen accelerates oxidation, carbon dioxide retards it

The control of oxidative rancidity is a major problem with the freezing of high fat fish (those over 5 percent fat). The results from a number of research investigations on herring, mackerel, salmon and other species indicate that rancidity can be kept to a minimum by the following conditions:

**Rapid chilling**    Spoilage starts immediately after a fish dies and the rate of spoilage is mainly temperature dependent. The sooner the fish is cooled, the better. Use of small ice flakes gives the ice greater contact with the fish and removes heat faster than large ice chips. Small ice flakes are superior for rapid chilling (181).

**Short time to freezing**    The longer the times between harvesting, chilling and freezing, the greater the oxidation of fats upon freezing (166).

**Temperature of freezer storage**    Studies with various species have shown increased storage time and preservation of quality with storage at $-30°C.$ ($-22°F.$) compared with storage at $-18°C.$ (zero F.) (166, 184). Home freezers usually do not reach temperatures as low as $-30°C.$ but are designed to reach temperatures between -15°C (+5°F.) and −20°C (−4°F.) (185). Many do not reach this range and vary in their holding temperature with defrosting cycles. Retail freezing units also vary widely in their temperature. Fluctuations in holding temperatures – even well below freezing – also increase oxidation as well as texture loss.

**Use of additives**   There are reports that the appropriate use of tripolyphosphates and ascorbic acid will reduce oxidative rancidity in some species of fish (152, 166). Most fish has been resistant to the beneficial effects of food antioxidants, although some success with ascorbic acid has been reported. It should be noted that the use of polyphosphates to improve the quality of mistreated fish is not effective (37, 172, 186, 187).

**Species**   In general, susceptibility to rancidity increases with the fat content of the fish. That does not mean, however, that low fat fish will not undergo oxidative rancidity. Pacific cod and walleye pollock are two examples of low fat fish that have oxidation problems during frozen storage (166).

**Spawning**   Prior to spawning, fish feed voraciously and increase their body fat content substantially. After spawning, their fat content is very low and the water content of the muscle high. These changes are particularly marked in Pacific salmon species which die after spawning. Such changes in composition make the quality of the flesh inferior. Even though the fat content is reduced, oxidative rancidity still occurs.

**Presence of red muscle**   Pigmented muscle is rich in iron and copper, two minerals that promote oxidative rancidity. Keeping time is therefore reduced, even under ideal storage conditions in such fish. This applies mainly to tuna, swordfish and bluefish.

**Bleeding**   Fish that have been bled prior to freezing exhibit superior keeping qualities. This is partly due to the removal of blood with its iron-containing pigments that foster lipid oxidation. Bleeding fish as soon after catch as possible results in a higher quality product all around and is a strongly recommended handling procedure.

In summary, there is no more appropriate recommendation than that of Dr. Donald Kramer: "If I were to pick the two most important points which should be stressed to fishermen, they would be early bleeding and early chilling" (166).

# Vacuum Packaging

## Conditions in the Vacuum Package

Thanks in part to the development of sophisticated packaging materials and processing equipment, and a better understanding of the causes of fish spoilage, vacuum packaging is becoming a viable technology in seafood processing. It is widespread in the meat industry for fresh, processed and cured products, but has faced difficulties in its application to seafood. The major obstacle to its use in seafood is the potential for the growth under low-oxygen conditions of *Clostridium botulinum*, a ubiquitous bacterium that produces a deadly toxin, type E toxin -- botulism poisoning.

Vacuum packaging brings about several changes: a drastic reduction in oxygen content, an increase in carbon dioxide and an increase in acidity. The concentration of carbon dioxide is not as great as that created in modified atmosphere packaging, but it is enough to increase the shelf life of fish (188). If the packaging material is a very good barrier to oxygen, which it must be to obtain adequate shelf life extension, then the growth of a variety of spoilage organisms is substantially decreased. But microbial growth is not prevented entirely, and this is the crux of the problem. If harmful organisms are present and the holding temperature of the package rises above 38°F. (3°C.) for any length of time, then spoilage and toxin production can occur. It should be noted that most domestic refrigerators are above 40°F.

In vacuum sealed packages, carbon dioxide increases as a result of bacterial activity and cellular metabolic activities. Carbon dioxide discourages the development of the normal spoilage bacteria, yeast and molds but does allow the development of other types of bacteria (188). These surviving flora usually result in less objectionable changes in the fish – those less readily detected by the nose.

There remains a major worry, however, in packages with little or no oxygen. Such an environment is just what the bacterium that causes botulism, *Clostridium botulinum*, needs to flourish. In such an environment other spoilage organisms may not thrive, allowing the production of the deadly toxin before the product becomes noticeably unpalatable. Normal spoilage organisms in fish serve as an early warning system about bacterial activity, and their malodorous products alert the consumer to discard the product. Botulinus toxin is destroyed by normal cooking so the major risk is with ready-to-eat products.

It is the possibility of undetected botulism activity which makes vacuum packaging of some types of fish risky. The presence of spices, smoke flavors and perhaps only mild signs of spoilage may mask the extent of *C. botulinum* activity. Smoked fish products are among the most susceptible seafoods because they present virtually all the conditions necessary for botulism toxin to be produced. These conditions are:

- presence of the organism – *Clostridium botulinum* is everywhere in the seafood processing environment;

- processing has not destroyed the organism or its spores – Clostridium can survive many smoking and marination procedures;

- *Clostridium botulinum* must be able to grow in the food – temperature above 38°F. (3°C.) is necessary (and frequently occurs in home and retail refrigerators); it requires anaerobic (oxygen-free) conditions, but its development has been observed in unpackaged foods where anaerobic conditions can be created just below the surface of the food (188).

In smoked fish products, the presence of carbon dioxide, smoke compounds, salt and other substances like sodium nitrite all act to discourage toxin production, although they do not guarantee its absence. Spoilage and toxin production are also favored the longer the time after harvest that packaging occurs (188). It appears that vacuum packaging with increased carbon dioxide levels is not, by itself, the only answer to discouraging harmful microorganisms.

Exposure to temperatures above 38°F. (3°C.) can permit toxin production in vacuum packed products without any other signs of bacterial activity. The presence of sodium nitrite (100-200 parts per million), a high level of salt (over 3.5 percent in the presence of nitrite, 4.5 percent without), or potassium sorbate, plus storage below 38°F. (3°C.) will inhibit *Clostridium botulinum*. The bacteria's spores need even higher salt levels for destruction: 8.2 percent to 10.5 percent (189). The problem with relying on temperature is that storage temperature during many phases of transport and distribution can seldom be guaranteed. At the present time, it may be stated that the general use of vacuum packaging in smoked fish products that are marketed unfrozen should be discouraged (188).

Vacuum packaged fresh fish, using materials that are highly impermeable to oxygen, held either refrigerated or frozen, retain their quality longer than fish in overwrapped packages. Spoilage occurs more rapidly at higher temperatures regardless of packaging material. Vacuum packaging by itself does not ensure freedom from microbial activity. One serious problem with vacuum packaging is that there are no normal visual or other sensory indicators relating to the quality of the fish. Vacuum packed fillets show no loss of translucence (sheen) and no odors are detectable through the packaging. If the product is spoiled by mishandling, the consumer can have a real surprise when the pack is opened at home: fish spoiled under anaerobic conditions produce amazingly noxious odors.

Vacuum packaging has the additional disadvantage that the oxygen impermeable materials required are relatively expensive and appropriate equipment is needed. Until some guarantee of freedom from botulinum toxin can be assured, the method will be slow in taking hold in the marketplace.

## Packaging Materials

Packaging protects food from environmental contamination and conversely shields the surroundings from the package contents. The latter is especially important with seafood because fluid losses can promote spoilage, facilitate the development of odors and diminish consumer acceptance (190). We are used to thinking of packages as benign and inert, but such is not always the case.

Packaging affects the nutritive value of seafood by controlling exposure to light, water, heat, oxygen and bacteria. Package material may also interact with the package contents, a possibility that has many implications for seafood preservation and nutritional quality. The effects of these factors will be considered as they pertain to seafood.

**Light**    Both visible and ultraviolet light can affect nutrients. The length of exposure, the wavelength and intensity of the light and the permeability of the package to the light all affect whether or not nutrients will be destroyed. Those nutrients most susceptible to photo-destruction are riboflavin, ascorbic acid, vitamin A, fats, sulfur-containing amino acids and other B vitamins in the presence of riboflavin. Except for vitamin A and ascorbic acid, all these nutrients are present in important amounts in seafood and need to be protected from unnecessary or lengthy light exposure.

Light also catalyzes or promotes the autoxidation of polyunsaturated oils in fish (172). Fast turnover in the retail case and the rotation of packages will minimize the adverse effects of light on photo-sensitive nutrients. Packages for products with long shelf lives are better made from opaque materials.

**Temperature**    The type of packaging material greatly affects the rate at which heat is transferred to and from the food. This is important for both refrigerated and frozen seafood. Insulating containers like styrofoam food trays greatly reduce the transfer of heat to the fish, but will retard cooling if the packaged fish is not already very cold. The problem of packaged fish in self-serve refrigerated seafood counters is complex. Cooling takes place by conduction and convection while heat is generated from fluorescent and other light fixtures and transmitted by radiation. The thermal properties of the seafood wrap may be especially important for retarding heat uptake by the package (191).

Package materials also affect the rate of freezing and thawing. In freezing the type of process is critical, and factors associated with package material may be less important than other considerations. On the other hand, package materials which retard the uptake of heat in frozen food are important in maintaining cold temperatures and hence in preserving nutrients.

**Oxygen**    The presence of excessive amounts of oxygen promotes seafood deterioration through the oxidation of fats, the degradation of some amino acids and the destruction of certain vitamins. The effects of oxygen are related to the pressure of the environment, the humidity and the temperature. Exposure of the package contents to oxygen may occur through loose closure, puncture and/or diffusion through the packaging material itself.

Considerable research has been conducted into the gas permeability of different packaging materials and the subsequent keeping qualities of the contents. Permeability considerations apply not only to oxygen, but also to other gases like carbon dioxide, nitrogen and water vapor. Initial research focused on oxygen permeability and oxidative and bacterial damage, but the development of modified atmosphere packaging has made the consideration of the movement of other gases a practical matter.

Seafood processors have available to them a variety of materials of different oxygen permeability for use in fresh and frozen seafood packaging. The selection of the most appropriate form, however, also depends on the type of packaging used. For example, a highly impermeable material is not likely to be as effective in seafood overwrapping as it is in vacuum packaging. The nature of the material and the type of packaging are related.

The permeability to oxygen of some common packaging materials is shown in Table 4.1. The larger the number, the more permeable the material.

*Table 4.1    Oxygen Permeability of Various Packaging Materials at 25-30°C.*[a]

| Material | Permeability Range[b] |
|---|---|
| Silicon rubber | over 250,000 |
| Polyvinyl chloride film, household | 13,000 - 14,000[c] |
| Conventional polyethylene | 6000 - 15,000 |
| Coated and wax papers | 100 - 15,000 |
| Cellulose acetate | 1000 - 5000 |
| High density polyethylene | 1500 - 3000 |
| Pliofilm | 200 - 5000 |
| Plain cellophane | 20 - 5000 |
| (Poly)-Trifluorochloroethylene | 50 - 1000 |
| Saran | 10 - 350 |
| Mylar | 50 - 100 |

[a] Data from Harris and Karmas, Nutritional Evaluation of Food Processing (196).
[b] Measured in (Cc).(Mil).(Day-1).(M-2).(Atm-1)
[c] Reference (201).

Table 4.1 makes it clear that the common household plastic films like polyethylene, wax paper and plastic wraps are among the more permeable materials available. Saran, on the other hand, is highly impermeable and makes a desirable wrap for home freezing uses. Its disadvantage is that it becomes brittle and is likely to crack in the cold. Overwrapping Saran covered seafood with aluminum foil gives added protection. Single-strength aluminum foil is not recommended by itself.

Studies with Cryovac® and other packaging materials have shown that the use of highly impermeable films in vacuum packaging is superior to the use of polyethylene or polyvinyl chloride (PVC) films in overwrapped packages for preserving the quality of both fresh and frozen fish (192). When the fillets were clean to begin with, there was essentially no odor development observed in the washed vacuum packed samples in the first six days of storage at 32°F. By contrast, the PVC packed fish had a noticeable development in odor and were given only a "fair" sensory rating of quality at the end of the same period. These comparisons, of course, include differences in both packaging materials and type of package, but they do reflect the kinds of options available in the marketplace. These studies and others suggest that vacuum packaging with suitable materials can increase the shelf life of both fresh and frozen seafood (169, 192).

Permeability is also affected by temperature and moisture. That means that some films may be better suited to freezer temperatures and others to refrigerator temperatures. Under freezing conditions, where humidity and moisture levels are high, the influence of water on the material is important. Films made from ethylene vinyl alcohol are especially sensitive to humidity and would be less suitable for freezer wraps than other barriers (193).

## Modified Atmosphere Packaging and Storage

As early as 1932, Coyne reported the beneficial effects of carbon dioxide ($CO_2$) in inhibiting the growth of bacteria from fish (194, 195). Bacterial growth was inhibited even after the cultures were removed to air, an observation that has been confirmed recently (188). Bacterial growth is not inhibited in atmospheres high in nitrogen (196). The beneficial effects of $CO_2$ have been discussed above in conjunction with vacuum packaging. They have also been applied to other storage systems, namely $CO_2$ saturated seawater and $CO_2$ enriched atmospheres.

Studies at the National Marine Fisheries Service in Seattle, Washington have demonstrated increased storage life of fresh fish and shellfish using refrigerated seawater saturated with $CO_2$ (196). The results appear to apply to a wide variety of species including fatty species of salmon, low fat rockfish and shrimp.

When the air surrounding the fish is changed in composition, usually by enriching it with $CO_2$, and the container then sealed, the atmosphere is said to be "modified". In such containers, the atmosphere can change owing to the activity of bacteria, tissue metabolism and permeability of the container. By contrast, if the atmosphere around the fish is subjected to a continuous flow of a specified gas mixture, then the atmosphere is described as "controlled" (196). Practical applications in seafood handling use modified atmospheres.

Several studies have demonstrated extended shelf life of seafood using modified atmospheres enriched with $CO_2$ (197-199). The optimal level of $CO_2$ is open to debate, since improvements are observed with levels as low as 11.5 percent $CO_2$ and as high as 80 percent $CO_2$ (196). Good shelf life extension has been reported with 50 percent $CO_2$ (169). The higher the level, the longer the shelf life extension, and the better the quality within the acceptability range.

Fish and shellfish from modified atmosphere storage have lower bacterial counts, greater acidity level, reduced trimethylamine formation and lower ammonia production (199). There is also a residual and positive effect on the keeping quality after removal from the $CO_2$ enriched environment. As with the vacuum packaging studies, however, temperature is a critical component of the effectiveness of $CO_2$. Temperature abuse results in bacterial spoilage and possible development of toxins.

Just how $CO_2$ exerts its beneficial effects on seafood shelf life is not known with certainty. Initially, fish exposed to $CO_2$ absorb the gas which becomes incorporated into cells making them and the surrounding fluid environment more acid. The tissues gradually counteract the effects of the acid by producing bicarbonate. $CO_2$ itself has powerful inhibitory effects on microbial activity; it alters the transfer of certain ions, especially potassium, across the cell wall and it may affect enzyme systems in the cells. The possible mechanisms for the action of carbon dioxide are discussed in (196).

There are two disadvantages to modified atmosphere packaging. One is the accumulation of unpleasant odors in the package, owing to the activity of anaerobic organisms. These odors are not the usual type of "fishy" odors produced by seafood, because of the different types of bacteria operating in the modified atmosphere. Once the package has been opened and left exposed to the air, the vapors dissipate and the fish is palatable. Fish held in controlled atmospheres do not accumulate these odors because the circulation of fresh gas removes them. At least one such controlled atmosphere system has been developed at Texas A & M University (197).

The second and more serious problem is the threat of *C. botulinum* activity. *C. botulinum* can operate in $CO_2$ modified atmospheres as well as in a vacuum pack. The major factor inhibiting its growth is cold temperature. Eklund has observed *C. botulinum* growth in $CO_2$ modified atmospheres at temperatures as low as 42°F. (5°C.), so that unless temperatures can be held consistently below 38°F. (3°C.), botulinum activity cannot be ruled out (188). It is likely that other off odors would be produced under the conditions permitting botulinum activity, but this is not certain either.

What other conditions might discourage *C. botulinum*? Besides temperature control below 38°F. (3°C.), at least three substances are known to inhibit toxin formation. These are salt, sodium nitrite and sorbate. Other substances like sodium hypophosphite, liquid smoke, sulfur dioxide gas and chlorine have been, or currently are being, investigated. Also, the organism cannot tolerate too much acid. A pH value below 4.5 (neutrality is pH 7.0) will not support botulinum growth so pickled or marinated fish is not a risk. An outline of the situation with regard to these substances follows:

**Salt**   High levels of salt, 5-6 percent, will inhibit the growth of C. botulinum (188, 189). If salt is used along with sodium nitrite, less is required – 4.5 percent water-phase salt. With sodium nitrite, a level of 3.5 percent is sufficient. The problem with these levels is that they are above consumer acceptability. Even if such products were consumed, the sodium content would greatly exceed recommended amounts. Salmon jerky, containing about 30 percent moisture and 16-18 percent water-phase salt, is not susceptible to *C. botulinum* and thus does not need sodium nitrite either (188). Its extremely high sodium content compromises the nutritional value of the product, however, and calls into question the use of such products.

**Sodium nitrite**   This substance appears to be one of the most effective inhibitors of *C. botulinum* known. It is effective at concentrations of 100-200 parts per million (10-20 mg/100 g). FDA approved a higher level of 260 ppm for smoked chub (189). It is commonly used in processed meat products and in some smoked fish products to remove the threat of *C. botulinum* but does not always appear on the label. Its presence can be suspected in very brilliant, intensely orange-red smoked salmon. Nitrite may also produce undesirable color changes in some fish, causing white fleshed fish to turn pinkish red and some cooked products to turn greyish red

(200). Nitrites in the presence of free amines can produce nitrosamines which are potential carcinogens. Consumer pressure against the use of nitrite and alleged association with cancer makes the use of nitrite less desirable. The alternative of high salt is equally, if not more, unappealing. Nevertheless, high quality smoked fish can be produced without either nitrite (201) or excessive salt.

**Sorbate**    Dr. Lindsay at the University of Wisconsin has conducted studies on the effects of sorbate in conjunction with tripolyphosphate for the inhibition of botulinum activity. His results indicated that in a $CO_2$ modified atmosphere 5 percent potassium sorbate with 10 percent tripolyphosphate used as a dip for 30-60 seconds resulted in a delay of botulinum growth in samples held at room temperature or higher (21° and 27°C.) (200). In all cases where toxin had been produced, there were noticeable signs of spoilage. This "worst case scenario", analogous to leaving fish out on a hot summer day, was used to demonstrate that even under adverse conditions sorbate can be useful. It should also be noted that the use of tripolyphosphate improves the uptake of sorbate by the fish. Sorbate rapidly penetrates the flesh and becomes uniformly distributed throughout the flesh. This is important for protection against the bacteria.

The procedure of dipping is not without its hazards. It has the potential for cross contaminating the fish, possibly resulting in increased bacterial loads. Using sprays or a flow through system gets around this problem, but introduces others: cost and equipment outlays.

Sorbate is known to reduce bacterial growth in seafood and prolong shelf life (202, 203). Whether it has effects on the taste or sensory properties of seafood is debated: some effects were reported in (200) while others have found none (200, 203). The range of sorbate concentration found effective in dips is 2.5-5.0 percent, with the higher amount giving greater protection.

**Sulfur dioxide gas**    In this procedure, sorbate dipped fish is exposed to sulfur dioxide in a modified atmosphere for a brief period, a few seconds to a few minutes, and then flushed with an inert gas or $CO_2$ enriched atmosphere. Samples treated with sulfur dioxide and then innoculated with *C. botulinum* and held at room temperature remained non-toxic for three days (200). Bleaching is a side effect that occurs at higher concentrations of the gas. This work is in the experimental stage of development, but holds much promise.

**Sodium hypophosphite**    When incorporated into fish dips, this substance inhibited *C. botulinum* growth, but also resulted in textural defects (200). It too is experimental, and is being investigated for use in smoked fish products.

**Liquid smoke**    This substance is being studied at the National Marine Fisheries Service laboratory in Seattle for use with hot-smoked fish. When the internal temperature of the smoked fish exceeds 150°F. (65°C.), *C. botulinum* spores, the most resistant form of the bacterium, become injured and more sensitive to salt (188, 261). This vulnerability may make the use of lower levels of salt in smoked fish a possibility instead of a wish. Let us hope so.

**Chlorine**    Long used as a sanitizing agent, chlorine is lethal to botulinum organisms and spores. When it is present in food, however, it is rapidly inactivated and cannot be relied upon to destroy bacteria. It should be used for maintaining sanitary handling facilities, thus reducing the likelihood of contaminating the fish.

---

## Canning

Canning is a well established technology for preserving foods. Because the product is cooked by heat, harmful microorganisms, including the deadly *Clostridium botulinum* and its spores, are destroyed, and the product is given a long shelf life at room temperature.

There have been many concerns, however, about the effect of canning on nutrient retention. There is no question that certain nutrients are greatly diminished in canned foods, while some minerals are increased. The destruction of nutrients by canning is related to the heat sensitivity of the nutrient as well as the handling procedures, acidity, and time/temperature conditions of canning. The primary concern with the canning of seafood has been the destruction of *C.botulinum*.

The nutrients most affected by canning are thiamin and ascorbic acid. Other B vitamins like riboflavin, niacin and vitamin $B_{12}$ show greater losses in canning than in freezing or usual cooking procedures, but the losses are not as great as for thiamin and ascorbic acid (205). Fish are only moderate sources of thiamin, but the destruction of as much as 70 percent by canning is a detriment. Some fish also possess an enzyme that destroys thiamin, and its activity prior to the canning process may reduce the initial vitamin level (206, 207).

Canned fish have an advantage not available with most other forms of processing: any bones present are edible. During heat treatment the bones of such species as salmon, sardines and mackerel become softened and thoroughly digestible. This represents an important source of calcium in the diet, especially for people intolerant to the consumption of dairy products. The recent development of marketing canned salmon as a boneless (and skinless) product carries with it the nutritional disadvantage of the loss of calcium. Table 4.2 illustrates the vast differences in calcium content between fresh, raw and smoked salmon and different species of canned salmon.

It has been questioned whether canning destroys certain amino acids. The portion of the contents closest to the walls of the can are subjected to the greatest rigors of treatment and some amino acids like arginine, threonine, cystine and cysteine may be partially destroyed in the low acid environment of canned fish. Overall, however, there does not appear to be any appreciable decrease in the nutritive value of the fish protein, which is the main concern (176).

The last category of nutrients affected by canning is minerals. Canning results in an increase of several nutrients as a result of migration of metals from the lining of the can to its contents. Thus, the composition of the lining of the can may affect nutritive value. The availability of nutrients from the can itself is affected by the acidity of the contents, and is greater in acidic foods. Canned fish

**Table 4.2 Calcium Content of Canned, Raw and Smoked Salmon[a]**

| Species | Calcium Content mg/100 grams |
|---|---|
| Sockeye, fresh, raw | 5.5[b] |
| canned | 251.5[b] |
| canned | 259 |
| smoked | 14 |
| King, canned | 154 |
| Pink, canned | 196 |
| Coho or silver, canned | 244 |
| Chum, canned | 249 |

Note: Additional data on calcium in canned salmon report a value of 22 mg/100 grams (234). Although the authors did not comment, it is clear that the sample tested was bone free.

[a] Data from Reference (232) unless otherwise indicated
[b] Data from Reference (233)

is low in acid, yet enrichment of certain minerals is observed (205). The minerals most affected by canning are lead, iron, zinc, copper, tin and some other trace elements.

In a recent study carried out by the National Food Processors Association for the National Marine Fisheries Service, the nutrient composition of several species of fish and shrimp was compared for samples collected in different seasons and processed in different ways (205). Data for two species that were canned are available. To illustrate how canning affects nutrient content, values from this study can be compared with the values for raw and broiled salmon. Table 4.3 illustrates the uptake of zinc as well as the sensitivity of thiamin and vitamin $B_{12}$ to cooking and canning.

The figures in Table 4.3 indicate that zinc migrates from the can to the solid contents. (The widespread commercial use of aluminum cans and special bonded can linings obviates this problem). There is loss of both sodium and potassium when the canning fluid is discarded. The instability of vitamin $B_{12}$ is important, but the analyses also showed greater variation than for the other B vitamins. Protein and fat content appear to increase but that is the result of loss of moisture from the flesh and is not a real increase. The study also documented an increase in arsenic, but this finding was attributed to variability of the method of analysis when values approach the limits of reliable detection (205).

Because of concern over the levels of hazardous trace elements in the food supply, monitoring the amounts of trace elements in fish and shellfish is a public health priority. Seafood is a major source of heavy metals in the diet, and is by far the largest single source of dietary arsenic (107). Any increases in heavy metals as a result of food processing are a worry.

*Table 4.3  Effects of Broiling and Canning on Selected Nutrients in Sockeye Salmon[a]*

| | Proximates | | Vitamins | | | | Minerals | | | |
|---|---|---|---|---|---|---|---|---|---|---|
| Preparation | Pro-tein | Fat | Thia-min | Ribo-flavin | Nia-cin | Vit $B_{12}$ | Iron | Zinc | Sod-ium | Potas-sium |
| | *g/100 g* | | *% Retention[b]* | | | | *% Retention[c]* | | | |
| Raw salmon | 22.3 | 5.6 | 100 | 100 | 100 | 100 | 100 | 100 | 100 | 100 |
| Broiled | 26.4 | 7.2 | 91 | 100 | 99 | 72 | 100 | 96 | 97 | 102 |
| Canned | 23.5 | 6.3 | 20 | 97 | 83 | 62 | 108 | 207 | 86 | 87 |

[a] Data are means of 11 samples taken from 2 studies conducted over 3 years calculated from Ref (182); canned samples represent drained solids.

[b] % Retention is calculated:

$$\frac{\text{nutrient content in cooked fish}}{\text{nutrient content in raw fish}} \times \% \text{ Yield}$$

[c] % Yield is calculated:

$$\frac{\text{weight of fish after preparation}}{\text{weight of fish before preparation}} \times 100$$

# Irradiation

## Applications of Irradiation to Seafood

One of the peaceful uses of atomic energy is the application of ionizing radiation to foods. The words "ionizing" and "radiation" are rather frightening to most people and conjure notions of radioactive foods. Overcoming this misunderstanding and fear is one of the major challenges to the seafood industry on the brink of useful applications. The question most people want answered is, what harm, if any, is there if I consume irradiated foods? From the information available today based on extensive food analyses, feeding studies, biochemical tests and the experience of populations in at least 24 countries with some 40 irradiation-processed foods, the answer appears to be that no harm will result.

The United States withdrew from its active involvement with irradiated foods in the 1970s, with the exception of the US Army's studies on the wholesomeness of irradiated or sterilized foods. International studies were undertaken under the general aegis of the Food and Agricultural Organization (FAO) and the International Atomic Energy Authority (IAEA). As a result, wholesomeness studies involving 24 countries were conducted on low-dose irradiated cod and ocean perch. Based on the findings from this work, provisional acceptance was given to these products (208).

Ionizing energy in food processes is measured in energy units or "Grays", which in turn are based on rads – units of "radiation energy absorbed" (209). Both terminologies are used. The conversion between Grays and rads is shown below:

$$1 \text{ Gray (Gy)} = 100 \text{ rads}$$
$$1 \text{ kiloGray (kGy)} = 1000 \text{ Grays} = 100,000 \text{ rads}$$
$$10 \text{ kiloGrays (kGy)} = 1 \text{ Megarad (Mrad) or one million rads}$$

Ionizing energy can be used in four different kinds of applications in seafood. Each will be listed and described in order of the amount of energy required to achieve the desired effects.

**Destruction of insect eggs and larvae**    Recommended for use with dried fish products in tropical countries. Practical dose range is 100,000 rads (1 kGy).

**Radiation pasteurization**    Also known as radurizaton. This is the application usually referred to as "low dose" radiation. It applies to fresh finfish and shellfish. It extends refrigerated shelf life by inactivating or killing most spoilage organisms and makes it possible to ship chilled unfrozen seafood from coastal regions to inland locations in top condition. It will not destroy the larvae of anisakis, a roundworm found in herring and in some fish used in sashimi. Practical dose range is 75,000 to 250,000 rads (0.75-2.5 kGy).

**Radiation sanitization**    Also called radicidation and can be applied to dried and frozen seafoods. This technology has been tested in frozen shrimp, fish fillet, minced fish blocks and dehydrated fish protein products. It kills disease-producing bacteria that do not form spores, such as salmonella, an organism responsible for many outbreaks of food poisoning. Its effects on *Clostridium botulinum* are equivocal. It has been used in Holland for many years to clean up Far Eastern shrimp and froglegs rejected in the USA. Practical dose range is 0.25-0.5 Mrads (2.5-5.0 kGy).

Radicidation is a substerilization procedure; that is, it does not kill every living organism in the tissue. The possibility that some botulinum spores remain viable after this treatment cannot be definitively ruled out (188). Part of the reason for this is that the studies designed to see whether irradiated fish will support botulinum growth use rather artificial conditions. They do so on the "worst case" assumption and include an abusive environment. The procedures in well handled, temperature controlled systems appear to be safe (178).

It should be noted that *C. botulinum* and other organisms are more susceptible to radiation treatments in the cold and do not germinate and grow as readily and at as low a temperature as their nonirradiated counterparts (210, 211). Furthermore, irradiated fish products would be cooked, a process that destroys the toxin and the organism. For an amusing yet cogent discussion of the use of irradiation technology in seafood products, the reader is urged to consult reference (210). References (209, 212) also present timely reviews.

**Radiation sterilization**    Also known as radappertization. This is used to prepare fishery products for long-term storage without refrigeration. Such products will keep for years provided that the package is not punctured or corroded. In order to avoid undesirable changes in texture, color, flavor or odor, the seafood is first "cooked" by pretreating with heat to an internal temperature of 70-80°C. (210). This also inactivates enzymes that would otherwise cause tissue breakdown. Final packaging is done to exclude oxygen so that oxidation does not occur. The product is sterilized while frozen at -40°F. (-40°C.) to minimize off odors. Radiation sterilization kills *C. botulinum* spores. Practical dose range is 3-4 Mrads (30-40 kGy).

The advantages of radiation sterilization are long shelf life, dry packaging to conform to the shape of the contents and no risk of botulism, since the spores are killed at this dose. The procedure has not yet been approved for use in the USA outside of the manned space program.

## What is a Wholesome Irradiated Food?

As consumers, we need some assurance that "wholesome irradiated" food is not a contradiction in terms. Wholesomeness, as used by the World Health Organization (WHO) Joint Expert Committee and the Institute of Food Technologists Expert Panel, includes four main aspects:

- is the irradiated food radioactive?

- have pathogenic (disease-causing) organisms been destroyed?

- are toxic radiolytic products produced?

- is nutritive value retained?

The answer to the first question is no. Radioactivity occurs naturally in all foods but at such low levels that there is no health hazard. Irradiation by cobalt-60 or electron beam produces gamma rays which do not make other materials radioactive. Any radioactivity in the food will be there as a result of "background" radiation.

With low dose radiation applications (radiation pasteurization) most, but not all, disease causing organisms are inactivated or killed. As with vacuum packaging and modified atmosphere storage, there is a change in the types of organisms that predominate. The spoilage organisms tend to be wiped out, meaning that the first signs of spoilage may go undetected by the nose. *Clostridium botulinum* is not destroyed, but may be sufficiently injured to be ineffective. As with the above mentioned packaging techniques, proper handling at refrigerator temperatures is required to ensure the inhibition of microbial growth. Botulinum spores do not germinate below 38°F. There is no substitute for good handling practices from catch to consumer.

It is interesting to note that in the WHO discussion of the microbiological aspects of irradiated cod and ocean perch the report said that "consideration is restricted to fresh teleost (bony) fish . . .(they) are far less likely to harbor organisms pathogenic for man than are fish caught near the shore" (208). Certainly the initial microbial load affects the likelihood of bacterial growth, but the comment omits reference to the possibility of cross contamination at various stages of fish handling prior to irradiation. Good sanitation is, as always, essential.

The subject of radiolytic products is controversial and remains a suspicion among consumers, advocacy groups and others. The Institute of Food Technologists Expert Panel on Food Safety and Nutrition has stated that,

"The absence of toxic products resulting from food irradiation has been established on scientifically firm ground. The chemistry studies, animal feeding studies, tests for mutagenicity and tests for teratogenicity have revealed no confirmed negative evidence as to the wholesomeness of radiation preserved foods. Significantly, whenever adverse findings were originally reported in the literature, re-testing failed to confirm the original adverse reports. In fact, in some instances, analysis showed that the reports of unusual findings were *not* the result of factors specifically related to the irradiation proposed for commercial application" (209).

Animal feeding studies involving cod, ocean perch, shrimp and tuna have failed to detect any problems of carcinogenicity or toxicity from the irradiated seafood (212). Although the quantity of radiolytic products increased with the irradiation dose, products remained qualitatively similar (213). In the absence of convincing evidence of harmful radiolytic products and the positive results from feeding studies in animals and among free living populations of people, it would appear that low dose radiation is no more more harmful than any other food preservation technique in use today.

## Effects of Irradiation on Nutrients and Palatability

**Effects on Protein and Amino Acids**    The general observation seems to be that irradiation does not cause any greater losses of nutritive value than that of other accepted processing methods (212). This cautious statement is based on the studies of Josephson and coworkers who found no significant reduction in the nutritional quality of the protein, lipid, carbohydrate and mineral constituents of the foods examined (214). Other workers have confirmed these findings for the protein and amino acids of a variety of seafoods (215, 216). It seems that in terms of nutrient retention, irradiation is superior to freezing or canning.

The earlier techniques of irradiation did result in some protein degradation, ammonia production and the destruction of certain amino acids, particularly the ones containing sulfur, cystine and cysteine. Degradation of amino acids is apparently different in different fish species as well (178). The breakdown products that result from changes in amino acids have been associated with unpleasant changes in taste and texture (217). Nowadays, irradiation is carried out at extremely low temperatures in an inert atmosphere and with lower doses than before, so that the destruction of amino acids is avoided. It has also been observed that the presence of moisture in foods protects against protein destruction (217).

**Effects on Carbohydrates**    Irradiation may cause some changes in carbohydrates similar to those resulting from heat processing. The effects depend on the temperature, moisture content and dose. Starches may be partly broken down, reducing their thickening properties, and surface browning may occur (217). Most fish has a negligible amount of carbohydrate, but breaded products and prepared entrees or snacks may have substantial amounts of carbohydrate present.

**Effects on Lipids**    The effect of irradiation on lipids is similar to autoxidation or the breakdown of the fish oil that occurs with prolonged storage and freezing. Like autoxidation, irradiation results in greater destruction when oxygen is present. Peroxides may be formed, but these have a fleeting existence because they are immediately broken down further, eventually to fatty acids (217). Because the double bonds in polyunsaturated fatty acids are the most susceptible to destruction by irradiation, the unsaturated fatty acids are the first to be affected by irradiation. Decreases in the omega-3 fatty acid content of cod and haddock have been reported (218). It has not been reported whether significant changes in omega-3 fatty acids would occur with low dose radiation. The chemical changes are minimized when foods are irradiated at low temperatures and in the absence of light and oxygen (219).

The effect of irradiation on fish oils also depends on the species. Nawar compared the effects of irradiation on mackerel oil with other oils and found the radiolytic pattern could be predicted by the fatty acid composition of the oil (220). Most of the studies on lipids have been conducted with doses of irradiation in the vicinity of 5 Mrad (50kGy), which is above the practical dose range for radiation sterilization (3-4 Mrads, 30-40 kGy) and greatly in excess of that used for low dose radiation (75,000 to 250,000 Mrads, 0.75-2.5 kGy).

The conclusion of several investigators is that irradiation of foods at the expected levels of no more than 5Mrad (50 kGy) does not lead to any significant loss in the nutritive value of food lipids.

**Effect on Vitamins**    The destruction of fat and water soluble vitamins is related to the nature of the vitamin itself, the dose of radiation and the type of food. The vitamins most sensitive to destruction by heat are the same ones most sensitive to irradiation. Thus losses of thiamin and ascorbic acid are the greatest. Vitamin destruction can be minimized by keeping the food frozen during radiation sterilization. At pasteurization doses, vitamin destruction is slight.

Substantial loss of pyridoxine has been reported in irradiated mackerel and clams. In the clams the greatest loss occurred in the samples receiving the highest dose of irradiation (219, 221). Pyridoxine retention was greater than 90 percent in the lower dose sample of clams and in both low dose samples of haddock studied (219).

Both riboflavin and niacin are stable under low dose irradiation with losses of 6 percent or less being reported (178, 219). Vitamin B$_{12}$ has been less frequently studied but retentions greater than 90 percent have been reported in clams and haddock for doses up to 450 Krad (4.5 kGy) (250). Others regard the stability of vitamin $B_{12}$ as intermediate (219).

The fat-soluble vitamins A,D,E and K have been less widely studied, probably because their levels in most fish are very low. Vitamin A and vitamin E, the antioxidant vitamin, are very sensitive to irradiation in the presence of oxygen (178). Information about vitamin E comes from irradiation studies in foods other than seafood since reliable data on seafood are unavailable. We know very little about the distribution of vitamin E in seafood, but existing information suggests that seafood is not a major source. In view of its importance as an antioxidant, its destruction by irradiation or other processing methods is a distinct disadvantage.

The effect of irradiation on mineral content is unknown. There is no reason to suspect any adverse effects.

Virtually every responsible scientific panel that has reviewed the data on the effects of irradiation in foods, particularly regarding seafood, has concluded that foods irradiated within the dose range up to about 5 Mrad (50 kGy), are safe and nutritionally sound. Nutrient losses or alterations can be minimized by using the lowest dose possible to achieve the desired effect, by irradiating in the absence of oxygen and by treating products in the frozen state. There seems to be no convincing evidence to quarrel with the data accumulated so far.

**Effect on Palatability**    Because irradiation may affect the sensory qualities of some foods, especially seafood, special attention has been paid to procedures that will minimize unpleasant effects. A review of the sensory changes that occur was recently published (222). Low dose irradiation of seafood usually does not produce changes in appearance or texture, but some alterations in flavor or odor may occur (212). There are, of course, exceptions to the general rule.

There is a threshold dose for each species beyond which the odor and flavor are affected. The method of preparation can affect the threshold at which changes may be detected. Not surprisingly, deep-frying tends to mask off-flavors while steaming and baking will reveal them. Changes may be masked in smoked fish products.

Some light colored fish may darken slightly with irradiation, but salmon becomes bleached at sterilization doses because of pigment oxidation. It is not clear how well salmon responds to low dose radiation (212).

## Summary

The use of ionizing radiation in the treatment of seafood has been extensively studied. Irradiation offers the possibility of increased shelf life for freshly caught seafood, as well as frozen and smoked fish products and vacuum packaged seafood. Destruction of *Clostridium botulinum* spores cannot be guaranteed at doses that keep seafood palatable and wholesome, but some injury to the bacterium and decreased likelihood of its activity have been demonstrated. Irradiated seafood (and other foods) does not become radioactive, and many harmful microorganisms are inactivated. There is no evidence of harmful radiolytic products being produced at the levels of radiation suitable for the treatment of food.

Seafood irradiated with low dose radiation retains nearly all of its original nutritional value except for some loss of thiamin content. Polyunsaturated fatty acids, which are abundant in several species, and possibly vitamin E, may also be undermined by the treatment. Rancidity is not prevented and may be accelerated.

Less than 10 percent of each of the other water-soluble vitamins studied may be lost, with the possible exception of pyridoxine and vitamin $B_{12}$. Effects on minerals have not been reported but no losses of any consequence would be anticipated. Irradiation treatment at sub-freezing temperatures in the absence of oxygen and light are the best conditions for retaining nutritive value and minimizing the destruction of nutrients and prevention of off odors and flavors.

Extension of shelf life of irradiated seafood is dependent upon having top quality product at the outset, treatment being applied as soon after harvest as possible, and storage as close to freezing temperature as possible after irradiation. Shelf life diminishes quickly as the storage temperature increases.

It can be concluded that irradiation of seafood under top quality handling conditions can be a promising means of delivering fresh, frozen and processed seafood products safely to all parts of the country. Substerilizing radiation does not undermine the safety of the food supply and can be a useful way of improving its quality. It remains for FDA to approve the procedure as a process instead of an additive so that appropriate regulations can be established to permit the safe application of this technology to seafood.

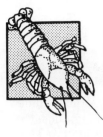

*Chapter Five*

# Nutrition Aspects of Cooked and Processed Seafoods

## Minced Fish

A major concern in the seafood business is the relatively low yield of edible product from the fish harvest. Estimates of the yield of fish fillet from whole fish are in the neighborhood of 30 percent with recent figures ranging from 26 to 37 percent (40, 223-225). These estimates include both hand and machine filleting procedures. By contrast, the yield of minced fish obtained from mechanical bone separators is about half as much again. Estimates range from about 40 to 50 percent (40, 184, 223, 225).

The issue facing the minced fish business is how to make the product acceptable to the consumer. There are several possibilities. One is to use the mince for products like imitation crab meat. Frozen mince provides the starting material for making seafood products of varied flavors, shapes, textures and appearances. Another possibility is to use the mince directly, or in combination with other seafood ingredients to make such items as cutlets, sausages, fish sticks and so on (184).

The preparation and handling of the mince is important in determining the final composition and nutritional value of the product. Mince made from whole headless frames is higher in fat, cholesterol and calcium than mince made from fillets, but the protein content is similar (80). Others have reported that washing the mince removes blood, pigments, fat and soluble protein (223, 225).

The question of changes in amount and kind of protein is important because the primary contribution of fish to the diet is its protein. A study by Adu and others showed the amount of protein in washed rockfish mince was half that in the fillet or unwashed mince (223). Others have reported much smaller losses (225). The protein remaining, however, appeared to have high nutritional value, so that it is primarily the quantity of protein that is affected by washing, not the final nutritional quality. One might add that the tests used to evaluate protein quality are of questionable validity, but the comparisons with the control values suggest that the conclusions are appropriate.

The amount of nutrients lost varies directly with the washing procedures, the initial levels present in the mince and the severity of the mince preparation procedures. The values reported in the literature are sufficiently different from each other that no accurate generalizations can be made.

Changes in the cholesterol content are intriguing. Mince made commercially from skin-on fillets and whole headless frames had significantly more cholesterol than those prepared from fillets or prepared by hand (83). This observation held for whiting and cod preparations but not for red hake. It may be suggested that because the mechanical procedures are more drastic than hand ones more of the cholesterol may have been extracted into the mince. Mince made from starting material composed of parts of the fish usually discarded may also be higher in cholesterol. Kryznowek's observations indicate that careful monitoring of the composition of fish mince products is necessary to ensure they do not acquire nutritional characteristics not expected of them.

Kryznowek et al. have reported large increases in the calcium content of mechanically prepared whiting and have suggested that the presence of small amounts of fish scales may be responsible (80). Certainly the presence of bone or bone fragments as is possible with mechanical bone separators would also increase the calcium content appreciably. The calcium content in mechanically minced cod increased enormously on a percentage basis, but unimportantly on a total quantity basis. In these studies, both moisture and estimated protein content were similar to the skinless fillet samples.

Adu and colleagues have also reported on the changes in mineral composition in washed and unwashed rockfish mince. Phosphorus, potassium and sodium levels were reduced while iron, copper, zinc and chromium levels were increased in the washed mince compared with the unwashed mince. Iron was substantially greater in both washed and unwashed mince compared with the fillet, suggesting that the composition of the processing equipment, the acidity of the wash and the presence of salts may all affect the final mineral content. Undoubtedly the presence of salts or additives in the wash water will affect the mineral composition of the mince as well.

Fish mince technology has other side effects that influence the palatability and keeping qualities of the fish mince. The development of off-odors and flavors has been reported in fish mince and may be influenced by the nature of the mince at the outset, the use of additives and the development of rancidity (40, 223). Color of the mince and changes during frozen storage may diminish the acceptability of mince from some species.

Fish mince offers the potential for greatly increasing the edible yield from fish and for using species of fish not widely consumed at present. The possibility of developing palatable nutritious products with nutritional qualities equivalent or superior to the fresh or frozen form is feasible. Standards of nutritional quality and care in processing will help ensure the development of high quality foods. As Keay and Hardy suggest (184) the evolution from "codfish tennis balls" to "cordon bleu" fish pate indicates both the potential and the possibilities of this technology.

# Surimi

Surimi is a Japanese word describing deboned, minced and washed fish. Surimi is made by mechanically deboning fish flesh, washing the resulting mince with water and mixing it with substances to improve its stability to freezing (226, 227). Minced fish is similar to surimi, but has not been washed and has poorer freezer storability. The substances added to the surimi to improve its stability during freezing are called cryoprotectants. The additives used for this purpose are sucrose (sugar), sorbitol, a sugar alcohol, and polyphosphate(s). Cryoprotectants prevent the muscle proteins from denaturing or becoming too rubbery and help preserve desirable textural properties. Cryoprotectants may be omitted if the surimi is not expected to be frozen.

The art of making surimi goes back to 1100 A.D. when the Japanese began preserving their excess fish harvest by mincing it, mixing it with salt and water and then cooking it (228). The various ways of cooking surimi have defined particular surimi products, but nowadays the term kamaboko has taken on the generic meaning of Japanese-style fish cake or any cooked surimi product. Strictly speaking, kamaboko refers to those products that are steamed; chikuwa are prepared by broiling and satsuma-age by deep frying. Descriptions of various kamaboko products and of surimi technology have been published (226, 229). The successsful development of freezing methods for surimi has paved the way for a whole new market of processed seafood. Surimi is now being produced in America as well as Japan.

Surimi can be made from a wide variety of fish with only minor modifications in the processing techniques to accommodate the differences in fish proteins and fat content. Some sixty different species have been used but only a few are processed on a commercial scale (226). Pacific pollock is the major species used at present. High quality surimi is being produced by processing aboard ship where the fish can be treated as soon as it is caught. Shore plants also produce surimi, but the fish is necessarily several days older before it is processed.

The final step in surimi processing is the formation of consumer-ready surimi-based products. These are made by extruding the surimi paste or gel into various shapes using molds, forming thin sheets that are partially heat set, or by making emulsions (226). Products resembling crab legs, crab salad meat, scallops and shrimp have been marketed and fish sausages are being developed. The freshness and age of the fish, the parts of the fish used and the number of washings all affect the quality and amount of fish protein. The whitest product with the most desirable gelling properties comes from fish processed immediately after harvest, where the tail, backbone and belly flaps are not used. The temperature of frozen storage and fluctuations in storage temperature also affect quality. Holding temperatures below -20°C. (-4°F.) are superior (230).

Quality of surimi is assessed by measuring the color, viscosity and gel-forming ability of the surimi with objective tests. The Japanese have developed a grading system for surimi and modifications of their system suitable for U.S. conditions have been proposed (224, 226).

A variety of ingredients is usually added to the surimi to achieve certain product characteristics. In addition to the salt, sugar and polyphosphate used to extract the protein from the flesh, starch and/or egg white may be added to improve texture and water binding properties. Potato or wheat starch increases the gel strength and elasticity of the surimi. Egg white may be added to enhance gel strength and to make the product whiter and glossier (226). Final products may contain in addition vegetables, monosodium glutamate, other fish and shellfish, artificial or natural coloring and/or flavors, lard, oil, cream and sorbic acid.

## Nutritional Properties of Surimi

The marketing of surimi-based products has received wide consumer and food service acceptance but has encountered certain labeling difficulties. The problems involve both nomenclature and nutritional quality. The law says that if a product is a substitute for another food, and is of inferior nutritional quality, it must be labeled "imitation". On the other hand, if it resembles another food, is not nutritionally inferior to it and is properly labeled, it need not be called imitation. The difficulty with surimi is in demonstrating that it is nutritionally equivalent to the products it resembles.

There are several aspects to this challenge. One is the selection of the appropriate basis for comparison. Should surimi be compared in nutritional quality to the fish from which it is prepared (perhaps walleye pollock) or should it be compared to the seafood whose flavor and/or shape it assumes (crab meat, for example)? What about the negative attributes of the product it resembles – perhaps its cholesterol content? How many nutrients should the comparison include? What percent of the content in the original product is considered equivalent? There are more questions but these illustrate the dilemma.

These questions have not yet been fully answered but it appears that the FDA recognizes the advances made in food technology and the development of new categories of food products. FDA may be willing to consider substitute foods as something other than imitation foods if they are nutritionally equivalent to traditional foods and are clearly labeled with contents and identity. It is incumbent upon manufacturers then to describe, label and market their products so as to avoid consumer deception. FDA has issued a Compliance Policy Guide for blended seafood products that states that the names of the components or the word "fish" must appear on the label, along with the specific names of all seafoods and other ingredients in the product (231). Judiciously selected product names, clear ingredients statements and nutrition labels can provide the information needed. Surimi based products may well be able to stand on their own merit without having to look like other foods.

The term surimi is unfamiliar to many consumers at present but is rapidly becoming the generic name for a group of foods containing minced boneless fish protein. Once people learn to identify surimi as a major food constituent, surimi will have its own identity in the marketplace. Then the need will be to establish minimum standards of nutritional quality for surimi so that a variety of seafoods could be used as the starting material. Such standards protect the consumer and food manufacturer from potential abuses of a high quality product.

The current unofficial standards of nutritional quality established for vegetable proteins may be unsuitable for high quality surimi proteins. In fact, if these standards were adopted, surimi would have to be fortified with more protein, several B vitamins, iron and possibly other nutrients. It is important to maintain both the high quality and quantity of protein in seafood products, for these foods are used primarily as a protein mainstay in the diet. Just what level of protein can be considered high or sufficient is debatable. Setting "optimal" nutritional standards rather than minimal ones for surimi would give the product a competitive as well as health advantage which is ultimately in the best interests of everyone.

As mentioned earlier, FDA recently issued a Compliance Policy Guide for processed and/or blended seafood products (231). In addition to the definition of imitation, the compliance guides specify that a statement of product identity must appear on the principal display panel, that the specific names of all seafoods used in the product must appear in descending order of predominance in the ingredient statement and that products used in the preparation of surimi, like sugar and phosphates also be listed in the ingredient statement. The compliance guides do not address the issue of nutritional quality except as included in the definition of the term imitation.

Other processed foods such as processed cheese and luncheon meats that are used mainly for protein vary widely in their protein content and quality as well as their other nutritional attributes. These foods are not subject to nutritional quality standards. Food manufacturers, nutritionists and policy makers need to share in the important decisions regarding nutritional quality standards. An excellent discussion of the issues involved in regulating protein quality in meats and poultry has been published (232). The discussion needs to include seafood products as well.

The nutrient composition of surimi varies with the manufacturer, the procedures and the ingredients used. Nutrient values for four different surimi products are shown in Table 5.1. The variability in nutrients represents differences between products and does not reflect the variability within the product itself. There are some interesting observations to be made from this table.

The four samples shown in Table 5.1 differ in protein content from 12 to 15 grams of protein. These differences may not appear large, but could be important if, for example, surimi were to be used as the primary source of protein in a child feeding program. This amount of protein is substantially less than the amount present in pollock or shrimp, but not crab. If the serving size were 3 ounces, the amount of protein in the surimi would range from 10-13 grams. This level falls short of meeting one third of the U.S. RDA for protein of 15 grams (U.S. RDA for high quality protein in a day is 45 grams). One might reasonably expect to consume one third of daily needs in a meal. Since the nutrient needs of children are less on a quantitative basis, this difference in protein content may be less

**Table 5.1** *Approximate Nutrient Content of Different Samples of Surimi*

| Nutrient | 1[a] | 2[b] | 3[c] | 4[d] |
|---|---|---|---|---|
| | Sample Number | | | |
| | Amount per 100 gram | | | |
| Calories, kcal | 87 | 73 | 93 | 96 |
| Protein, gm | 13.0 | 12.0 | 11.7 | 15.2 |
| Fat, gm | 0.1 | 0.7 | 0.9 | 0.9 |
| Carbohydrate, gm | 8.6 | 4.7[e] | 9.5[e] | 6.8 |
| Cholesterol, mg | <1 | N/A | N/A | 30 |
| Calcium, mg | 12 | 626 | 35 | 9 |
| Phosphorus, mg | N/A | 106 | N/A | N/A |
| Iron, mg | 0.2 | 0.6 | 0.4 | 0.3 |
| Sodium, mg | 1085 | 725 | 640 | 143 |
| Vitamin A, I.U. | 50 | 90 | N/A | N/A |
| Thiamin, mg | 0.06 | 0.03 | N/A | 0.02 |
| Riboflavin, mg | 0.04 | 0.06 | N/A | 0.02 |
| Niacin, mg | 0.38 | N/A | N/A | 0.22 |

[a] Simulated crab legs, courtesy of Jac Creative Foods, Los Angeles, CA.

[b] Sea Legs, courtesy of D.B. Berelson & Co., San Francisco, CA.

[c] Sea Stix, simulated crab legs, courtesy of Kibun Products International Inc. Pasadena, CA.

[d] Reference 244.

[e] Estimated by difference.

important. (Of course other foods in a meal, especially milk, also contribute protein, so that it is unrealistic to demand that the total supply come from a single food).

The quality of surimi protein is high, just like most other animal proteins. This means that a little goes a long way and that its nutritional contribution to a meal is probably greater than its analytical value suggests, because it enhances the poorer quality proteins present in other foods. The quality and quantity of protein in surimi-based foods is one of its most important nutritional features.

The fat content of surimi is very low, sometimes even less than that found in the original fish species. Surimi-based products, however, may have fat added to them and this feature changes the nutritional profile of the food substantially. The amount and kind of added fat needs to be evaluated. Lard and vegetable oil have been used in surimi-based products and one is hard pressed to condone the addition of animal fats or highly saturated vegetable ones to our already excessive intake of these substances. Nevertheless, if the total amount of fat is small, and the total calories from fat less than 20 percent, for example, the nutritional value of the product may not be compromised.

The cholesterol content of foods is an issue for some people. Most seafood, including shellfish, does not have high levels of cholesterol. Certain methods of surimi preparation may increase the amount of cholesterol present and cholesterol could become an issue in foods where it had not previously been expected. One way to handle the situation is to require cholesterol labeling of surimi-based products. The variability in the four samples shown in Table 5.1 illustrates the point, even though the maximum reported was low.

The iron content of surimi varies from 0.2 to 0.6 mg per 100 grams. This is similar to the variation and amount observed in fish and shellfish and suggests that both processing techniques and equipment as well as the source of the fish are important in determining the final iron content. Obviously other foods added to the surimi might affect the total iron content, not only in terms of amount but also by providing substances that might interfere or compete with the iron during digestion and absorption.

There is also substantial variation in the amounts of B vitamins. Fish is an important source of niacin, and to a lesser extent riboflavin. Losses in niacin are great. Thiamin is usually fairly low in fish owing to its ease of destruction and the presence of an enzyme in some fish that breaks down the vitamin. Losses of these and other water soluble vitamins are not surprising because of the washing procedures used to prepare surimi. Vitamin A levels are low as expected.

Two other nutritional aspects of surimi warrant comment. The first is the large increase in sodium content in surimi compared with fish and shellfish. This undoubtedly comes from the sodium tripolyphosphate, salt and sometimes sodium glutamate added during processing. The level in one sample is over one gram, and in another sample over 700 milligrams. These amounts are clearly nutritionally excessive and render the product vulnerable to strong criticism. The data in Table 5.2 do not adequately represent the wide range of sodium values observed in different surimi products (Table 5.1) nor do they reflect the sodium added to fish during home preparation or at the table. It is generally true, however, that surimi-based products are much higher in sodium than unprocessed fish and shellfish. The levels of sodium observed in commercial surimi products (Table 5.1) bear this out. Such high sodium levels will preclude the use of surimi products by thousands of people with high blood pressure who are trying to restrict their sodium intake and might otherwise enjoy the convenience and appeal of surimi.

The second feature is the presence of sugar (sucrose) and sorbitol, a sugar alcohol that is less sweet than sucrose but of equivalent caloric content. These ingredients, added to improve the stability of the surimi to freezing, increase the calorie content of the product without enhancing its nutritional worth. As there is less than one gram of carbohydrate naturally present in pollock, and not very much more in king crab legs, the amounts in surimi represent a substantial contribution to the calorie content of the product. They also give it a sweet taste which is objectionable to some. Apart from the contribution of these sugars to the technological processing of surimi, there is nothing to recommend their presence. That they are important to the final stability of the product justifies their

***Table 5.2   Comparison of the Nutrient Content of 100 grams
Walleye Pollock Surimi with Baked Pollock, Boiled Shrimp and
Raw Alaska King Crab Legs***

| Nutrient | Surimi[a] | Baked Pollock[b] | Boiled Shrimp[b] | Raw Alaska King Crab legs[a] |
|---|---|---|---|---|
| Calories /100g | 96 | 106 | 102 | 80 |
| Protein g/100g | 15.2 | 22.4 | 21.1 | 15.4 |
| Fat g/100g | 0.9 | 1.0 | 1.2 | 1.6 |
| Carbohydrate g/100g | 6.8 | <1 | — | 1.0 |
| Cholesterol mg/100g | 30 | 95 | 226[c] | 42[d] |
| Thiamin mg/100g | .02 | .08 | .03 | .04 |
| Riboflavin mg/100g | .02 | .07 | .04 | .04 |
| Niacin mg/100g | .22 | 1.6 | 2.6 | <1.1 |
| Vitamin $B_{12}$ mg/100g | — | 5.0 | 1.4 | — |
| Iron mg/100g | .26 | .26 | .54 | 0.6 |
| Sodium mg/100g[f] | 143 | 108 | 299 | 836[e] |
| Potassium mg/100g | 78 | 374 | 209 | 204 |

[a] Data from Reference 244.

[b] Data from Reference 205.

[c] Kryznowek has reported a value of 90 mg for cooked white shrimp.

[d] A value of 60 mg has been reported (83).

[e] Sidwell lists a value of 70 mg for raw King Crab (3).

[f] Sodium content varies widely – see Table 5.1

presence, but manufacturers should be encouraged to add as little sugar as is consistent with good storage properties.

A final perspective on the nutritional value of surimi is given in Table 5.2. This table shows the nutrient content of one sample of surimi compared with baked pollock, boiled shrimp and raw king crab legs. Comparison with cooked seafood is appropriate, for that is how each is consumed. The data on raw crab legs are included because data for cooked king crab are not available.

The comparisons in Table 5.2 show that surimi is lower in protein, cholesterol, thiamin, riboflavin, niacin and potassium than baked pollock or boiled shrimp. Losses in protein, vitamins and potassium occur mainly as a result of washing of the fish mince. Iron content is equivalent to that of baked pollock but is half that found in shrimp and crab. It is doubtful that many people eat shrimp or crab often enough to meet much of their iron needs from this source, so the iron content does not represent a meaningful loss of dietary iron.

The lower cholesterol value is apparent only by comparison with the natural shellfish which have more cholesterol than pollock. The value for pollock seems relatively high compared with surimi because of the loss of moisture during cooking. Others have observed an increase in cholesterol content in fish mince which they attributed to the extraction procedures and the composition of the starting material (80). There are insufficient data at present to conclude anything about the final cholesterol content of surimi products. Clearly the cholesterol content of the starting fish fillet is an inadequate base for predicting final cholesterol content.

## Salted Fish

High concentrations of salt have been used for centuries to preserve fish, meat and poultry. In many parts of the world, salt cod is still used. In large amounts, salt inhibits bacterial activity and in low concentrations it enhances flavor. In the salt preservation of fish, salt is added in the dry form sprinkled directly on the dressed fish or the fish is soaked in a brine solution. A rapid salt-curing technique for ground fish has also been described but to what extent it is used is not known (233).

The result of salting is that water and some water-soluble proteins are drawn out and sodium migrates into the flesh in its place. As the sodium content increases, the proteins become less soluble or are "salted out". Brined fish are usually stored in brine solution until used, while dry salted fish are air-dried and stored in crates or frozen (185).

Fish proteins are denatured by salt but it is not known whether this affects their digestibility. Nutritive value and essential amino acids are apparently unaffected (234). It is generally thought that salting has little effect on protein quality.

The effect of salting on vitamin and mineral content is difficult to assess because of the lack of comparative data. It is expected that some of these nutrients would be drawn out of the flesh along with water and dissolved proteins. A reduction of 50 percent of the B vitamins in heavily salted herring has been reported (235). Sodium content is of course greatly increased.

Salt increases the oxidation of lipid in fish and the salting of fatty fish must proceed quickly if the degrading effects of rancidity are not to outweigh the preservative effects of salt. Fatty fish like herring are brined immediately after harvest to minimize the chances of oxidation.

## Smoked Seafood

We tend to think of smoked foods as dating back to the cave man era, but "traditional" smoked fish was developed mainly in the early 19th century (236). In 1843 the famous kipper was invented in Northumberland, England. 19th century British fish curers followed a distinguished tradition established by the *harengeres* in Europe who were the twelfth century aristocrats of fish dealers selling mediaeval snob food (237). While smoked fish may remind some people more of a red herring than a delicacy, the development of modern kilns that allow control of temperature, humidity and air flow enable the production of high quality smoked seafood that is both safe and tasty.

Smoking used to be an important form of seafood preservation. It still is in some parts, but it is more important these days as a means of flavoring seafood. For preservation purposes, refrigeration, freezing and sometimes additives give a superior product.

Smoked fish are generally prepared in one of two ways: cold smoked where the temperature does not exceed 85° F. and hot smoked where the temperature reaches 140-150° F. Cold smoked fish are more moist but need to be cooked before eating, while hot smoked fish are completely cooked but drier. Examples of cold smoked fish are kippered herring and finnan haddie; smoked oysters are a well known hot smoked item.

The effects of smoking on the nutritional characteristics of seafood have not been thoroughly studied. There is loss of moisture and water-soluble nutrients during the brining prior to smoking, and additional water is lost during the actual smoking process. The gloss that develops on cut surfaces of fish that have been brined is mainly due to the swelling of the protein and the drying of the surface, not to additives (236).

Smoked fish may be coated with or packed in oil to preserve moisture and texture. The oil used for this purpose is usually soybean or other vegetable oil. While its use may maintain palatability, it also adds calories.

The nutritional content of some Norwegian smoked fish is presented in Table 5.3. The table shows that smoked seafood is an excellent source of protein, iron and vitamin $B_{12}$. Canned sardines, like canned salmon, are rich in calcium because the small bones are retained and softened during the canning process. Smoked seafood is also high in niacin and contains a respectable amount of riboflavin. Smoked seafood contains modest amounts of pantothenic acid (data not shown).

The fat content of smoked seafood is high, largely because moisture is lost

### Table 5.3 Nutritional Content of Some Norwegian Smoked Seafood[a]

| Seafood | Calo- ries | Pro- tein | Fat | Thia- min | Ribo- flavin | Nia- cin | Vit. $B_{12}$ | Iron | Cal- cium |
|---|---|---|---|---|---|---|---|---|---|
| | kcal | gm | gm | mg | mg | mg | mcg | mg | mg |
| Smoked mackerel | 180 | 21.5 | 10.6 | — | 0.38 | 6.6 | 12.0 | — | — |
| Smoked salmon fillet | 160 | 21.4 | 8.4 | 0.11 | 0.19 | 5.0 | 7.0 | — | — |
| Kippered herring | 205 | 21.1 | 13.4 | — | 0.37 | 4.8 | 1.5 | 0.7 | — |
| Brisling sardines in oil[b] | 340 | 18.6 | 29.6 | 0.03 | 0.32 | 6.7 | 10.8 | 1.5 | 250 |
| Brisling sardines in tomato sauce[b] | 195 | 16.8 | 14.3 | 0.03 | 0.32 | 5.7 | 11.7 | 2.7 | 250 |
| Sild sardines in oil[b] | 355 | 18.3 | 29.2 | 0.04 | 0.27 | 4.4 | 9.9 | 1.9 | 350 |
| Sild sardines in tomato sauce[b] | 180 | 17.1 | 12.2 | 0.04 | 0.29 | 4.1 | 10.9 | 2.9 | 360 |
| Greenland halibut[b] | 135 | 13.4 | 8.8 | — | 0.17 | 1.5 | 0.6 | — | — |

[a] Data per 100 gm from Ref. 178
[b] Canned

during the smoking process. High fat fish are usually the best varieties for smoking although lean fish are sometimes smoke-cured.

Two concerns about smoked fish are the presence of nitrites and polycyclic aromatic hydrocarbons (PAH). Both substances have been associated in some way with cancer. It is common practice to use nitrites in smoked fish to develop flavor and color and to deter the growth of harmful microorganisms (especially *Clostridium botulinum*). Its use is widespread but not essential for producing a top quality safe product. If nitrite is used, its presence is supposed to be listed on the ingredient statement. For further discussion of nitrites, see Chapter Three.

Polycyclic aromatic hydrocarbons comprise a family of complex organic molecules found in woodsmoke or the condensate from woodsmoke. They have been detected in smoked and cured meats, cheese, barley malt, beer and fish (238, 239). It is not clear whether these compounds are formed in the smoldering wood and deposited in or on the fish during smoking, or whether compounds in the smoke trigger the formation of PAH in the fish. There is some evidence that it is the latter.

One study looking at the role of woodsmoke in N-nitrosothiazolidine* formation in bacon provided evidence that the smoke itself did not contain NTHZ. Even when nitrite was added to the smoke condensate, the nitrosamine was not detected. The authors suggested that it is the presence of other compounds in the woodsmoke, possibly the formaldehyde or acetaldehyde in woodsmoke, that react with cysteamine or other amino acids to form the nitrosamines (240). This supports the observations of Connell et al. who provided evidence that extracts of woodsmoke were not mutagenic in bacteria but that those from the outer layer of smoked fish were (239). It seems clear that nitrosamine and PAH formation is related to the smoking process, but the chemical reactions are not completely understood.

Nitrosamine formation also uses products that result from the browning reaction between sugar (glucose) and amino acids. Sugar added during the salting or smoking process may increase the possibility that nitrosamines be formed.

The formation of potentially harmful hydrocarbons during the smoking process is also related to the type of chips used for smoke and the time and temperature of the smoking procedure (240). Wood that has been treated with fungicides and insecticides such as chlorophenols is also a source of potentially harmful hydrocarbons (239). The chemicals themselves or derivatives of them are a cause for concern. Concentrations of PAH are greater in heavily smoked fish than in lightly smoked samples.

Connell and coworkers reported in 1981 the first evidence that extracts of the surface layer of smoked fish caused changes in the genes (were mutagenic) in bacteria whereas extracts from the skin were not (239). On the

---

*NTHZ is a N-nitrosamine found in raw and fried bacon derivatives and is thought by some to be mutagenic i.e., causing changes in the genes, of certain bacteria; its mutagenicity is disputed by others. It belongs to a family of compounds of known carcinogens.

other hand, it has been suggested that the skin may act as a barrier to the uptake of many such compounds (235). Just what the health implications of these findings are is not clear, for mutagenicity by itself does not prove that a substance is harmful in man.

Changes in the gene structure of bacteria do not mean that there will be changes in the gene structure of man's cells. The simplified conditions of the laboratory are rather far removed from the complex situation in human tissues. There can be, however, a good correlation between a substance being mutagenic in bacteria and its being carcinogenic in laboratory animals.

In addition, we need to consider the conditions of exposure. Just because a mutagen is found in a food, it does not mean that there is any risk to our eating the food. The substance may be present in such small amounts and our liver in such good working condition that consuming the substance in small amounts from time to time may pose no measurable risk to health. In all probability, we are faced with this situation every day. At the same time, the presence of mutagens is a useful warning sign.

The implications of smoked seafood and health are currently difficult to assess because of the scarcity of data. It seems safe to recommend not eating the charred or outer skin of smoked seafood. Lightly smoked products are probably less risky than heavily smoked ones, but we cannot be certain of this.

There is the possibility that using liquid smoke products may confer desirable flavor characteristics without incurring health risks. Many dietary recommendations advise against frequent consumption of smoked meats and fish, presumably because of the danger of nitrosamine formation and the possible presence of potentially toxic organic compounds. Because the materials and methods used to prepare smoked seafood vary so widely it is important to obtain more information about the hazards of consuming these foods. Smoked seafood is a gourmet and ethnic item with the potential for providing a delicious source of omega-3 fatty acids from fish that might not otherwise be consumed. Its safety and nutritional merit warrant much more investigation.

## Breaded Seafood Products

Many varieties of frozen breaded seafood items are available in the supermarket and from food service organizations. They are portion controlled and developed to specification so that variation between servings is minimal. They consist of a certain proportion of seafood flesh plus a coating of batter or breading. The whole portion is often fried and then frozen. Products differ in the source of the seafood, the amount of coating and whether or not they are precooked.

A major issue for the buyer is the amount of seafood and the amount of coating a product contains. Amounts of breading in excess of 50 percent by weight are not unusual. Breaded seafood products that are USDC inspected must conform to minimum flesh requirements, so that purchasing products with the PUFI or Grade A symbol is one guarantee of a minimum standard. The current minimum flesh requirements for standardized and nonstandardized breaded and battered products in shown in Table 5.4.

Some companies have distinguished themselves and their products from the crowd by developing and marketing lightly breaded seafood items with just 14 percent breading (241). This remarkable departure from convention is successful with consumers and nutritionists alike and may set standards for nutritionally superior breaded seafood.

Coated seafood may be covered with batter or breading. Batters usually contain flour, starch, dry milk, eggs and seasonings. Since starch-based batters adhere better to the fish than flour based ones, they are more widely used. Breading mixtures may contain wheat cereals, cracker meal, potato flour, soy flour, starch or bread crumbs. The formula used depends on whether the product is precooked. Products cooked by the consumer must brown more slowly and so have breadings that do not reach final color until the product is completely cooked (242). Cooked products are fried prior to packaging and then frozen, whereas raw items are frozen after coating.

The nutritional aspects of breaded fish products mainly have to do with how much fish, coating and fat the product contains. Coatings made from enriched flour and bread products would be expected to have more B vitamins and iron than those made with either unenriched starch products or very little coating. As the proportion of coating goes up, the amount of fish decreases, resulting in a product with less protein, vitamins and minerals than might be expected on the basis of total weight.

Frying in oil greatly increases the total fat content and, depending on the fat used, may increase the saturated fat content as well. Unless the package label gives nutrition information and the ingredient statement declares unequivocally the source of the fat, the buyer has no way of assessing either the amount or kind of fat in breaded and fried seafood products. Tables of food composition give generic information about "fish sticks" which shows that these products may contain nearly 9 grams of fat per 100 grams, for a contribution of 45 percent of the total calories from fat (243)! That is no basis for a positive nutritional recommendation. Since most of us consume too much fat already, such convenience fried seafood offers no health advantage.

Manufacturers need to be encouraged to develop high quality, convenient, precooked or raw seafood items with a minimum of tasty topping or coating that has not been fried and is not recommended for frying. Bake, broil, microwave, steam or stir-fry items have all the advantages of quick cooking or heating without the disadvantages of added fat. Consumer preparation instructions should omit the suggestion to deep fry and encourage the use of only small amounts of oil in preparing or heating the product. In that way, the flavor and inherent nutritional advantages of seafood will not be compromised.

## Fish on the Fast Food Menu

Fast food restaurant chains have become a way of life in the United States, offering their patrons quick service, economy and standardized menu items.

### Table 5.4   Minimum Flesh Content Requirements for USDC Inspected Products

| Products | USDC Grade Marks* | PUFI Mark* |
|---|---|---|
| *Fish Fillets* | | |
| Raw breaded fillets | —[a] | 50% |
| Precooked breaded fillets | — | 50% |
| Precooked crispy/crunchy fillets | — | 50% |
| Precooked battered fish fillets | — | 40% |
| *Fish Portions* | | |
| Raw breaded fish portions | 75% | 50% |
| Precooked breaded fish portions | 65% | 50% |
| Precooked battered fish portions | — | 40% |
| *Fish Sticks* | | |
| Raw breaded fish sticks | 72% | 50% |
| Precooked breaded fish sticks | 60% | 50% |
| Precooked battered fish sticks | — | 40% |
| *Scallops* | | |
| Raw breaded scallops | 50% | 50% |
| Precooked breaded scallops | 50% | 50% |
| Precooked crispy/crunchy scallops | — | 50% |
| Precooked battered scallops | — | 40% |
| *Shrimp* | | |
| Lightly breaded shrimp[b] | 65% | 65% |
| Raw breaded shrimp[b] | 50% | 50% |
| Precooked crispy/crunchy shrimp | — | 50% |
| Precooked battered shrimp | — | 40% |
| Imitation breaded shrimp[c] | — | No minimum flesh content Encouraged to put % on label |
| *Oysters* | | |
| Raw breaded oysters[d] | — | 50% |
| Precooked breaded oysters[d] | — | 50% |
| Precooked crispy/crunchy oysters[d] | — | 50% |
| Precooked battered oysters[d] | — | 40% |
| *Miscellaneous* | | |
| Fish & seafood cakes | — | 35% |
| Extruded and breaded products | — | 35% |

[a] Means no USDC grading standard currently exists.

[b] FDA standards of identity require that these products contain a minimum of 50% shrimp flesh by weight and if labeled "lightly breaded" must contain not less than 65% shrimp flesh.

[c] Any product with a standard of identity which contains less flesh than the standard calls for must be labeled imitation.

[d] Flesh content of oyster products can only be determined on an input weight basis during production.

Source: USDC/NOAA/NMFS

*For definitions, see p. 147.

Originally developed on the hamburger theme, fast food chains have diversified their menu offerings to include salads, entrees and seafood. It may be surprising to see what has happened to the nutritional value of "traditional" foods now served in a box.

Table 5.5 gives the content of several major nutrients in five common fast food menu items. The data were compiled by USDA and are average values for several fast food chains. The items shown in the table were selected to illustrate popular alternatives of approximately equivalent calorie value. There are two entrees (one chicken and the other fish) and three sandwich selections.

The most important observation from Table 5.5 is that fish is no longer a lean item compared with chicken or hamburger. In fact, it is higher in fat than either a 4 ounce hamburger or a light meat chicken entree. The fish sandwich is nearly one third lower in protein than the other items shown. The fish items are lower in niacin than the other selections and are intermediate in terms of riboflavin. All items are high in sodium.

In fast food establishments, the seafood offering can be higher in fat and even higher in cholesterol than a 4 ounce hamburger and lower in protein than some of the popular alternatives. What has happened to bring about this change is the breading and frying that increases the total carbohydrate and fat content at the expense of protein. The B vitamins are difficult to compare because a good share of them is supplied by the enriched flour used to make the rolls. Iron in fish is lower than in red meats, so there is no real change. Fish, with its potential for being superior or at least nutritionally equivalent to its protein rivals, is offered instead as a vehicle for fat, carbohydrate and sodium. We can and must do better.

## Cooking and Changes in Nutrient Content

Cooking seafood renders it both palatable and digestible. It can, however, diminish its nutritive value if care is not taken to handle and cook the item to minimize nutrient losses. In general, nutrients are well retained by most methods used to cook seafoods, but a few nutrients may be substantially reduced.

Nutrients are lost after cooking either because they are chemically destroyed by the cooking conditions or because they are contained in parts of the fish or fish juices not consumed. Stability of nutrients during cooking procedures depends on the nutrient itself and on the nature of the cooking conditions such as time, temperature, acidity and the portion of the fish and cooking juices that is consumed.

Some nutrients present in fish are also not available to us because we do not eat the part of the fish where the nutrients are concentrated. This is the case with the liver and viscera of fish. For example, the liver of many (but not all) species may be high in vitamins A and D (See Tables 2.9 and 2.10 in Chapter Two). Vitamins and minerals tend to be higher in the dark muscle of fish than in the white muscle; other body parts may also be rich in nutrients.

Solubility in water increases nutrient losses because moisture is lost during thawing of frozen seafood and in most cooking procedures. Seafood

Table 5.5 *Nutrient Content of Selected Fast Food Items*[a]

| Fast Food Item | Calories kcal | Protein gm | Fat gm | Carbo-hydrate gm | Cholesterol mg | Thiamin mg | Riboflavin mg | Niacin mg | Vitamin B$_{12}$ mcg | Iron mg | Sodium mg |
|---|---|---|---|---|---|---|---|---|---|---|---|
| Fish Entree | 269 | 14.4 | 15.6 | 16.2 | — | 0.07 | 0.06 | 1.6 | 1.0 | 0.3 | 458 |
| Fish Sandwich, large | 276 | 10.6 | 15.7 | 24.2 | 53 | 0.20 | 0.14 | 2.1 | 0.9 | 1.3 | 365 |
| Chicken Entree, light meat | 263 | 14.8 | 14.2 | 18.9 | 95 | 0.08 | 0.10 | 6.7 | 0.2 | 0.6 | 430 |
| Hamburger, 4 oz. patty | 255 | 14.3 | 12.1 | 21.6 | 41 | 0.22 | 0.22 | 4.5 | 1.3 | 2.8 | 438 |
| Cheeseburger, 4 oz. patty | 270 | 15.5 | 16.2 | 20.4 | 54 | 0.17 | 0.25 | 3.8 | 1.2 | 2.3 | 631 |

[a] Data for 100 grams from Reference (245)

prepared so that the cooking juices are consumed with the seafood has higher nutrient content. Both vitamins and minerals may be lost in cooking fluids, although minerals are stable under most cooking conditions.

A summary of the general stability of nutrients in food preparation is shown in Table 5.6.

---

### Table 5.6   General Stability of Nutrients in Food Preparation

| Highly Unstable | Somewhat Unstable | Generally Stable[a] |
|---|---|---|
| Ascorbic acid | Vitamin A | Minerals |
| Thiamin | Vitamin D | Carbohydrates |
| | Vitamin E | Lipids |
| | Pyridoxine (vitamin $B_6$) | Protein |
| | Folic acid | Niacin |
| | Vitamin $B_{12}$ | Vitamin K |
| | Riboflavin | |
| | Pantothenic acid | |

Data from Reference 246.

[a] Equal to or more than 85 percent retention.

---

Two nutrients are highly unstable to nearly all cooking conditions: ascorbic acid (vitamin C) and thiamin. Ascorbic acid is readily destroyed by heat and oxygen and losses may be as great as 100 percent. The vitamin C content of fish is so low that the issue as far as seafood is concerned is largely academic. There is little vitamin C to lose and even less remaining after cooking.

Thiamin is even more unstable than vitamin C. It is readily destroyed by heat, alkali and by the action of the enzyme thiaminase, found mainly in fresh water fish and occasionally in marine species (33, 247, 248). Because it is water-soluble, thiamin can be leached into cooking juices, lost in washing procedures as in the preparation of surimi and lost with the moisture or drip during thawing. With so many vulnerabilities, it is not surprising that thiamin losses may be as high as 80 percent in canned seafood (249). On the other hand, in household seafood cookery thiamin is well retained, usually 85 percent or more (Tables 5.7 and 5.8).

More detailed information about the losses of vitamins in cooking is presented in Table 5.7 (249). It should be pointed out that the majority of studies on cooking losses and nutrient retention have been conducted on foods other than seafood, particularly fruits and vegetables. There is no reason to assume, however, that similar losses would not occur from seafoods cooked or handled under similar conditions. There is a great deal we do not know about nutrient stability in food and that means we are limited in our ability to predict the

## Table 5.7 Summary of Vitamin Losses in Cooking [a]

| Vitamin | Sensitive to: | Cooking losses | Primary Factors |
|---|---|---|---|
| Vitamin C | oxygen<br>heat<br>alkaline pH<br>water | 0-100% | 1. leaching into water, esp. from cut surfaces<br>2. oxidation<br>3. heat destruction |
| Thiamin ($B_1$) | water<br>heat<br>alkaline pH | 30-70% veg<br>0-80% meat<br>0-50% baking | 1. leaching<br>2. heat destruction |
| Riboflavin ($B_2$) | water<br>alkaline pH<br>light | 9-39% animal<br>10-30% plant | 1. leaching<br>2. use of chocolate in baking (increases alkalinity)<br>3. exposure to light |
| Niacin | water | 3-27%[d] | 1. leaching |
| Pantothenic Acid | heat<br>water<br>alkaline pH<br>acidic pH | 7-56%[d] | 1. leaching<br>2. heat destruction |
| Pyridoxine ($B_6$) | water | 30-82%[d] | 1. leaching |
| Folic Acid | heat<br>oxygen<br>alkaline pH<br><br>acidic pH | 46-95% fish/pork<br>33-95% var. meats<br>29-70% egg yolk, liver, chicken<br>0-50% vegetables | 1. heat destruction<br>2. loss of protective ascorbic acid in product |
| Vitamin $B_{12}$ | alkaline pH<br>oxygen<br>heat | 0-20% | 1. leaching (meat drippings) |
| Biotin | oxygen<br>alkaline pH | 0-50% | |
| Vitamin A[c] | oxygen<br>heat<br>light | 0-60% | 1. exposure to light (sunlight or artificial) |
| Vitamin D[d] | oxygen<br>light | 0-40% | 1. exposure to light |
| Vitamin E | oxygen<br>UV light | 0-60% | 1. oxidation |
| Vitamin K | light<br>oxygen | insufficient data | 1. exposure to light<br>2. oxidation |

[a] From Reference 249
[b] Generally good recovery in cooking liquids
[c] Present as beta carotene and other provitamin A carotenoids in vegetables
[d] As added to milk

**Table 5.8  Percent True Retention of Selected Nutrients in Different Seafood Prepared in Various Ways.**

| Preparation Method[b] | Seafood[c] | Protein | Fat | Cholesterol | Thiamin | Riboflavin | Niacin | Vitamin B$_{12}$[k] | Iron | Zinc | Sodium | Potassium |
|---|---|---|---|---|---|---|---|---|---|---|---|---|
| Baked[d] | Flounder[c] | 98 | 100* | 96 | 94 | 96 | 93 | 82 | 94 | 98 | 98 | 100 |
| | Pacific pollock[c] | 93 | 95 | 98 | 84 | 96 | 88 | 100* | 90 | 96 | 79 | 84 |
| | Pacific whiting[c] | 94 | 100* | 96 | 100 | 96 | 100* | 93 | 94 | 95 | 87 | 94 |
| | Sockeye salmon[c] | 100* | 100* | 100* | 92 | 100* | 100* | 78 | 100* | 100* | 96 | 100* |
| | Atlantic mackerel[c] | 96 | 100*l | 100* | 94 | 100* | 100 | 100* | 100 | 100* | 88 | 94 |
| | Tropical shrimp[c] | 100* | 100* | 100* | 100* | 100* | 100* | 100* | 100 | 100* | 95 | 97 |
| Broil[d] | Flounder | 99 | 99 | 95 | 94 | 100* | 100* | 84 | 89 | 98 | 96 | 100 |
| | Pacific pollock | 93 | 96 | 92 | 80 | 92 | 88 | 100* | 88 | 91 | 82 | 85 |
| | Pacific whiting | 97 | 100* | 98 | 96 | 100 | 96 | 96 | 96 | 100 | 94 | 99 |
| | Sockeye salmon | 100* | 100* | 100* | 91 | 100 | 99 | 71 | 100 | 96 | 97 | 100 |
| | Atlantic mackerel | 94 | 100*l | 94 | 96 | 100* | 96 | 100* | 98 | 100* | 97 | 90 |
| Microwave[d] | Flounder | 96 | 92 | 95 | 94 | 100 | 96 | 94 | 90 | 92 | 91 | 100 |
| | Pacific pollock[e] | 98 | 95 | 95 | 77 | 86 | 92 | 96 | 90 | 97 | 85 | 88 |
| | Pacific whiting[e] | 95 | 100 | 99 | 100* | 98 | 100* | 96 | 97 | 96 | 86 | 97 |
| | Sockeye salmon | 100* | 100* | 100* | 100 | 100* | 100* | 84 | 100* | 100* | 100* | 100 |
| | Atlantic mackerel | 98 | 100*l | 100* | 100* | 100* | 100* | 100* | 100 | 100* | 89 | 95 |
| | Tropical shrimp[e] | 100* | 100* | 100* | 94 | 94 | 92 | 100* | 98 | 96 | 92 | 93 |
| Bread & Fry[d] | Pacific pollock | 97 | 460f | 96 | 92 | 97 | 96 | 94 | 98 | 96 | 90 | 92 |
| | Pacific whiting | 100* | 355f | 94 | 86 | 98 | 100 | 92 | 98 | 100* | 99 | 100 |
| | Tropical shrimp | 100* | 470f | 96 | 94 | 100 | 97 | 88 | 94 | 96 | 96 | 100 |
| Boil[d,m] | Tropical shrimp | 96 | 100 | 100* | 89 | 71 | 87 | 71 | 93 | 100* | 66 | 66 |
| Canning[n] | Sockeye salmon[g] | 93 | 100* | 99 | 25 | 78 | 84 | 60 | 94 | 273h | 86 | 85 |
| | Atlantic mackerel[d] | 90 | 97 | 100 | 27 | 79 | 78 | 100* | 100 | 118*h | 71 | 74 |
| | Tropical shrimp[d] | 87 | 100* | 100* | 30 | 50 | 52 | 37 | 100* | 118*h | 390i | 40 |

k Retention figures for Vitamin B$_{12}$ are more variable than for the other vitamins in part because of the variability of the analytical method (microbiological assay) and because the vitamin becomes bound to protein during cooking and is difficult to extract (205)

l Fat retention in mackerel greater than 100% may have been due to the migration of fat from the skin to the muscle during cooking as the fish was not skinned prior to cooking (205)

m Vitamin and mineral retention values are lower than those of other cooking methods because water soluble nutrients are leached into the cooking water and lost.

n Retention values for vitamins and minerals are lower than for cooking methods because water soluble nutrients are leached into the canning liquid, which is generally not consumed. Thiamin losses are large owing to destruction of the vitamin by heat processing.

a Data from 1982, Ref. 182
b For a description of the preparation methods see Appendix 1
c For a description of the sample see Appendix 2
d Based 11 samples
e Based on 6 samples
f Retention is greater than 100% because of uptake of fat during frying
g Based on 5 samples
h Retention is greater than 100% because of migration of zinc from the can to the contents
i Retention is greater than 100% because salt was added to the canning fluid.
j % True Retention = $\dfrac{\text{wt. of nutrient in cooked} \times \text{\% yield}}{\text{wt. of nutrient in raw}}$
* Calculated retention greater than 100% but for practical purposes, retention is reported as 100%.

true nutrient content in cooked foods. Two excellent summaries of this topic were published by Borenstein (246, 250).

Certain general principles apply to the conservation of nutrients in seafood. These are outlined below. Maximum nutrient availability from seafood occurs when:

- drip from thawing is incorporated into the cooking procedures

- cooking juices are consumed

- cooking time is kept to a minimum

- holding time after cooking is kept to a minimum

- alkaline substances like baking soda and baking powder are avoided

- the entire edible portion is consumed

- the bones in canned fish are consumed

- both the light and dark muscle of fish are consumed

- seafood dishes are not reheated, or are reheated for as short a time as possible

## Estimating the Nutrient Content of Cooked Seafood from Data on Raw Portions

One of the most important uses of nutrient composition data is to estimate the nutrient content of foods as consumed. Seafood is nearly always consumed cooked, but most of the nutrient content information available is based on raw seafood. In order to estimate the nutrient content of cooked seafood, the data on raw seafood must be adapted. To do this, both cooking yield and nutrient retention data are required. Several sources of such data for seafood are available (205, 251-3). Nevertheless, complete data are not available for every species and for all cooking methods. This situation forces us to make certain assumptions about the seafood item as purchased: its yield - that is, how much is left after storage, handling and cooking, and the amount of nutrients remaining after cooking. If yield data are not available, we can sometimes impute values from similar species or procedures. Estimating nutrient retention is more difficult and may be impossible for several nutrients where no retention data are available.

Another caution about nutrient data is its level of accuracy. The analytical methods are subject to certain measurement errors. Estimates of food consumption are not precise. Even serving portions that are weighed, as is done in many research studies, give only approximate estimates of the amount consumed. Plate waste, handling losses and other factors introduce errors into measurements. These inaccuracies mean that quoting nutrient values to several decimal places is inappropriate. A level of accuracy to one decimal point is usually the most suitable degree of accuracy for most data. Vitamin data may be expressed to two decimal places but rounding to a single place after final calculations is probably the most useful procedure.

There are two main situations where nutrient content has to be estimated:

1. known portions of seafood after they have been cooked and

2. nutrient content in a given portion of cooked seafood.

In the first instance the initial information is based on a given weight of raw seafood. In the second, the initial information is the weight of the cooked serving. In most instances, estimates of nutrient content must be derived from data on raw edible portions of seafood. If reliable data are available from the analysis of cooked seafood, it is preferable to use these data rather than derive estimates from data on raw portions. Each of these applications of nutrient composition information will be discussed separately.

## 1. Information About Yield

The yield of a portion of seafood is the amount remaining after it has been processed. It reflects change in weight and gives no indication about change in nutrients. In this section, processing refers to different cooking procedures. The starting form is the seafood as purchased, usually a fillet, steak or dressed fish. In most instances, the losses that occur from cooking are those attributable to heat destruction, loss of cooking liquids and handling losses. For some forms of seafood, like live lobster, the major losses are the shell and body parts.

Yield is calculated as follows:

$$\text{percent Yield} = \frac{\text{Weight of seafood after cooking}}{\text{Weight of seafood before cooking}} \times 100$$

Information about the yield of seafood through different stages of preparation from the time the fish leaves the water (round) to the final stage of edible meat has been published for many varieties of seafood (252). The data for these yield figures were obtained under laboratory conditions and the yields obtained in commercial practice are probably less. A sample calculation showing the different yields at each stage of preparation is given in Table 5.9

The yield data for cooking fish and shellfish in different ways are summarized in Tables 5.10 and 5.11 using figures from Agriculture Handbook No. 102 (252). Yield tables are useful for two kinds of estimates:

1. how much of a portion remains after cooking

2. the initial raw weight from a given weight of cooked seafood

If a particular species is not listed in the yield tables, the best one can do is estimate the yield using figures for the species most closely resembling the seafood desired. Similarity of species is gauged by zoological family and sometimes by fat content.

### Table 5.9  Sample Calculations to Determine Yield During Preparation of Striped Bass[a]

| Form Before Preparation | Preparation | % of Yield [f] | Calculation | Finished Product (gm) |
|---|---|---|---|---|
| Round (Whole fish)[b] | None | 100 | — | 100 |
| Round | Drawn[c] | 94 | $100 \times .94$ | 94 |
| Drawn | Dressed[d] | 70 | $94 \times .70$ | 66 |
| Dressed | Fillet w/skin[e] | 65 | $66 \times .65$ | 43 |
| Fillet w/skin | Broil | 80 | $43 \times .80$ | 34 |
| Broiled fillet w/skin | Meat only | 90 | $34 \times .90$ | 31 |

[a] Adapted from Reference 252

[b] Whole fish as taken from the water

[c] Whole fish with entrails removed.

[d] Whole fish eviscerated and scaled with head, tail and fins removed.

[e] Sides of fish cut lengthwise away from backbone; flesh is practically boneless.

[f] Yields may be higher than those obtained under commercial conditions.

If there are no yield data for the cooking method used, then estimates may be based on the most similar method for which data are available. Without such data, estimates are usually impossible. If yield data from widely differing methods are similar, then an average is a reasonable estimate for a given cooking method. If data from only one method are available, then yield estimates may not be possible.

A recent study on the effects of cooking and canning on the yield and nutrient retention in six varieties of seafood was conducted by the National Food Processors Association (NFPA) for the National Marine Fisheries Service (205). This study provides the most recent data we have on nutrient changes in seafood after different cooking procedures and canning. These data permit nutrient estimates from a wider range of cooking methods than was previously possible. The yield figures for four different cooking methods and canning from this study are presented in Table 5.12.

In baking, broiling, poaching, steaming and stir-frying there is a net loss of weight after cooking. This change is primarily due to loss in water, which may carry with it small amounts of protein and water soluble vitamins. Table 5.12 shows a range of cooking yields from 69 percent for broiled pollock to 94 percent for breaded and fried Pacific whiting in the NFPA study. These yields appear to be somewhat higher than those reported by USDA (Tables 2.10 and 2.11). A small amount of fat may be lost, but in general fat is well retained during cooking. When seafood is fried there is a net gain in fat from the oil used.

Indeed, especially with deep frying and breading plus frying, there may be an actual increase in yield owing to the uptake of fat during cooking. There is some loss of moisture and whether this is offset by the uptake of fat depends on the actual cooking conditions. The uptake in fat is probably responsible for the

**Table 5.10   Yield of Finfish after Various Methods of Preparation.**

| | Form before preparation | Form after preparation | Percentage yield[a] |
|---|---|---|---|
| Anchovy | canned | drained solids | 73 |
| Black sea bass | skinless fillet | bake/broil | 82 |
| Bluefish | skinned fillet | broiled | 85[c] |
| | dressed[d] | baked/broiled | 69 |
| | skin-on fillet | baked | 75 |
| | skin-on fillet | broiled | 71 |
| | skin-on fillet | deep-fried | 73 |
| | skin-on fillet | pan fried | 82[e] |
| Cod | frozen, raw | baked, uncovered | 76 |
| | thawed, raw | baked, covered | 83 |
| | thawed, raw | baked, uncovered | 69 |
| | thawed, raw | broiled | 72 |
| | thawed, raw | pan fried | 81 |
| | thawed, raw | poached | 88[e] |
| | thawed, breaded, raw | baked | 83 |
| | dry salted, raw | soaked | 119 |
| | dry salted, soaked | cooked[f] | 64 |
| Croaker | skinned fillet | broiled | 69[c] |
| | dressed, raw | baked | 86[e] |
| | fillet, small fish[g] | baked | 79 |
| | fillet, large fish | baked | 97 |
| Flounder | skinned fillet | broiled | 79[c] |
| | dressed, raw | baked | 75[e] |
| | fillet | baked | 72 |
| | fillet | broiled | 73 |
| | breaded fillet | deep fried | 88[e] |
| | breaded fillet | pan fried | 111 |
| Haddock | skinless fillet | baked | 78 |
| | skinless fillet | broiled | 82 |
| | breaded fillet | oven fried | 85 |
| | breaded fillet | pan fried | 77[e] |
| | steak | baked | 81[e] |
| | steak | microwave | 94[e] |
| Halibut | steak, thawed | baked | 84 |
| | steak, thawed | broiled | 73 |
| Herring | canned, plain, canned | drained solids | 71 |
| | kippered, canned | drained solids | 87 |
| Mackerel | dressed, raw | broiled | 80 |
| | fillet | baked | 86 |
| | fillet | broiled | 77 |
| | canned | drained solids | 84 |

**Table 5.10** *Yield of Finfish after Various Methods of Preparation. (Continued)*

| | Form before preparation | Form after preparation | Percentage yield[a] |
|---|---|---|---|
| Ocean perch | skinless fillet | poached | 75 |
| | skinless fillet | baked | 79 |
| | skinless fillet | broiled | 81 |
| | fillet, frozen | poached | 69 |
| | fillet, breaded, fried, frozen | heated in oven | 97 |
| Pollock | frozen fillet | cooked[f] | 57 |
| | thawed fillet | cooked[f] | 64 |
| Red snapper | dressed | baked | 75[e] |
| | dressed | broiled | 76[e] |
| | skin-on fillet | baked | 72[e] |
| | skin-on fillet | baked | 70[e] |
| Salmon, "Pacific" | dressed, stuffed | baked | 81 |
| | thawed steak | baked | 89 |
| | thawed steak | broiled | 83 |
| Salmon, all varieties | canned | drained solids | 81 |
| | drained solids | boneless solids | 98 |
| Sardines | | | |
| Atlantic | canned | drained solids | 87 |
| Pacific | canned | drained solids | 81 |
| Japanese | canned | drained solids | 83 |
| Norwegian | canned | drained solids | 85 |
| Portuguese | canned | drained solids | 85 |
| Swedish | canned | drained solids | 89 |
| Sea bass | skinned fillet | broiled | 78[c] |
| Sea trout | skinned fillet | broiled | 90[c] |
| weakfish | dressed | baked | 69 |
| | skin-on fillet | broiled | 65 |
| | skin-on fillet, breaded | pan fried | 87 |
| Shad, white | dressed | baked, covered | 76 |
| | dressed | baked, uncovered | 71 |
| | skin-on fillet | baked | 91 |
| | skin-on fillet | broiled | 81 |
| | skinless fillet | broiled | 69 |
| Smelt | fillet, french fried, frozen | baked | 79[e] |
| Sole, unspecified | skinless fillet | broiled | 69[e] |
| | fillet, breaded raw | deep fried | 88[e] |
| | fillet, breaded, fried, frozen | baked | 91 |
| Spot | skinned fillet | broiled | 93[c] |

***Table 5.10    Yield of Finfish after Various Methods of Preparation.
(Continued)***

| | Form before preparation | Form after preparation | Percentage yield[a] |
|---|---|---|---|
| Striped bass | fillet, skin-on | baked/broiled | 80 |
| | fillet, skin-on | pan-fried | 89 |
| | skinless fillet | broiled | 76 |
| | dressed | baked | 62[e] |
| | dressed | broiled | 84[e] |
| | dressed | pan-fried | 89[e] |
| Swordfish | steak | baked | 73 |
| | steak | broiled | 71 |
| Trout, brook and rainbow | eviscerated | baked | 91 |
| | skin-on fillet | broiled | 77 |
| | skin-on filllet, breaded | fried | 94 |
| Tuna, canned | chunks in brine | drained solids | 79[e] |
| | chunks in oil | drained solids | 100[e] |
| | flakes in oil | drained solids | 94 |
| | solid pack in oil | drained solids | 82 |
| Unspecified | frozen battered | baked | 90 |
| | fish sticks, breaded | broiled | 87 |
| | fish sticks, breaded | pan fried | 97 |
| Whitefish | skin-on fillet | baked | 80 |
| White perch | dressed | broiled | 78 |
| | skin-on fillet | broiled | 85 |
| | skinless fillet | pan fried | 67 |
| | dressed, breaded | pan fried | 81 |
| | fillet, breaded | pan fried | 81 |

[a] Reference 252 unless otherwise specified.

[b] Percentage yield calculated as: % yield = $\frac{\text{weight after cooking}}{\text{weight before cooking}} \times 100$

[c] Reference 251.

[d] Dressed = without head, tail, fins, entrails, scales, skin and bones.

[e] Limited data available. Reference 252 also gives yield data from dressing and boning.

[f] Cooking method not specified.

[g] Less than 1 pound.

*Table 5.11 Yield of Shellfish after Various Methods of Preparation.*

| | Form before preparation | Form after preparation | Percentage yield[a] | Ref |
|---|---|---|---|---|
| Abalone | raw whole | raw muscle | 42 | 252 |
| Clams | raw meat | broiled | 59.4 | 251 |
| Crabs: | | | | |
| Blue | whole | boiled | 24.0 | 251 |
| Blue | whole, live | boiled | 17[b] | 252 |
| Dungeness | eviscerated, | boiled | 93 | 252 |
| | boiled | total meat | 24 | 252 |
| King | cooked in shell | total meat | 25 | 252 |
| | frozen | total meat, raw | 51 | 252 |
| | canned | drained | 77 | 252 |
| Lobster | live | boiled | 92 | 252 |
| | boiled | body | 7 | 252 |
| | boiled | claw | 11 | 252 |
| | boiled | tail | 10 | 252 |
| | thawed tail in shell | cooked meat | 55 | 252 |
| | frozen tail in shell | cooked meat | 53 | 252 |
| | canned | drained solids | 70 | 252 |
| Oysters | raw meat | broiled | 61 | 251 |
| | canned | drained solids | 92 | 252 |
| Scallops | thawed raw | boiled | 50[c] | 252 |
| Shrimp, all sizes | | | | |
| (unspec) | thawed in shell | boiled | 76[d] | 252 |
| | shelled, deveined, raw | boiled | 73[e] | 252 |
| | fantailed, breaded, raw | deep fried | 64 | 252 |
| Spiny lobster | thawed tail with shell | boil/broil | 90 | 252 |
| (crayfish) | cooked tail in shell | meat | 65 | 252 |
| | cooked tail without bottom shell | meat | 72 | 252 |

[a] Percentage yield calculated as: $\% \text{ yield} = \dfrac{\text{weight after cooking}}{\text{weight before cooking}} \times 100$

[b] Edible meat.

[c] Limited data available.

[d] Range for different sizes 70 - 82 percent.

[e] Range for different sizes 67 - 76 percent.

high yield figures for breaded and fried fish in Table 5.12.

In cooking methods where ingredients are added to the fish before cooking as in breading or stuffed dressed fish, the appropriate calculation of yield uses the weight of the raw fish plus stuffing or breading, rather than

**Table 5.12    Yield of Different Seafoods Prepared in Various Ways[a]**

| | Method of Preparation[b] | | | | |
| Seafood[d] | Bake | Broil | Microwave | Bread & Fry | Canned |
| | | | % Yield[c] | | |
| Flounder, skinless fillet | 84 | 80 | 85 | —[e] | — |
| Pacific pollock, skinless fillet | 72 | 69 | 74[f] | 88 | — |
| Pacific whiting, skinless fillet | 83 | 78 | 84 | 94 | — |
| Sockeye salmon, skinless, boneless steak | 88 | 80 | 87 | — | 85[g] |
| Atlantic mackerel, skinless fillet | 86 | 80 | 90 | — | 80 |
| Tropical shrimp, mixed species, headless, peeled & deveined | 86 | 82 (boiled) | 80[f] | 88 | 77[g] |

[a] Data from National Food Processors Association study, Reference 205. Means of 11 samples unless indicated otherwise.

[b] For details of preparation, see Appendix 1.

[c] % Yield $= \dfrac{\text{weight of seafood after cooking}}{\text{weight of seafood before cooking}}$

[d] For details of sample, see Appendix 2.

[e] Dashes denote lack of data.

[f] Mean of 6 samples.

[g] Mean of 5 samples.

weight of the raw fish only, as shown below:

$$\text{Percent Yield} = \frac{\text{Weight of cooked stuffed fish}}{\text{Weight of raw stuffed fish}} \times 100$$

## 2. Nutrient Retention

Nutrient retention refers to the amount of a particular nutrient that is left after cooking or processing. Calculation of nutrient retention depends on two sets of measures: the change in weight after cooking, or the yield, and the determination of the amount of nutrient in both the raw and cooked form. It is determined as shown below:

$$\% \text{ True Retention} = \frac{\text{Weight of Nutrient in Cooked Portion}}{\text{Weight of Nutrient in Raw Portion}} \times \% \text{ Yield}$$

It should be pointed out that nutrients are not gained during cooking procedures unless they come from the cooking utensils (iron skillets) or added

136

ingredients (cheese topping, deep frying). Cooking does not increase nutrient content*.

Tables that show an increase in a nutrient after cooking compared with the amount before cooking are showing increases in concentration as a result of loss of moisture. Stated differently, tables frequently compare nutrients in raw and cooked seafood on an equal weight basis, not according to how much nutrient remains in a portion after cooking. It is easy to misinterpret tables of nutrient composition by overlooking the effects of cooking on nutrient concentration.

The calculation of nutrient retention is also sensitive to small differences in amounts of nutrients, especially at low values. When the amounts of nutrients observed are close to the limits of detection, then small differences are nearly meaningless. The result is that the calculated retention can be misleadingly low (or high). The following example from the NFPA study illustrates this problem.

The iron content of raw pollock was observed to be 0.17 mg and that in cooked pollock 0.15. The yield was 70 percent. Then,

$$\text{True Retention} = \frac{.15}{.17} \times 70 \text{ percent} = 62 \text{ percent}$$

Sixty-two percent retention suggests that 38 percent of the iron was lost, whereas both .15 and .17 are within the error of the analytical method and are probably not different from each other.

Nutrient retention has been determined for a number of vitamins and minerals in a wide variety of foods and the most recent data have been published by USDA in a Provisional Table on Percent Retention of Nutrients in Foods (253). The figures from this table that apply to seafood are presented in Table 5.13.

There are also nutrient retention data from the recent NFPA study not only for several vitamins and minerals but also for protein, fat and cholesterol (205). The average nutrient retention values from the NFPA study are presented in Table 5.14. The values in this study compare well with the USDA figures and show that there is very little nutrient loss with most cooking methods. Microwave cookery is especially efficient in conserving nutrients.

When cooking methods are compared with canning, it is clear that the heat processing involved in the canning procedure is very hard on several nutrients. About 70 percent of the thiamin is destroyed (as expected); niacin losses may reach 50 percent; and vitamin $B_{12}$ losses may exceed 50 percent. The variability in the data for some nutrients was quite large (not shown), making it difficult to predict the average nutrient retention with much confidence.

*Cooking may lead to apparent increases of certain nutrients that become available as a result of the cooking conditions, but this occurs infrequently. A well known example of this phenomenon is the release of bound niacin from corn (maize) cooked with lime. The bound niacin is present before the cooking, but is released and becomes available to the body only in the presence of alkali and heat.

*Table 5.13   Provisional Table on Retention of Nutrients in Seafood Preparation[a,b]*

| Food and method of preparation | Vitamins | | | | | | | Minerals | | | | |
|---|---|---|---|---|---|---|---|---|---|---|---|---|
| | Thiamin | Riboflavin | Niacin | Pantothenic Acid | Vitamin B6 | Folic Acid | Vitamin B12 | Iron | Zinc | Phosphorus | Sodium | Potassium |
| | Percent | | | | | | | | | | | |
| Lean Fish[c] – less than 5% fat | | | | | | | | | | | | |
| Baked or broiled | 90 | 95 | 95 | —[d] | — | — | 90 | 100 | 100 | — | 100 | 100 |
| Breaded, deep fried | 85 | 95 | 100 | — | — | — | 90 | 100 | 100 | — | 100 | 100 |
| Fish with 5-15% fat – e.g. catfish, sablefish, salmon, rainbow trout baked or broiled | 95 | 100 | 100 | — | — | — | 75 | 100 | 100 | — | 100 | 100 |
| High Fat Fish – more than 15% fat e.g. eel, herring, lake trout, mackerel, spot baked or broiled | 90 | 100 | 95 | — | — | — | 95 | 100 | 100 | — | 100 | 100 |
| Shrimp[e]: baked | 95 | 100 | 95 | — | — | — | 100 | 100 | 100 | — | 100 | 100 |
| Boiled | 90 | 75 | 75 | — | — | — | 60 | 100 | 100 | — | 65 | 65 |
| Deep fried | 85 | 95 | 95 | — | — | — | 85 | 100 | 100 | — | 100 | 100 |
| Crab[e]: Boiled | — | — | — | — | — | — | — | 80 | 100 | 70 | 100 | 75 |
| Steamed | — | — | — | — | — | — | — | 80 | 100 | 75 | 100 | 90 |

[a] Percent retention is calculated as follows:
$$\frac{\text{Nutrient content per gm cooked food} \times \text{gm food after cooking}}{\text{Nutrient content per gm raw food} \times \text{gm food before cooking}} = \text{\% True Retention}$$

[b] Adapted from Reference (253)

[c] See Table 2.3 for examples of species with less than 5% fat.

[d] Dashes denote lack of reliable data

[e] Species not given

If the retention of a nutrient is known, the amount of the nutrient remaining in the seafood after cooking is easy to calculate, as shown in the example below:

To determine how much protein there will be in a 4 oz. portion of raw flounder after it is baked, knowing that:

Retention of protein after baking is: 98 percent (Table 5.14)
A 4 oz. portion of raw flounder has 19.2 grams protein (calculated from Table 9.1) Then,

19.2 grams × .98  =  18.8 grams protein remaining after baking the flounder portion.

## Applications of Yield and Retention Data

The examples in the preceding two sections have shown how yield and retention data are calculated and how they may be used. In this part some additional examples are given, related to practical situations.

Example 1. Determine how much raw cod fillet will provide four 6 oz. servings, broiled.

Yield after broiling skinless cod fillet: 72 percent (Table 5.10) Therefore,

$$\frac{4 \times 6 \text{ oz.}}{.72} = 33.3 \text{ oz. of raw cod. Two pounds should do it.}$$

Example 2. Estimate the amount of fat in a 4 oz. serving of pan fried bluefish. Yield after pan frying: 82 percent (Table 5.10)
Fat content of raw bluefish: 2.9 gm/100 gm (Table 9.1). Therefore,

$$\frac{4 \text{ oz. cooked}}{.82} = 4.9 \text{ oz. raw}$$

Convert oz. to gm: 4.9 oz. x 28.4 = 139.2 gm raw bluefish

$$\frac{139.2 \times 2.9}{100} = 4.0 \text{ gm fat in 4.9 oz. raw bluefish}$$

The mixing of units of measure, grams and ounces, in this example reflects the habit of measuring small amounts like nutrients in grams (which give whole numbers) and serving sizes in ounces (which are familiar units in food service).

There are no data on fat retention in bluefish after pan frying. To estimate a reasonable retention figure, consider two features: the effect of method of cooking on fat retention, and the effect of species on fat retention. The data in Table 5.14 present the average retention values from the NFPA study for 11 nutrients broken out by cooking method. It can be seen from this table that fat is completely retained during canning and the four cooking methods studied when the six species of fish and shrimp were averaged. Fat

*Table 5.14 Average Nutrient Retention Values For Different Cooking Methods and Canning of Six Species of Seafood*[a,b]

| Nutrient | Bake | Broil[d] | Microwave | Bread &Fry[d] | Canned[f] |
|---|---|---|---|---|---|
| | | Cooking/Processing Method[c] | | | |
| Protein | 98 | 97 | 99 | 100 | 90 |
| Fat | 100 | 100 | 100 | 428 | 100 |
| Cholesterol | 99 | 97 | 100 | 95 | 100 |
| Thiamin | 95 | 91 | 95 | 91 | 27 |
| Riboflavin | 100 | 100 | 98 | 98 | 69 |
| Niacin | 98 | 96 | 99 | 98 | 71 |
| Vitamin $B_{12}$ | 100 | 93 | 98 | 96 | 69 |
| Iron | 98 | 94 | 98 | 97 | 100 |
| Zinc | 100 | 98 | 99 | 98 | 170[h] |
| Sodium | 90 | 97 | 91 | 95 | 78 |
| Potassium | 96 | 95 | 96 | 99 | 67[i] |

[a] Data from Reference 205.

[b] Average values for samples of: flounder, pollock, whiting, sockeye salmon, mackerel and shrimp; most analyses were based on 11 samples of each species.

[c] For descriptions of the cooking methods, see Appendix 1.

[d] Data include all species except shrimp.

[e] Data from pollock, whiting and shrimp.

[f] Data from salmon, mackerel and shrimp.

[g] Retention greater than 100% because of absorption of fat.

[h] Retention greater than 100% because of migration of zinc from the lining of the can to the contents.

[i] Retention low because of very low values for canned shrimp for which there is no apparent explanation; retention calculated without these values is 80%.

retention for breading and frying is much greater than 100 percent owing to the uptake of fat. It seems reasonable to assume, then, that fat retention in pan fried bluefish would be at least 100 percent. Calculating, 4.0 x 100% retention = 4.0 gm fat in cooked bluefish.

The other feature in this example not accounted for by the above calculations is the effect of the fat in the pan on the final fat content of the fish. Unless the example gives an indication of how much oil was used to fry the fish, there is no way of knowing how much oil would be taken up by the fish. Fat uptake is less without breading because breading increases the surface area of the fish and hence the fat uptake. There are two options in this example. One is to ignore the influence of the fat in the pan and report the estimated fat content as an underestimate because of the lack of information about the cooking conditions. The other option is to make a guess about what might have been done and increase the estimate of the fat content. If you explain the assumptions you make in deriving an estimate for the frying conditions, the final result might be acceptable. Either way, the estimate leaves something to be desired.

Example 3. Estimate the cholesterol content in 100 grams of raw clams from the data on the cholesterol content of cooked clams.

Yield of cooked clams from raw meat: 59% (Table 5.11) Soft shell clams have 40 mg cholesterol/100 gm cooked meat; hard shell clams have 65 mg cholesterol/100 gm cooked meat (Table 2.8) Therefore,

$$\frac{100 \text{ gm cooked}}{.59} = 169 \text{ grams raw clams}$$

Raw soft shell clams have: $\dfrac{100 \times 40}{169} = 23.7$ grams cholesterol/100 gm

Raw hard shell clams have: $\dfrac{100 \times 65}{169} = 38.5$ grams cholesterol/100 gm

# Chapter Six

# Seafood Labeling: More Than Just a Name

---

## What's in a Name?

Seafood names are a sensitive issue. One reason is that many fish have several names. For example, porgy is also known as scup or sea bream. Another is that the same name may refer to more than one species. Whitefish may refer to any white fleshed fish such as cod and flounder (144); it may refer to Atlantic wolffish (254) or lake whitefish (144); or, it may refer to ocean whitefish, otherwise known as tilefish (144, 254). Anyone buying "whitefish" should know what he is doing and ask plenty of questions.

A third difficulty with seafood names is that the same name may have different meanings in different parts of the country and may refer to different species. Snapper is a case in point. A variety of fish may be called snapper, but the most common reference is to red snapper. Most snappers come from the Atlantic and Gulf coasts, although a few varieties are found on the West coast. California, however, has a red rockfish, which is legally called Pacific red snapper within California (144). Outside that state and the state of Washington the same fish is a rockfish and the name snapper is unlawful. A snapper may depend on where you are!

Names of fish can be misleading as well. Take the term "Boston bluefish", which is no bluefish at all. It is young pollock. And how many people know what scrod or schrod is? A scrod is a size designation for a variety of white-fleshed fish below certain weights (144). Scrod may be haddock, cod, pollock or even cusk. Most frequently, though not always, it is haddock.

Then there are aesthetic difficulties with seafood names. How many people think dolphinfish is actually the mammal dolphin? Use of the alternative Hawaiian, name mahimahi removes this confusion and adds a touch of the exotic too. The obstacles to consumer acceptance of unfamiliar fish with names like grunt, wolffish and rat tail are obvious. The temptation to call in the ad agency to create a new name must be nearly irresistible.

## Food Labeling

The Food and Drug Administration (FDA) is responsible for ensuring that a spade is called a spade. Except for meat and poultry, FDA governs the labeling of all foods. In 1973, FDA made final a set of regulations governing the labeling of food, stating the kinds of information that were required on food labels and defining the meaning of terms (255). The regulations also prohibit certain kinds of claims (256). For the names of fish, FDA relies on the American Fisheries Society publication, *List of Common and Scientific Names of Fishes from the United States and Canada* (394,) together with some definitions included in the Code of Federal Regulations and various rulings and customs. A definitive list of "market names" is being prepared by FDA and the National Marine Fisheries Service. In general, it is illegal to use a misleading, incomplete or incorrect common name on a package.

Food labels must contain the following information: name of the product; net contents or weight, including packing liquid; name and address of the manufacturer, packer or distributor; and the ingredients listed in descending order of content by weight. The ingredient statement can be omitted when a product conforms to "standards of identity" (see below). To protect the consumer further from misleading labeling practices, Congress enacted the Fair Packaging Act in 1966 which requires that information for consumers use ordinary language and be placed prominently on the label (258, 259). The seafood industry must also comply with these labeling regulations. An excellent summary of the contents of food labels is contained in a reprint from *FDA Consumer* called "A Consumer's Guide to Food Labels" (260).

In addition to the required information for all food packages, manufacturers may also include other items. Nutrition information with appropriate explanatory statements may be given. Open dating, grading symbols, preparation instructions, recipes, code dating for shelf life, universal product code and other defined symbols may also be included. Explanations of this information follow. The explanations are not exhaustive and readers wishing to devise product labels are advised to consult the Code of Federal Regulations for details (21).

### Name of the product

It may seem self-evident that the name of a product should tell the purchaser what the product is. That is fine when the name is clear, like cod fillets. But does the consumer know what surimi or kamaboko is? Because the opportunity to mislead the consumer occurs readily, and because manufacturers succumb to the temptation to do so, FDA issues rulings on product definition as the need arises. The recent rulings about the description of surimi and products derived from surimi illustrate the point (see Chapter Five).

The name of a product must also be its common or usual name. The reasoning behind this rule is that if a product resembles that which it is not, the consumer ought to be able to tell the difference. The point is self-evident.

FDA has made several rulings about the naming of fish, seafood and their products. Whenever possible, common names of fish are derived from the zoological name of the species. The most recent rulings have defined capelin, crabmeat, kippers, red snapper, lobster, langostino, crawfish, caviar, Pacific whiting, Greenland turbot, bonito and certain processed seafood products. These definitions are described in (261).

## Net contents or net weight

Any package must state the net weight of the contents, meaning the weight of the contents alone, without the jar, can or box. The net weight includes the liquid, if present. The weight of canned fish includes both the solids and liquid present. Certain seafood products, like cooked lobster, shrimp and mussels in brine, must declare the drained weight of the contents (261). Although a statement of drained weight is not mandatory for all products, many manufacturers will include this information or give some other indication of the quantity of the contents. For example, canned artichokes may state how many artichoke hearts the consumer can expect. The principle would seem to apply to many seafood products such as whole herring, sardines and clams, but the rulings appear to be inconsistent. Fortunately, the marketplace usually takes care of those manufacturers who try to sell more clam juice than clams in the can.

## Manufacturer location

The name and place of business of the manufacturer, packer or distributor must be on all food labels. In most instances, sufficient information is given to allow a consumer to contact the manufacturer. It is sometimes not clear from the information on the label who the manufacturer really is. A reputable firm has nothing to gain by being devious on his food label about his whereabouts.

## Ingredients listing

Many consumers do not know that the list of ingredients on a food label must be stated in descending order of content. That means that the ingredient present in the greatest amount by weight appears first. Any additives in the product must be listed, but colors and flavors do not have to be listed by name. The fact that artificial colors or flavors are added must be declared, but the specific names of the colors and flavors are not normally required.

The ingredients listing can be very informative. It indicates the primary component of an item, which may be in doubt for such items as breaded shrimp. It also reveals whether fat, sugar or starches have been added to foods, like seafood, where one might not expect such components to be present naturally.

Furthermore, if fat or oil has been added, the ingredient statement must indicate specifically which fats or oils have been added. The point of this requirement is to permit consumers to identify foods which have certain fats that they may wish to select or avoid. Manufacturers have made it rather difficult for consumers to exercise such choices, however, because they are allowed to state that a product may contain either one fat or another. If either fat is of concern to the consumer, he had best avoid the product.

## Standards of identity

The exception to the rule governing ingredients listing is products conforming to mandated formulas, known as standards of identity. These standards dictate the kinds and amounts of ingredients certain products must contain as well as permissible optional ingredients. Products not conforming to these standards cannot be called by their familiar name, e.g. mayonnaise.

There is no ready way for a consumer to know which foods are included in the standards of identity. Also, manufacturers of such foods may choose to put an ingredients statement on the label. Some examples of foods covered by the standards are: cocoa products, flour, corn (grain) products, macaroni and noodle products, bread, milk, cream and cheese products, frozen desserts, food flavorings, dressings like mayonnaise, canned fruits and juices, fruit jams, jellies, preserves and butters, table syrups, soda water, eggs and egg products, margarine, nuts, frozen and canned vegetables, tomato products such as catsup, and meat and poultry products.

The standards of identity that pertain to the seafood industry are given in Title 21 of the Federal Code (165).

## Open dating

Confusion reigns supreme in the realm of package dates. FDA does not regulate whether or not a manufacturer or retailer must put a date on his package, but consumer and retailer pressures have encouraged manufacturers to disclose some kind of shelf life information. The result is a variety of dating practices, not all consumer friendly. The term "open dating" is a catch-all phrase including a variety of concepts. Some dates favor the retailer so that he can better rotate the products on his shelves; others favor the consumer because they imply freshness and/or safety; others are uninterpretable. The basic ideas in open dating are:

**Sell by or pull date**   is the last day a product should be offered for sale. It implies that the product has been stored and handled properly up to this date and allows for some safe storage time at home. The main problem with sell by dates is that the consumer has no way of knowing how long product safety or quality is assured after that time. But the consumer faces the same issue without sell by dates. Examples of products with sell by dates are self-service fish, milk, refrigerated dough products and cold cuts.

It is germane to note that the Food Marketing Institute, a trade association of food wholesalers and retailers, has issued a position statement advocating the voluntary use of the sell by date. They also support the use of "best if used by" information when it is linked to the sell by date. An example might be: "best if used within seven days after the date stamped on the bottom of the container" (262).

**Best if used by date**    is the date which indicates the duration of peak quality. It does not mean that the product is not safe to eat after the date marked, but rather that the manufacturer will not guarantee its quality. Breakfast cereals are a familiar example using such dates. Obviously an opened box of cereal will still be good to eat after the best if used by date, especially if it has been tightly sealed between uses. Some manufacturers and retailers are reluctant to use best if used by dates because handling after purchase is unknown.

**Expiration date**    is the last date the food should be eaten or used at home, assuming proper home storage. It is often confused with the "best if used by" date and means much the same. The confusion stems from the question, once the date has elapsed, should I throw the product out? In some cases, the product may still be safe to eat; that is, it will not make you sick, but its quality and flavor may have declined noticeably. Expiration dates may appear on baby food, dough products and yeast. They are not widely used because of the negative safety connotations suggested above.

**Pack date**    is the date of manufacture, processing or packaging and tells how old the product is when you purchase it. It usually appears as a series of numbers and/or letters and may appear anywhere on the label or can. Pack dates are most often used with products having a long shelf life, like canned goods, cake mixes and oils. Manufacturers are sometimes reluctant to reveal pack dates because of perceived consumer misgivings about products several months old. Furthermore, there are differences in opinion about the optimum shelf life of such products (263, 264).

Pack dates often appear in code so that the consumer cannot easily determine what the date is. There may be additional information of interest to the retailer or manufacturer combined with the pack date code, such as the plant and shift where the product was packed. This makes it more difficult to determine the pack date. Most of the time pack dates are not of concern to consumers; however, during instances of product recall, pack dates and codes can be crucial. Information about deciphering pack codes is contained in (265). A useful set of examples of actual pack codes has been compiled by the New York State Consumer Protection Board (266).

**Freshness date**    is similar to a sell by or best if used by date and may appear on bakery products. After this date, bakery products are sometimes sold at reduced prices.

The bottom line about open dating is that it makes it easier for the merchant to sell your product and more reassuring for the consumer to buy it. Tell the consumer two facts:

- the best purchase period for your product, that is, a sell by date; and

- how long you think its quality will be retained, i.e., a "best if used by" date.

If quality is dependent on storage conditions, as it is with fresh seafood, tell the purchaser how to store it, at what temperature, and for how long to do so. The advantages of openness are consumer confidence and manufacturer credibility, two assets in marketing.

## Grading

Some foods have a grade symbol or description set by USDA or by state health departments. Not all foods have grading standards and the words, symbols etc. are not the same across all products. Meat, potatoes, fruits and dairy products are all different. Products are graded only at the request of the manufacturer, so that not all brands or foods within a category may be graded. Because of the many inconsistencies of the grading system, consumers tend to be poorly informed about the meanings and kinds of grades.

The unifying concept with USDA grades is quality. Grades are hierarchical with terms like prime, No. 1 and Grade A indicating the highest quality. Except for the meat grades of prime and choice, the descriptive terms make these quality levels clear, but do not indicate how the quality differs between grades.

Federal inspection and grading standards exist for processed fish products, but participation in the program is voluntary (261). Seafood that has been processed under the appropriate conditions may use the approved grade mark on its container or label. The appropriate conditions are that it:

1. has been packed under inspection according to the Code of Federal Regulations;

2. has been certified by an inspector as meeting the requirements of the grade (267).

The grades for fishery products are:
**Grade A:** top quality, uniform in size, virtually free from blemishes and excellent flavor characteristic of the species

**Grade B:** good quality but may not conform in size or blemishes as uniformly as Grade A

**Grade C:** fairly good quality; just as wholesome and nutritious as Grades A and B

*Note:* Grade B or C products are usually marketed without any grade designation and almost never appear in the retail marketplace (261).

In the business of unprocessed seafood, the term grade often has nothing to do with product quality. Grading refers to sorting fish according to size. Size includes length, thickness and weight. Moreover, grading classifications vary for different species. The adherence to any grading system varies with the operation of local markets and auction systems. Chaos prevails.

Grade marks look like this:

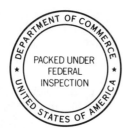 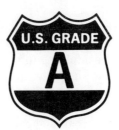

The USDC has also established general grade standards for fresh or frozen fish fillets of any species suitable to eat (261). It is not known to what extent fish processors adhere to these standards. The standards represent a useful start toward establishing national quality control assurances.

The Canadian government has proposed grading standards for certain kinds of fish (268). No uniform code exists in the USA. There are movements by some parties in this direction, but no consensus has been reached.

## Inspection

Whereas grade may refer to a level of quality or size in seafood, inspection refers to the conditions under which the product was produced. There are two levels of inspection for fish processing operations. The first is that required by the FDA and applies to all processing plants. The second is a voluntary federal inspection conducted by licensed or appointed inspectors of the U.S. Department of Commerce (USDC).

Products packed under USDC inspection are entitled to display the PUFI symbol, which means "packed under federal inspection".

The PUFI mark means that the product is clean, safe and wholesome; that it has been produced in an acceptable establishment; and that it meets specified quality or grade classifications (261, 267). While inspection does not certify grade, in practice the two operations go hand in hand. PUFI symbols may be used on many products for which Grade Standards have not been established.

The symbols for grade and inspection may be combined.

Several circumstances have limited the use of both grading and inspection systems on processed products. The first is the shortage of inspectors. There simply are not enough trained and licensed inspectors to go around. The second is cost. The processor bears the cost of federal inspection and, if demand for quality assurance is low and the program optional, processors are unlikely to add to their burdens. Add to this situation widespread consumer confusion over grading symbols and nomenclature and one may marvel that any system exists, much less is ever implemented. Nevertheless, over 70 percent of all frozen seafood products come from participating plants. Clearly, producers feel there is a market benefit.

## UPC Code

The universal product code (UPC) has become synonymous with technology in food retailing. The series of parallel lines on a food package is a form of machine-readable language containing information about that product. When the series of lines passes across the light beam of an electronic scanner, the information contained in the lines is translated into the numbers found below the lines. These numbers identify the item, its price and the manufacturer. The UPC code contains 10 numbers and is specific to the manufacturer and the product. Price information is adjusted by changing the meaning of the numerical code in the retailer's computer scanning system.

A number of problems exist with UPC codes which cause them to be rejected by the scanning equipment. Rescanning an item costs money: millions of dollars for major supermarket chains. In a major study by Pathmark Supermarkets in New Jersey, more than a third of their UPC symbols failed to conform to the UPC Council's specifications (269). Among the most flagrant abuses were: poor location of the symbol on the package, shortened bars, symbols running in the least preferable direction for scanning and poor color contrast. The point is that, when designing packages for seafood or other foods, it is false economy to scrimp on the UPC code.

More information about UPC codes can be obtained from the Uniform Product Code Council (270).

## Price

Food labels also tell the consumer how much the item costs. The total cost is the retail price. Unit price is the cost for each "unit" in the package, where a unit may be an ounce, pound, pint, quart, gallon, count (as in number of tea bags) or square feet. Unit price enables the buyer to compare the cost of different brands or choices within the same product category. Unit pricing is not required by federal law, but some states, counties and cities require it.

## Consumer guidance

Some food labels offer suggestions for handling, storing, preparing and serving the product. Recipes may be included on the face of the label, on the back, inside the package, or as a stick-on label. Consumer guidance is especially important with seafood to encourage successful cooking, promote new preparation ideas and ensure satisfaction with the product. A variety of adhesive labels giving preparation and handling tips for different species and retail forms of fresh fish may encourage trial of new products and generate interest in the products. As an example, instructions for storing, thawing and using frozen vacuum packed seafood would be useful.

## Symbols

Certain letters and symbols may appear on a food label without explanation. The following are the most common:

®     means that the trademark used on the label has been registered with the U.S. Patent Office

©     the copyright symbol means that the literary and artistic content of the label is protected under the laws of the Copyright Act

Ⓤ     means that the food complies with the Jewish dietary laws as authorized by the Union of Orthodox Jewish Congregations

**Kosher**     indicates that the food has been prepared according to the Jewish dietary laws (271).

**Pareve**     identifies kosher foods that are neutral and may be used with either meat or dairy foods.

Other symbols may appear on a package as the logo of a particular company, brand, trade group or organization. The use of brand or company logos is widespread and the clever use of artwork with logos can sometimes be misleading.

## Nutrition Labeling

### Nutrition information on food packages

One of the tangible outcomes of the 1969 White House Conference on Food, Nutrition and Health was the development of a voluntary nutrition labeling system. In 1973 the FDA published final regulations describing the conditions under which manufacturers could present the nutritional merits of their products (255). The regulations covered three areas of nutrition: labeling, nutritional quality guidelines and imitation foods. Additional regulations have been passed governing health claims, sodium labeling and a variety of other nutrition-related issues (21, 272). Full details from what must be declared to what may not be said, including the size of type to be used, are given in the Code of Federal Regulations, Chapter 21 (21).

Nutrition labeling is a voluntary program designed to educate people about the nutritional content of foods and to protect consumers against fraudulent health claims. Nutrition information is mandatory only on foods where nutrients are added, like enriched flour, or those making a health claim, like weight control products. Since its inception, nutrition labeling has been

---

### FDA POLICY ON HEALTH CLAIMS AND LABELING.

The following is an extract from a speech made by Joseph P. Hile, FDA Associate Commissioner for Regulatory Affairs, on March 5, 1985 to the Food and Drug Law Institute (355): The Agency has drawn on its experience of the past and has reached several conclusions that can form the basis for a listing today of principles leading to the possibility of allowing health messages on food labels.

First, FDA supports the disease prevention programs of the Public Health Service. We are prepared to favorably consider ways by which food labeling might be used as a means of conveying health messages so long as our ability to regulate health fraud is not diminished or compromised.

Health messages on food labels do now, and will if formally provided for, represent labeling within the meaning of the Food, Drug and Cosmetic Act and would be within the jurisdiction of FDA.

Third, the public's interest demands that:

a. Any studies used as a basis for health messages be recognized by qualified experts as valid and supportive of such messages;

b. The messages emphasize that good nutrition is a function of total diet and therefore the messages should *ordinarily* appear on foods that are part of a total dietary plan;

c. The wording of such messages must be reasonably uniform, product to product, to protect consumers from misleading claims; and

d. There must be order in the marketplace to guard against dietary "power" races.

We think it is appropriate that any health message used generally on food labeling be subjected to the scrutiny of the PHS as a whole.
Labeling should provide a means by which the consumer can compare products bearing health messages (e.g. by requiring nutritional labeling).

In the interim, firms contemplating the use of health messages should consult with FDA so that the firm is fully aware of the Agency's position regarding their proposed labeling.

Finally, any language used that is outside a scientifically accepted health message wording would be subject to action by FDA as representing the product as a drug because it bears medical claims.

---

controversial, initially because of its cost to manufacturers and later because of its shortcomings and mixed consumer response. The controversy has not subsided, which is probably good, but nutrition labeling has been adopted by more manufacturers every year.

FDA defines "labeling" to mean "all labels and other written, printed, or graphic matter upon any article or any of its container or wrappers, or accompanying such article" (273). That means not only material on the package, but package inserts, point-of-purchase materials, signs, brochures and the like.

A nutrition label must include the following information in a standard format (21):

**Serving size**   "serving" means a reasonable quantity of food as would be consumed as part of a meal by an adult; a "portion" means the amount of a food customarily used only as an ingredient in the preparation of a meal component (e.g., ½ cup flour).

**Servings per container**   the quantity in the container divided by the serving size.

**Calorie content**   calorie content per serving is rounded to the nearest 2 calories up to 20 calories, rounded to the nearest 5 calories between 20 and 50 calories, and to 10 calories above 50 calories per serving; claims about calorie content must conform to the following:

"low calorie": no more than 40 calories per serving nor 0.4 calories per gram;
"reduced calorie": contains a reduction in calories of at least one-third compared to the equivalent unmodified food; states specifically the foods being compared; and is not nutritionally inferior to its higher calorie equivalent.

**Protein content**   number of grams of protein per serving rounded to the nearest gram if above 1 gram per serving; below 1 gram per serving, the label may say "less than 1 gram."

**Carbohydrate content**   number of grams of carbohydrate in a serving expressed to the nearest gram if above 1 gram; below 1 gram per serving, the label may say "less than 1 gram."

**Fat content**   number of grams of fat in a serving rounded to the nearest gram, except if a serving contains less than 1 gram where the phrase "less than 1 gram" may be used instead. In addition, total fat may be expressed as a percent of the total calories along with the phrase "percent of calories from fat."

**Fatty acid content**   is optional and may be included only if the food contains 10 percent or more fat on a dry weight basis and not less than 2 grams of fat in an average serving; fatty acids calculated as triglycerides may also be expressed in grams as "polyunsaturated" and "saturated" fat; note that the sum of the polyunsaturated and saturated fat will not always equal the total fat because of the presence of monounsaturated fatty acids.

**Cholesterol content**   is optional, but if used follows the statement on fat content; cholesterol content is given in milligrams per serving rounded to the nearest 5 milligrams.

NOTE: When either fatty acid or cholesterol content is given, the following statement must appear on the label either immediately following the values given or footnoted at the end of the label: "Information on fat and/or cholesterol content is provided for individuals who, on the advice of a physician, are modifying their dietary intake of fat (and/or cholesterol)."

**Sodium**   Since April 1984, sodium content has been a mandatory part of nutrition labeling. Sodium content, expressed as milligrams per serving, must appear on the label immediately following the statement of fat content (and fatty acid/cholesterol content, if given). Sodium content may be given without full nutrition labeling, but the converse does not hold.

Sodium content is expressed as zero when the content is less than 5 milligrams per serving. Values are rounded to the nearest 5 milligrams when the amount is between 5 and 140 milligrams and to the nearest 10 milligrams for amounts greater than 140 milligrams.

Furthermore, FDA has defined the meaning of certain claims made in conjunction with sodium content. The following terms may be displayed on the label, provided the sodium content is in compliance:

1. Sodium free: sodium content less than 5 milligrams per serving;

2. Very low sodium: sodium content between 5 and 35 milligrams per serving;

3. Low sodium: sodium content between 35 and 140 milligrams per serving. FDA describes this range as "less than 140 milligrams" (35);

4. Reduced sodium: foods that have been formulated as direct replacements for foods containing at least four times the sodium content, i.e., 75 percent reduction.

Note that FDA does not define "high" sodium. As a result it is the responsibility of nutrition educators and health professionals to make people aware of those foods which have large amounts of sodium. To do so in print, however, could risk being out of compliance with the FDA regulations. People do need to be able to recognize those foods which have high levels of sodium.

Unprocessed seafood has the nutritional advantage of low sodium content. It behoves manufacturers to maintain this benefit and take advantage of the marketing opportunity to flaunt it. Nutrition labeling permits such declarations and puts those manufacturers with nutrition labels on their seafood products in the forefront.

**Salt**   Salt is not synonymous with sodium. Salt is sodium chloride, of which 40 percent is sodium. The major source of sodium in foods is salt. Food labels may contain the claim "no salt added" or "unsalted" provided that: no salt is added during processing; the food it resembles normally has salt added; and sodium content is declared as required.

**Potassium**  Declaration of potassium content is voluntary. Where it is provided, FDA requires that it follow the statement on sodium and that the content be expressed in milligrams per serving, rounded as for sodium.

Presently, relatively few foods have potassium content on the nutrition label. While potassium values are usually obtained at the same time as sodium analysis, obtaining the additional information increases the cost to manufacturers. FDA believes that there is insufficient concern about potassium intake among the general population to warrant its inclusion in nutrition labeling. Its presence, however, is helpful to many dietitians who counsel thousands of people with high blood pressure.

**Percentage of U.S. Recommended Daily Allowances (U.S. RDA) of the following nutrients**  protein, vitamin A, vitamin C, thiamin, riboflavin, niacin, calcium, and iron, rounded as follows: 2 percent increments up to and including 10 percent; 5 percent increments above 10 percent up to and including 50 percent; and, 10 percent increments above 50 percent. Nutrients present in amounts less than 2 percent of the U.S. RDA may be listed as zero, or by the following statement: "contains less than two percent of the U.S. RDA of this/these nutrient(s)". Note too that the order in which the nutrients are to be listed is that given above.

Other vitamins and minerals shall be included when they have been intentionally added to the product, and may be listed if they are naturally occurring. The amounts present are expressed in terms of percent U.S. RDA. Nutrients for which no U.S. RDA have been established may not be declared.

An example of a nutrition label for a processed seafood product (frozen flounder fillets) is shown below:

---

### NUTRITION INFORMATION PER SERVING

Serving size: 4 oz   Servings per container: 4

| | |
|---|---|
| Calories | 90 |
| Protein | 19 grams |
| Carbohydrate | 0 grams |
| Fat | 1 gram |
| Sodium | 35 mg |

#### % U.S. RECOMMENDED DAILY ALLOWANCES (U.S. RDA) PER SERVING

| | |
|---|---|
| Protein | 40% |
| Vitamin A | * |
| Vitamin C | * |
| Thiamin | 4% |
| Riboflavin | 2% |
| Niacin | 4% |
| Calcium | * |
| Iron | 2% |

*Contains less than 2 per cent of the U.S. RDA of these nutrients

---

### Table 6.1   U.S. Recommended Daily Allowances (U.S. RDA)

| Vitamins, Minerals and Protein | Unit of Measurement | Infants | Adults and Children 4 or More Years of Age | Children Under 4 Years of Age | Pregnant or Lactating Women |
|---|---|---|---|---|---|
| Vitamin A | International Units | 1,500 | 5,000 | 2,500 | 8,000 |
| Vitamin D | International Units | 400 | 400[a] | 400 | 400 |
| Vitamin E | International Units | 5.0 | 30 | 10 | 30 |
| Vitamin C | Milligrams | 35 | 60 | 40 | 60 |
| Folic Acid | Milligrams | 0.1 | 0.4 | 0.2 | 0.8 |
| Thiamine | Milligrams | 0.5 | 1.5 | 0.7 | 1.7 |
| Riboflavin | Milligrams | 0.6 | 1.7 | 0.8 | 2.0 |
| Niacin | Milligrams | 8.0 | 20 | 9.0 | 20 |
| Vitamin $B_6$ | Milligrams | 0.4 | 2.0 | 0.7 | 2.5 |
| Vitamin $B_{12}$ | Micrograms | 2.0 | 6.0 | 3.0 | 8.0 |
| Biotin | Milligrams | 0.5 | 0.3 | 0.15 | 0.3 |
| Pantothenic Acid | Milligrams | 3.0 | 10 | 5.0 | 10 |
| Calcium | Grams | 0.6 | 1.0 | 0.8 | 1.3 |
| Phosphorus | Grams | 0.5 | 1.0 | 0.8 | 1.3 |
| Iodine | Micrograms | 45 | 150 | 70 | 150 |
| Iron | Milligrams | 15 | 18 | 10 | 18 |
| Magnesium | Milligrams | 70 | 400 | 200 | 450 |
| Copper | Milligrams | 0.6 | 2.0 | 1.0 | 2.0 |
| Zinc | Milligrams | 5.0 | 15 | 8.0 | 15 |
| Protein | Grams | 18[b] | 65[b] | 20[b] | 45 + [c] |

[a] Presence optional for adults and children 4 or more years of age in vitamin and mineral supplements.

[b] If protein efficiency ratio of protein is equal to or better than that of casein, U.S. RDA is 45 g. for adults, 18 g. for infants, and 20 g. for children under 4.

[c] The 1980 R.D.A. suggests an **additional** protein intake of 30 gm/day for pregnant women and 20 gm/day for lactating women.

Source: U.S. Department of Health and Human Services, Public Health Service, Food and Drug Administration

## Other descriptive terms relating to nutrition

**Imitation**   The negative connotation of this word has long annoyed food companies and others. Its use on a label implies that the product is inferior to that which it resembles, but it is not clear in what way it is inferior. Imitation vanilla, for instance, may have virtually undetectable differences from the pure extract. Imitation fruit drinks, on the other hand, may be substantially different from the pure juices they imitate (258). In partial redress of these discrepancies, FDA now requires that the word imitation be used on a label only if the product is nutritionally inferior to the food imitated. Establishing nutritional inferiority is contentious, to say the least.

Such a definition of imitation seemed sensible in the days when food technology and nutrition concepts were less sophisticated than they are today. Now, if you make a product and remove what may be considered to be negative components, like fat, one could argue that the resulting product is nutritionally superior, even though it is required to be called "imitation". Low fat margarine, which may have as much as 40 percent of the fat removed, is a case in point (274). Surimi based seafood products may be another example. With labeling, it is useful to know not only what the product is, but also what it is not. Study the label of a non-dairy creamer as an eye opener.

**Natural**  used in conjunction with meat or poultry, the term means "minimally processed and contains no artificial ingredients." Its use otherwise does not come under Federal regulation. The term is self defined but its use is not without peril: it means whatever the manufacturer or consumer thinks it means. Such kinds of ambiguity ultimately result in enormous confusion and often in backlash against the manufacturer. Even if your advertising agency tells you the word "natural" will help sell your product, avoid it unless you carefully define its use for the consumer. Even then, resisting the temptation is usually wise.

**Sugar-free, sugarless, no sugar**  may be used only if the food is labeled "low calorie" or "reduced calorie" (see above), or if it is accompanied each time it is used by the statement, "not a reduced calorie food," "not a low calorie food," "not for weight control," or "useful only in not promoting tooth decay."

**Dietetic, diet, artificially sweetened, sweetened with non-nutritive sweetener**  such terms may be used only if the food is labeled "low calorie" or "reduced calorie" or claims special dietary usefulness.

**Dietary supplement**  refers to a product to which has been added over 50 percent of the U.S. RDA of more than one nutrient.

## Other considerations of nutrition labeling

There are other aspects of nutrition labeling that seafood companies and others need to pursue if the conditions apply. For example, the labeling regulations for baby foods are covered separately and are not covered in this volume.

Foods for special dietary use, including those with nutrient supplements exceeding 50 percent of the U.S. RDA (e.g. fortified breakfast cereals), must conform to specific labeling requirements. There are regulations governing the labeling of saccharin and its salts, and the use of non-nutritive substances.

Health and nutrition claims are strictly regulated. For example, no claim may be made that a food is a significant source of a nutrient unless that nutrient is present in excess of 10 percent of the U.S. RDA in a serving. Likewise, no food may be described as nutritionally superior to another unless it contains at least 10 percent more of the U.S. RDA of the claimed nutrient (21).

Another area of key concern to food companies is the definition of compliance. Standards of compliance for nutrient content differ according to whether the nutrients are added (as in fortified or fabricated foods), or are naturally occurring. For products whose nutrients are not added during processing, compliance is generally $\pm 20$ percent of the amount stated on the label. Conditions under which nutrient content is determined are also specified (21).

## Nutrition labeling issues

As the reader will have guessed, nutrition labeling has not been enthusiastically embraced by everyone. Consumer advocates have supported its development and implementation, but have criticized its complexity and omissions. The food industry objected to the costs of nutrition analyses and new labels. Industry has also been critical of the fact that consumers appear to have poor understanding of the labels and appear not to read them. Other problems with nutrition labeling include:

- the use of the metric measures of weight which are difficult for many people to understand;

- the imperfections of the U.S. RDAs;

- implied or real health claims;

- the omission of useful information both on the label and in promotional literature;

- the lack of guidance as to whether or not a food is "nutritious;"

- incomplete information about dietary fat.

An excellent discussion of some of these issues is contained in *Understanding Nutrition* by Whitney and Hamilton (258).

In 1982, FDA published the results of a survey of nutrition labeling conducted among nutrition professionals, food industry representatives and consumers (275). The study reported the following major problems with nutrition labels: complexity of the information presented; desire for more or different information from that currently available; and desire for information about food constituents people wish to avoid, like sodium, calories and cholesterol. The authors recognized the priority of making the label clear and understandable.

In spite of the shortcomings of the present nutrition labels, surveys show that consumers want nutrition information, that they support nutrition labeling, that they view nutrition as an important aspect of the foods they buy and that indeed they do not understand some of the information on the label. There is also evidence that FDA and consumer advocates are working to improve the present system by improving the clarity of the labels and the way information is expressed (276).

There have also been demands to improve the labeling of certain foods, particularly processed meats, to divulge the fat content (277). So long as nutrition labeling remains a voluntary program, some manufacturers will choose not to disclose the nutrient composition of their products, in spite of consumer and government pressures to do so. This appears to be the case with some meat processors, especially since their products have been criticized for their dubious nutritional merit. Both fat and cholesterol content are of key concern in good health, and it may be expected that demands for more product information will continue.

## Nutrition labeling in the seafood industry

The seafood industry is not as advanced as the meat industry in terms of the kind and number of processed products available, but this situation is changing rapidly. The widespread acceptance of processed fish such as surimi heralds new developments. Fish sausage, the palate pleaser of the 1984 U.S. Olympic team, can be expected for consumers soon. With these and other products entering the marketplace, the demand for nutrition information will equal, if not exceed, that for meat products. In order for seafood to capitalize on its healthful image and maintain its nutritional advantages, products will have to be developed with superior nutrition in mind and will need to proclaim their virtues on their labels and accompanying literature. Nutrition labeling cannot be ignored by the leaders in the seafood business.

Nutrition labeling of fresh seafood shares the same dilemmas as those of the meat and produce industries. Because the composition of the product varies with many environmental factors beyond the control of the fisherman or producer such as season, maturity and handling, it is cumbersome and expensive to obtain reliable analytical data on a representative sample of a species. USDA, whose responsibilities include obtaining data on the composition of foods, has worked with both the meat and produce industries to obtain generic data for meats and selected produce items respectively. USDA is currently updating its handbook of nutrient composition for seafood.

Reliable generic data is critical for providing nutrition and health information about seafood. With such data, package labels can be developed, guidelines established for the evaluation of the nutritional quality of processed seafood products, and data interpreted in a way that consumers can understand and use. It will also serve as a benchmark against which future changes in product can be compared. This last will become increasingly important as aquaculture supplies a greater share of the market.

The availability and interpretation of sound data is the basis for consumer education about the merits of seafood. Data are required to combat false information, faddism and quackery, and misleading advertising claims. Sound data will buttress aggressive marketing strategies and distinguish innovative companies from the pack. In short, the seafood industry needs to support not only the concept of nutrition labeling but also the acquisition of generic data. The most recent and reliable data currently available about the major nutrients in seafood is presented in Chapter Nine.

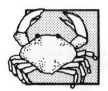

# Chapter Seven

# Seafood and Good Health

## Weight Control and Calories

One of the most popular promotions for fresh seafood is an appeal to the calorie conscious. Fish is low in calories because it has very little fat, for fat has more than twice the calories per ounce of either protein or carbohydrate. In fact, steaming lean fish fillets, like flounder, cod, pollock or sole provides a tasty entree with less than 1 percent fat. That is even less fat than broiled lean beef or roast chicken breast.

Most varieties of fish are lean. In general, the darker the color of the flesh, the higher the fat content. Table 2.3 (Chapter Two) shows the fat content of the most popular varieties of fish on a raw basis. Because most of the fat lies next to the skin, trimming the skin before eating will remove most of the fat.

Preparation and cooking can greatly influence the fat and calorie content of fish reaching the table. Both breading and the use of oil, butter or margarine add calories. What starts out as a weight watcher's delight may end up a caloric disaster. See what can happen to cod in Table 7.1.

Table 7.1 also illustrates the impact of fat on total calories in another way: the percent of calories from fat. Foods or meals considered low in fat and ideal for weight watchers will have less than 25 percent of their calories from fat. American diets, overall, have about 40 percent of their calories from fat which is too much. The current goal is to reduce this level to 30 percent. Some health professionals are striving for even lower levels like 20 percent (32).

While percent of total calories from fat is a quick way to gauge the caloric merit of a food or meal, this figure is usually not readily available. You have to calculate it. The way to do that is to multiply the amount of fat, usually given in grams, by 9 to convert it to calories. Then express this number, calories from fat, as a percentage of the total calories. Most consumers are not familiar with either the idea or the numbers associated with the concept of percentage of total calories from fat.

160

**Table 7.1   Differences in Calorie and Fat Content of Cod Prepared in Different Ways**

| Preparation | Calories | Fat/gm | percent Calories from Fat |
|---|---|---|---|
| Portion size: 100 gm (3½ oz) | | | |
| Cod, steamed | 97 | 0.8 | 1 |
| Cod in Spanish sauce | 97 | 1.4 | 13 |
| Cod fish sticks, raw | 132[a] | 0.4 | 3 |
| Cod, grilled with 2 tsp. butter[b] | 168 | 5.3 | 28 |
| Cod, batter fried | 172 | 7.5 | 39 |
| Cod fish sticks, fried | 193 | 7.7 | 36 |

Source: Sidwell (3)

[a] The additional calories come from the breading.

[b] Using 1 tsp. butter reduces the calorie content to about 133.

For example: Cod in Spanish Sauce has 1.4 grams of fat and 97 calories

1.4 x 9 = 12.6 calories from fat

$\frac{12.6}{97}$ x 100 percent = 12.99 or 13 percent calories from fat

The best ways to preserve the low calorie advantage of seafood:

• use cooking techniques which do not rely on batters, breading or large amounts of oil, butter or margarine;

• use very small amounts, like ½ to 1 teaspoon per serving, of oil, butter or margarine when in baking, broiling or stir-frying to enhance flavor and palatability while keeping the calorie level low;

• use vegetable sauces, as in the cod in Spanish sauce above, as another tasty way to escape calories.

Those most serious about keeping the fat out of their food will enjoy the flavor of fish steamed, poached in wine or bouillon, broiled, baked or barbecued or cooked by microwave. The use of herbs, citrus juices, wine, broth and vegetables can greatly enhance the variety and appeal of all seafood while keeping the calorie content low.

# Heart Disease, Fat and Cholesterol

Heart disease is America's leading cause of death. In most people, it is the result of processes which begin in youth and gradually undermine health. It is a complex disease with many factors working together for years to compromise heart and blood vessel function. Some aspects of heart disease we can do nothing about:age, sex and our genetic make-up. Others depend on us and the choices we make. These are: smoking, exercise habits, diet, stress, weight management and other health conditions like high blood pressure and diabetes. The current approach to heart disease prevention emphasizes the cultivation of "heart healthy habits" throughout life to discourage the build-up of fatty deposits in blood vessels, which eventually lead to heart attack and stroke. It is never too late to reduce one's "risk" of the disease.

People at risk of heart disease because of their family histories may require special interventions of medication and diet. These must be designed by a physician and dietitian. For most people, good diet is an important health promoting habit. There's no reason why it shouldn't be fun, easy and delicious as well. Using seafood is one of the ways to make healthful eating exciting and delicious.

There are at least five important aspects of diet which relate directly to heart health. These are: total fat content, type of fat, amount of cholesterol, sodium level and amount of fiber. The exact relationship of each of these factors to the development or exacerbation of heart disease is not clear and there is considerable debate over how much, if any, change should be recommended for the general public. The best approach is to offer sensible guidelines which have a scientific basis, are likely to be helpful and are known to be safe. Taken together with other healthful habits like not smoking, keeping a desirable body weight and getting regular, vigorous exercise, we can foster good health and less disease.

Seafood relates well to each of the diet-heart-health factors mentioned above.

**Total Fat Content**    Presently, about 40 percent of our daily food energy comes from fat. There are strong indications that lowering the total fat intake to 30 percent or less will reduce the risk of heart disease, and perhaps other diseases as well. Certainly, populations whose diets habitually have less than 40 percent of calories from fat also have lower rates of heart disease. Such people usually are different in other ways as well. But many health professionals are urging people to cut back on fat with the aim of curbing the usual American diet to 30 percent fat (31). For many people that means an intake of no more than 60-70 grams of fat per day – say 12-14 teaspoons or 4-5 tablespoons of fat daily.

Cutting back on fat means limiting the amount of fat-rich foods we eat and eating them less often. In their place we need to eat more fruits, vegetables and whole grains which have other nutritional advantages besides being low in fat. Eating lean fish, leaner meats and poultry also helps. The major sources of fat in the diet are oils, salad dressings and mayonnaise, butter and margarine, all fried foods, large servings of fat-rich meats, cheese and other dairy foods and fats used in baking and cooking. These are the foods to limit in order to reduce fat intake.

Seafood is inherently low in fat. There are relatively few varieties which are high in fat. (See Tables 9.1 and 9.2 and Chapter Two). Including fish in the diet regularly can substitute effectively for other, fattier foods. To be effective, however, it is most important to prepare and cook the fish adding as little fat as possible. Steaming, poaching, barbecuing, stir-frying, baking, broiling and microwave cooking are the best cooking methods to use for minimizing fat. By substituting low fat fish for richer meats and dairy foods on a regular basis, seafood will contribute positively and tastily to leaner living.

Another bonus from using lean seafood is that a low calorie serving still looks like an abundant portion on the plate. Keeping both eye and tummy appeal helps overcome the feeling that changing food habits means deprivation. Six ounces of many species can be scrumptiously prepared for just under 200 calories!

The advantages of lowering our intake of all types of fat, are:

- promotes lower blood lipid (fat) levels, thereby discouraging the accumulation of lipids in blood vessels;

- reduces the intake of saturated fat (animal fat);

- reduces cholesterol consumption, because foods high in fat are often (but not always) high in cholesterol too;

- promotes weight control by reducing calorie intake;

- favors the intake of more fruits, vegetables, cereals and grains which give us fiber, vitamins and minerals.


**Type of Fat**    Not all fats are created equal. They differ in the kinds of fatty acids they contain. Fatty acids are long chains of carbon atoms with hydrogen atoms attached to them. In some fatty acids, hydrogen atoms are missing, resulting in a "double bond" or "unsaturation". The more hydrogen atoms missing or double bonds there are, the more unsaturated is the fatty acid. Fats with unsaturated fatty acids are softer at room temperature than saturated fats, and many are liquid oils. Most vegetables, nuts and grains have substantial amounts of unsaturated fatty acids. Examples of unsaturated fats are corn and safflower oils. For a full explanation of fats and terms relating to fats, see Chapter Two.

Saturated fats do not contain any double bonds. They are firmer at room temperature than unsaturated fats. Animal fats, shortening and some hydrogenated margarines contain a high proportion of saturated fats. Some familiar examples are butter, cheese, lard and beef fat.

There are some important exceptions to the animal-vegetable rule of thumb for saturated and unsaturated fats. Avocados, coconut and palm oils (used widely in food processing and commercial frying), household and industrial shortening and some margarines are moderately high in saturated fatty acids (2).

Seafood is another important exception to the rule. Most seafood fats contain a substantial proportion of unsaturated fatty acids, making them oils. In addition, they contain a unique category of highly unsaturated fatty acids, called omega-3 fatty acids. The importance of fish oils is discussed below and in Chapter Two.

The type of fat we consume affects our blood lipid levels. The term lipid refers to substances that dissolve in organic solvents like nail polish remover and ether. The blood contains a variety of lipids including triglycerides or fat, lipoproteins and cholesterol. High blood lipid levels increase the risk of heart disease. Eating primarily saturated or animal fats tends to raise blood lipid levels, while including a good share of unsaturated fats, like those in vegetable and fish oils, tends to lower lipid levels.

As noted above, fish are exceptional animal foods in that, unlike meats and dairy foods, their fat contains a high proportion of polyunsaturated fatty acids. Moreover, many varieties of seafood have certain polyunsaturated fatty acids not found in most other foods. The molecules of the fatty acids, called "omega-3" fatty acids, are longer, and have more double bonds, five or six, than other vegetable and animal fats. Fish oils differ from animal fats and vegetable oils in the following ways:

- they have some fatty acids that are longer – 20 and 22 carbon atoms compared with 18 in vegetable oils;

- some fish oil fatty acids have more double bonds – five or six compared with the one or two for vegetable oils;

- the position of the double bonds is closer to the end of the molecule than it is in vegetable oils.

These omega-3 fatty acids are effective in lowering blood lipid levels, especially triglycerides. They may prove to be very helpful in reducing the risks of heart disease. Research into the metabolism of these fatty acids is currently very active and the outlook is most exciting and hopeful (see Chapter Two).

It is well to remind ourselves that no single food or food group determines overall health. The advantages of seafood can be erased by excessive consumption of fat from other sources, and by careless or lazy lifestyle habits. For example, the habitual smoker probably does more to undermine his health by smoking than he can ever gain in protection by wise eating.

**Cholesterol** Many studies have been conducted to determine the importance of dietary or food cholesterol in one's risk of heart disease. High blood cholesterol levels increase the risk of heart disease. In most people, eating substantial amounts of cholesterol contributes to high blood cholesterol levels. Furthermore, if you limit your intake of cholesterol, your blood cholesterol level will fall.

On the other hand, there are many factors besides dietary cholesterol which affect the level of cholesterol in the blood. Some which increase blood cholesterol are: high total fat consumption, high intake of saturated fat, obesity and lack of regular exercise. Eating foods rich in cholesterol along with substantial fat increases cholesterol uptake, while the presence of other sterols from plants or other sources decreases uptake (87). Blood cholesterol is lower among those consuming plenty of foods high in fiber (278). The situation is complex and generalizations tend to be overly simplistic.

How much cholesterol do seafoods have? Nearly all varieties of fish are relatively low in cholesterol, making them suitable for everyone. Some forms of seafood are moderately high in cholesterol and a few are very high. In some shellfish, there are plant sterols present as well, but very little is known about their uptake and metabolism. It is thought that the other sterols are not appreciably metabolized and that they reduce the uptake of cholesterol from seafood (87). Approximate amounts of cholesterol in seafood are shown in Table 2.7 and 2.8. in Chapter Two.

Most health professionals agree with the following suggestions to keep one's cholesterol level down:

---

**WAYS TO LOWER BLOOD CHOLESTEROL**

- eat no more than 300 milligrams of cholesterol each day;
- limit total fat and saturated (mostly animal) fat intake since these elevate blood cholesterol levels;
- achieve and maintain desirable body weight;
- have regular vigorous exercise;
- eat plenty of foods high in fiber: bran, whole grains, fruits and vegetables.

---

The effect of consuming diets high in seafood with cholesterol provided only from seafood is not what would be expected on the basis of similar feeding studies with other food sources of cholesterol. High levels of seafood cholesterol do not lead to an elevation in blood lipids or blood cholesterol (162) . However, in cholesterol sensitive individuals, blood lipids are increased. The reasons for these observations are not well understood and this is an active area of research. The metabolism of the omega-3 fatty acids in seafood is thought to be involved in the response to cholesterol in these studies, but it is not clear in what way. Furthermore, not all people respond to such diets in the same way. There is a great need for more data collected from larger numbers of subjects before we will understand what is happening. Further comments on this are contained in the section on omega-3 fatty acids in Chapter 2.

In summary, most forms of seafood are relatively low in cholesterol. Those with higher amounts do not lead to higher blood cholesterol levels in most people, in contrast to what would be expected. In addition, cholesterol-rich seafoods are seldom consumed in great enough quantity or sufficiently often to pose a serious risk for most people. The caution exists, however, for those individuals at high risk because of their particular blood lipid pattern.

**Sodium** The adverse effects of excessive sodium intake, which comes mainly from salt, are mediated primarily through an elevation in blood pressure. High blood pressure is a major risk factor for both heart disease and stroke and is discussed in the following section in this Chapter. The effects of sodium are also discussed in Chapter Two and sodium in processed seafood is covered in Chapter Three.

**Fiber**   Brief mention will be given to fiber, because it is related to heart health and many other clinical conditions. Its presence in the diet may also contribute to lower risk of breast and other cancers (32, 280). Dietary fiber is not found in seafood (except sea plants).

Dietary fiber is found only in plant foods: fruits, grains, vegetables, nuts and seeds. It consists of the undigestible portions of these foods and has several components. A simple definition of dietary fiber is the plant cell wall. It is that portion of plant materials that cannot be broken down by human digestion or be absorbed by human digestive enzymes. However, there are bacteria in the intestine that do break down most types of dietary fiber so that eventually energy is available to the body from the metabolism of dietary fiber (1, 281).

The components of dietary fiber are cellulose, hemicellulose, pectin, gums and lignin (1). Foods richest in dietary fiber are bran, whole grains, legumes, fruits, especially dried fruits, bran cereals, nuts and seeds.

Dietary fiber is exceedingly difficult to measure accurately because of the diversity of its components. It bears virtually no relationship to the amount of crude fiber listed in tables of food composition. Crude fiber values seriously underestimate the total dietary fiber in a food. Tables of dietary fiber content have been published (1, 282).

Fiber is relevant to the discussion of blood lipid levels and cholesterol metabolism because several feeding studies in people have shown that diets rich in certain types of dietary fiber lead to lower blood cholesterol levels (283-5). Not all kinds of fiber produce this effect, however (1). The most effective types of fiber are pectin, found mainly in fruit, and gum. Oat bran, unlike wheat or corn bran, also depresses blood cholesterol levels (284).

The typical American diet is low in dietary fiber. The National Cancer Institute and health professionals are urging everyone to consume more foods with fiber, or "roughage" as Grandma called it (32, 286). Unfortunately, seafood makes no contribution to this aspect of healthful eating. But seafood in combination with whole grains like brown rice, bulgur wheat, ground corn and whole grain bread, and vegetables like broccoli, celery, tomatoes, peas and many others, makes delicious heart-healthy fare.

## Summary:

Seafood is heart-healthy food from nearly every dietary perspective. Most varieties are low in fat, and when consumed regularly without the addition of extra fat, can help lower everyone's overall fat intake. Seafood species with more than 5 percent fat appear to be heart-healthy because of the beneficial effects of the omega-3 fatty acids they contain. Nearly all seafood is low in cholesterol and appropriate for people on both customary and low fat/low cholesterol diets. The oils in fish are rich in unsaturated fatty acids which tend to lower plasma lipids and cholesterol. The lower one's blood cholesterol, the lower the chance of heart disease. Diets rich in seafood or seafood oils do lower several blood lipids and affect other aspects of fatty acid metabolism, implying a uniquely beneficial effect of fish oils on heart health.

Fresh seafood also contributes to heart health because of its relatively low sodium content. Both marine and freshwater species are low in sodium (see Table 9.1). Most shellfish and crustaceans have more sodium than finfish, but their use seldom needs to be restricted because of this difference. Processed seafood, except for diet pack fish, is high in sodium and is a concern for people with high blood pressure. Package labels without nutrition labeling do not give the sodium content and may not indicate the presence of sodium containing additives. Where nutrition labels are present, however, sodium content must be declared.

And finally, some types of dietary fiber may be important in lowering blood cholesterol levels. Dietary fiber is found only in plants: fruits, vegetables, whole grains, nuts and seeds. Seafood contains no dietary fiber.

## High Blood Pressure and Sodium

Sodium is important because high intakes are associated with high blood pressure or hypertension. We know that high blood pressure greatly increases the risk of stroke and heart disease, yet it is one of the easiest conditions to control (287, 288). Because hypertension has few, if any, warning signs one needs regular blood pressure check-ups to detect it. Once discovered, it can be treated, usually with medication and diet. Maintaining desirable body weight also helps maintain normal blood pressure. Weight loss alone is frequently enough to bring high blood pressure under control (289, 290).

Likewise, reducing sodium intake can help many to control their blood pressure. Most of us consume anywhere from 2-7 grams or more of sodium each day, whereas the suggested intake is from 1-3 grams (7). Most of this sodium comes from salt added to foods, both in food processing and at the table. All of us would probably be better off if we tossed out the salt shaker.

Sodium and salt are not the same. Salt is composed of about 40 percent sodium; the rest is chlorine. If you want to convert an amount of salt to the equivalent amount of sodium or vice versa:

Weight of salt × 0.4 = Weight of sodium
Weight of sodium × 2.5 = Weight of salt

Most varieties of fish have about 60-100 mg sodium per 100 grams (3½ ounces) (3, 291). Most shellfish and crustaceans have more sodium, usually in the range of 200 – 400 mg per 3½ ounces (3, 291). Squid and scallops fall in between at about 160 mg (3, 291). These differences in sodium content among fresh seafoods are not a problem for healthy people trying to maintain a sensible intake of sodium. Only in severely restricted diets might certain varieties be limited. In fact, fresh seafood can be very important in building good food habits, in part because it has so little sodium.

Virtually all processed seafood has salt or other sodium containing ingredients added. Frozen fillets, and some fresh ones, may have sodium salts added if the fillets have been dipped in certain kinds of solutions prior to freezing. Information about the use of dip solutions is seldom on the retail label, although it is supposed to be (see Chapter Three for information on dips). Canned, smoked, dried and prepared fish products usually have large amounts of salt added and are very high in sodium. The exception is diet pack low sodium canned fish.

## Cancer and Diet

In 1982, the National Academy of Sciences issued a report called *Diet, Nutrition and Cancer*, in which it stated that "...most cancers [appear to] have external causes and, in principle, should be preventable" (292). The National Cancer Institute estimates that 35 percent of all cancer deaths may be related to the way we eat (293). Furthermore, the National Academy stated, "...by some estimates, as much as 90 percent of all cancer in humans has been attributed to various environmental factors, including diet. Other investigators have estimated that diet is responsible for 30-40 percent of cancers in men and 60 percent of cancers in women. Recently two epidemiologists suggested that a significant proportion of the deaths from cancer could be prevented by dietary means and that dietary modifications would have the greatest effect on the incidence of cancers of the stomach and large bowel and, to a lesser extent, on cancers of the breast, the endometrium, and the lung." (292).

The interrelationships between nutrition and cancer are in three major areas:

1. cause of cancer – specific nutrients as well as general food habits are implicated;

2. nutritional support of the cancer patient – many cancer patients are malnourished;

3. treatment of cancer – some cancers react specifically to individual nutrients; certain cancer treatments and drugs antagonize nutrients (294).

Three dietary components have especially strong associations with some types of cancer. These relationships are dietary fiber and colon cancer, dietary fat and colon cancer and dietary fat and breast cancer. Dietary fiber is discussed above, particularly as it relates to blood lipids and heart disease. Its relationship to breast cancer is superbly reviewed in reference (32).

High dietary fat intake has been implicated in the development of breast cancer in women. In Japan, women who consume on the average about 40-50 grams of fat per day, have only one fifth the incidence of breast cancer as women in America who consume, on average, three times as much fat (145 grams) per day (32). Studies among Seventh Day Adventist women confirm the association between high fat intake and risk of breast cancer (32). The sensible thing to do: eat less fat.

Laboratory studies on the development of mammary tumors in animals and work on tissues taken from breast cancer patients have suggested another association between dietary fat and breast cancer. It appears that certain types of fat, those in fish oil, may actually be helpful in preventing breast cancer. The

Information about diet and preventing cancer can be obtained from:

National Cancer Institute
Building 31,
Bethesda, MD 20205

Ask for: *Diet, Nutrition and Cancer Prevention.*

American Cancer Society
4 West 35th Street
New York, NY 10001. Phone 212/736-3030

Ask for: *Nutrition, Common Sense and Cancer.*
*Unproven Methods of Cancer Management.*
*Nutrition and Cancer: Cause and Prevention*

American Institute for Cancer Research
P.O. Box 76216
Washington, D.C., 20013

Ask for: *Planning Meals that Lower Cancer Risk:*
*A Reference Guide*

or call the Cancer Information Service:
1 - 800 - 4 - CANCER
in Alaska call: 1-800-638-6070
in Washington, D.C. call: 202-636-5700
in Hawaii, Oahu call: 808-524-1234

omega-3 fatty acids of fish oil appear to reduce the formation of certain prostaglandins – hormone-like substances produced mainly by platelets – and breast tumor cells. This reduction in prostaglandin synthesis appears to diminish tumor growth in laboratory animals and possibly discourage the development of tumors themselves (295). It is unknown to what extent, if any, fish oil consumption among women might be protective against breast cancer. The possibility is enticing.

The government acknowledges that we do not have all the information and answers we need to fully understand the causes, effective treatments and prevention strategies for various cancers, but it feels that sufficient evidence exists for offering advice on how we might lower our risk of cancer. The advice given is also consistent with recommendations for reducing the risk of heart disease and for building an all around, healthful diet. To summarize:

The National Academy of Sciences recommends that we:

1. Reduce our intake of fat, both saturated and unsaturated, from

the current average of about 40 percent of total calories, to 30 percent of total calories;

2. Increase our consumption of fruits, vegetables and whole grain cereals;

3. Minimize our consumption of salt-cured, smoked or charcoal-broiled foods;

4. Drink alcoholic beverages only in moderation.

Seafood relates to two of the four dietary guidelines above, numbers 1 and 3. Because most seafood is very low in fat, regular consumption of seafood is an effective and nutritious substitute for fattier meats and dairy foods. The few varieties which are relatively rich in fat can be substituted by many lean alternatives. The fatty varieties have the omega-3 fatty acid advantage, however, and appear to be an excellent substitute for other sources of fat in meals, like fatty meats, cheese and vegetable oils. Fish canned in water, vegetable sauce or broth is readily available for convenience uses, so that oil-packed fish has acceptable alternatives. Note that oil-packed fish is normally packed in vegetable oil, not fish oil, so the oil does not have the omega-3 advantage, although the fat in the fish itself does.

The third recommendation concerning salt-cured, smoked or charcoal broiled foods pertains to seafood, especially dried salted fish, smoked fish, charcoal and mesquite broiling and "blackened" fish preparations served in restaurants.

The salting of fish has a long tradition over many centuries as a staple over the winter and in long ocean voyages. Canadian and New England salt cod are available today and native Indian and Eskimo communities still use this method of food preservation. From a nutritional point of view, however, salting is discouraged because of the large amount of salt remaining after soaking and cooking. Excessive salt consumption results in excessive sodium intake with consequences linked to high blood pressure. Charcoal broiled and "blackened" fish may contain carcinogenic compounds produced by the "overheating" effect on the surface of the food.

Smoked fish contains other substances besides salt and whatever additives are used to prepare and flavor the product. Volatile substances in wood smoke are taken up by the fish. Some of these compounds, whether derived from the smoke or subsequently formed in the fish, may be harmful. The many different smoking methods and woods used and the great variation in final products make it difficult to obtain consistent data. Nevertheless, there has been sufficient concern about the carcinogenicity of substances found in smoked foods to warrant caution (235). This topic is discussed in more detail in Chapter Three.

# Allergies and Sensitivity to Seafood

The word allergy is a familiar term used popularly to refer to a variety of unpleasant effects in some people following exposure to certain substances. Many people claim allergies to foods, chemicals, pollen etc. The term has a precise meaning in medicine but a generally vague meaning outside science. Abuse and exploitation of the term has fostered the notion that food allergy is a common cause of illness. In fact, genuine food sensitivity reactions are relatively uncommon in adults and are caused by only a few foods, primarily milk, eggs, nuts and wheat (296). Allergies are more common in children than adults. Sensitivity to a variety of seafoods is well documented but is not widely prevalent.

In an effort to reduce the confusion about food sensitivity, the American Academy of Allergy and Immunology established definitions distinguishing among different kinds of adverse reactions to foods. A food allergy is defined as an "immunologic reaction resulting from the ingestion of a food or food additive" (297). The critical part of this definition is the term "immunologic," as this specifies the nature of the adverse reaction to a food. Immunologic means that antibodies, the body's defense proteins, are produced in response to an allergen or "provoking substance." Other adverse reactions to foods may involve biochemical or psychological responses. A food allergy, then, provokes an immunologic response.

The most common signs of food allergy involve the gastrointestinal tract or skin and occasionally the respiratory tract. Nausea, vomiting, hives, eczema, asthma and rhinitis are the most frequent symptoms (298). The basis for the symptoms is the reaction between a food protein and antibodies, which are specialized proteins produced by certain cells in response to the antigen. Reactions in highly sensitive individuals may be severe, even life-threatening. In most people, however, food allergies are unpleasant, not calamitous.

Allergic reactions to food usually involve the production of immunoglobulin E (IgE) which binds to certain cells called mast cells found in tissues and occasionally in the blood stream. Ingestion of the offending food or antigen causes the antigen to bind to IgE, a process that triggers chemical reactions in the mast cells leading to clinical symptoms (299, 300).

Sensitive individuals may react similarly to foods of different groups or to several foods within the same general group. For example, a person sensitive to shrimp may also be sensitive to other crustaceans like lobster; others may be sensitive only to shrimp. It is by trial and error that the sensitive individual determines these cross-reactions to different food proteins.

Allergenic foods may contain more than one allergen. Persons sensitive to a particular food may react to any or all allergens present in a food. For example, the major allergen in cod is a protein named allergen M. Cod also contains a minor allergen to which some people are sensitive (103).

Diagnosis of food allergy is a complicated process beginning with a thorough evaluation of a subject's historical experiences with various foods and clinical examination. Patient history is not enough, however, to confirm a diagnosis of food allergy and a variety of biochemical tests and food challenges may be required. The most commonly used diagnostic tests are skin testing, elimination diets, food challenges, and special tests for IgE (300).

Food allergy diagnosis is a popular arena for quackery and many worthless tests may be performed. People with serious concerns about food allergy should seek help from competent allergists and immunologists and avoid practitioners who use "cytotoxic" tests and food testing with "food drops" (298, 300).

The basis for treating food allergies is avoidance of foods containing the offending antigen. This treatment requires a knowledge of food composition and identification of the most likely sources of the problem food. When only one or two foods are involved, avoidance may be relatively simple. If the allergen is widespread and not always obvious in foods, as is the case with wheat proteins, avoidance diets may be difficult to devise. Pharmacologic agents, most commonly antihistamines, are useful in treating the symptoms after exposure to the antigen, but not in preventing the reaction.

Allergy to fish is classic in the history of food allergy. The problem is not common on a worldwide scale, but frequently occurs in fish-processing and fish-eating communities (302). Studies on codfish antigen have served as a model for understanding allergic reactions and the major allergen from cod has been isolated and purified (303-305). The major allergen in shrimp has also been identified (306). Allergens in fish are highly resistant to destruction. They are stable to heat, acid and enzymic destruction. That explains why raw, cooked, canned and other processed forms of seafood are still allergenic. Their exquisite ability to survive a variety of assaults is demonstrated by the fact that a sensitive breastfed infant can develop allergic symptoms after the mother has consumed fish. In order for a reaction to occur, the antigen has to resist cooking, passage through the mother's digestive system with its strong acid, protein degrading enzymes and bile, and then pass through several cellular membranes to reach the mammary glands. Furthermore, the antigen then has to resist the infant's digestive system and passage through additional membranes with their potential denaturing processes. In spite of all these opportunities for destruction, the codfish allergen has produced allergic symptoms in a sensitive infant each time the mother ate fish before nursing (302).

Most food allergies result from eating the problem food, but inhalation and contact can also produce symptoms. For example, the inhalation of steam from cooking fish or dust from dried fish material, including fish glue, can provoke allergic asthma in sensitive people (302, 307). Contact dermatitis (skin rash) has also been reported among fish processors (308).

Some allergens in food can be destroyed by processing, but others are remarkably resistant to destruction. For example, one of the minor shrimp allergens is destroyed by heat while the major one is heat stable (309). Allergen M in cod is quite resistant to heat, digestion and other denaturation procedures (305).

## Issues for the Seafood Industry

Sensitivity to seafood is well known but may be exaggerated and is frequently misdiagnosed. Educational materials pointing out the fact that true food allergies among adults are relatively uncommon may be helpful to consumers. It does not hurt to mention that some health care practitioners often diagnose food allergies inappropriately and that people who suspect sensitivity to seafood should have their misgivings verified by qualified medical allergists using several means of diagnosis.

Seafood processors need to be aware of the potential for allergic reactions among seafood handlers. There is a need to know the tolerance of individuals suspected of seafood allergies and the means of exposure. Industry should also insist upon reliable medical diagnosis of the sensitivity among seafood workers claiming allergies.

Food products containing seafood materials or derivatives require accurate labels describing all the sources of the ingredients. Processed seafood products made from a variety of ingredients including small amounts of different seafoods, other foods like soy protein, wheat starch and additives need explicit ingredient labels. Such statements as "may contain" one or other ingredients is a warning to sensitive consumers to avoid the product because the actual ingredients are equivocal.

Products containing fish oils and not fish proteins would not be expected to elicit allergic reactions in otherwise sensitive persons. Thus, the source and/or nature of the seafood ingredient is an important part of the ingredient description.

The ingredients statements on seafood items need to be explicit not only in regard to the fish proteins present, but also about the presence of other potentially allergenic substances like sulfite.

Explicit food labels are perhaps the best way to alert sensitive individuals to the presence of substances potentially hazardous to them. Successful food labeling also discourages the enactment of regulations forcing the elimination of certain substances from foods which are well tolerated by the vast majority of people (107). The recent experience with sulfites in shrimp and certain produce items, in which several people died, has led to FDA review of labeling requirements for sulfite and a renewed debate of regulation versus labeling (311, 312).

Ways of rendering seafood proteins non-allergenic offer the possibility of making seafoods available to sensitive people. This could be important in the development of processed seafood products. For example, would the extraction of various seafood proteins from fish, as in the manufacture of surimi, render them non-allergenic? With the present procedures used to make surimi one would not expect changes in the protein allergens. But who knows the type of processing and product developments on the horizon?

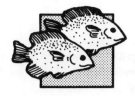

# Chapter Eight

# Marketing Seafood – the Nutrition Connection

Nutrition is an aspect of quality that can distinguish a product from its competitors. This is true for both processed and fresh products. As consumer concerns about health and fitness continue to increase, the awareness of a wholesome and nutritious diet increases also. Suppliers who know the nutritional advantages of their wares and can explain and promote these advantages are well positioned to expand their markets and strengthen their competitive position. Sodium is a good example. Most fish is naturally low in sodium. Prepared seafood products that limit the amounts of sodium-containing ingredients so that the final product has less than 140 mg sodium will still qualify to be called "low sodium." This property is a useful marketing tool to both the institutional and consumer markets.

The image of wholesomeness, good nutrition, health maintenance, heart health, updated nutrition concepts, wellbeing, modern lifestyles and other aspects of health can be integrated into the entire presentation of a product and a company. In seafood, as in some other food categories where many products are sold without brand identification, there is little generic promotion of the benefits of consuming seafood. Despite some small industry-wide or regional promotional campaigns, consumers are largely left to find out for themselves the advantages of eating seafood. This leaves room for retailers and restaurants, wholesalers, processors and others to develop awareness and information programs about seafood.

Consideration of the nutritional qualities of seafood products is appropriate to nearly all aspects of the seafood industry. Nutrition is, or should be, an important aspect of product development, especially concerning ingredients such as sodium, fat, sugar, carbohydrates and breading formulae. It is relevant to retailers as part of their promotional activities and to their interactions with consumers. Nutrition can also be important to wholesalers and distributors who service institutional and restaurant clients. Part of the impetus for writing this book is that consumer and industry awareness of nutrition is rapidly growing. This Chapter suggests some of the ways in which the seafood industry and its distributors can utilize the advantages of seafood's nutritional superiority to many other competing foods.

## Goals: What Are We Trying to Accomplish?

Whether or not an industry has any organized marketing program, there are often aspects of longer-term needs and objectives that are common to most of the members of that industry. These broad goals usually take months or years to achieve. Taking a look at the broad goals of the industry is a way of aiming the direction of an individual organization. Is the industry moving in a specific direction? Is that direction clear? Are a company's goals consistent with the direction of the industry or at odds with it? Is the company where it wants to be in terms of market share, type of products, product mix and base for expansion? The overall goals determine the paths a company takes either deliberately or by default.

It can be agreed that the general aim of the seafood business is to increase the consumption of fish, while the purpose of a particular seafood company is to increase the demand for its specific products. Defining the overall goals of the industry, as well as the particular aims of the company, can help in devising successful marketing strategies.

Increasing seafood consumption in total means getting more people to eat some seafood and encouraging those who do eat seafood to choose it more often. Normally, both strategies are needed. However, the separation of these issues is important in marketing because what you say to people who do not regularly consume seafood is sometimes quite different from what you say to those who are already familiar with using seafood. Goals need to be defined specifically in order to develop clear marketing plans and realistic expectations for both groups of the target market.

Fitting individual marketing programs to overall industry goals and programs is important. Let us assume that the overall goals of the seafood business are to:

1. *Increase the consumption of seafood and seafood products by a certain number of ounces per person per year.* Probably everyone would agree with this first goal, but each might have his own idea of how large the increase ought to or can be. The target should be set at a realistic level. The target groups must first be defined. They include consumers, food service managers, retailers, restaurant owners and anyone who plays a part in determining what people eat, whether in a restaurant or at home. The target group description will partly determine the approaches used to increase consumption. Marketing strategies are then designed to reach these people.

    Market research is needed to provide data against which changes can be assessed. Otherwise, you cannot know, even if there are changes in seafood consumption, whether or not your efforts had anything to do with the changes. Investing in well designed evaluation research can prevent you from wasting resources on marketing schemes which are not effective.

2. *Increase the proportion of people who enjoy eating seafood.* This second goal is clearly targeted toward consumers. Achieving it depends on knowing how consumers currently feel about seafood, where their reluctance is and what

problems exist as a barrier to enjoying seafood. Measuring changes in attitude is usually done by comparing the attitudes of people before and after marketing efforts, with appropriate control measurements of a similar group of consumers not exposed to the efforts.

   An analysis of seafood consumption during the same period indicates whether or not there is an association between attitude changes (if any) and seafood consumption. Such data do not allow conclusions to be drawn about marketing efforts causing changes in seafood consumption, but they can indicate whether or not your marketing efforts influence people's attitudes and whether your efforts are going in the desired direction.

3. *Increase consumer satisfaction with seafood products.* Improving consumer satisfaction is another goal targeted to consumers. Marketing efforts will be tailored to overcome existing consumer problems, suggest appropriate expectations, provide reliable advice, change the market supply or quality and so on. Happier customers come back for more and tell others about their good experiences. Such a goal requires working closely with retailers and food service users.

4. *Increase the availability of seafood products.* If the goal is to increase product availability, then data about the kinds and forms of products currently distributed in different market areas are needed. The target group is retailers and restaurants in the market areas of interest. Inquiries need to be made about what has been tried and how it fared and about the limitations of providing additional products and services. While it sounds basic, the answers are often surprising. Frequently, competitors have not done their homework. Your marketing strategies, superior services and expertise in working with retailers can influence the kind, quantity and quality of product available.

5. *Increase people's knowledge about the health advantages of seafood.* This may require working with a variety of groups. Getting retailers to provide point-of-purchase materials about seafood nutrition is one approach. Working with food editors and the press to feature seafood and its nutritional merits on a regular basis is another. Incorporating nutrition information as part of seafood packaging, recipes and point-of-purchase signs are ways to increase people's exposure to nutrition information. Sponsoring health professionals to talk about seafood nutrition on TV and radio shows is another means of reaching and educating consumers. Increasing knowledge usually requires sustained efforts, rather than "one shot" deals, and the time span to accomplish the changes is months or years rather than weeks.

6. *Increase the proportion of people who feel comfortable preparing seafood at home by $x\%$.* This last goal is also directed at consumers. As with some of the other goals, consumers may be reached through retailers, the media and advertising. The goal implies a need to raise consumer confidence, improve knowledge of cooking methods, provide reliable recipes and advice and target messages appropriately.

   Because many people lack confidence in their culinary skills with seafood, promoting reliable, easy and tasty fish preparation techniques can improve the cook's success and generate greater interest in seafood. Teach everyone not to overcook fish. Base your cooking advice on the Canadian cooking rule (see page 193).

Simple, seasoned recipes emphasizing the ease of baking, broiling or microwaving are effective. Suggesting a variety of flavor accompaniments besides the familiar lemon juice is helpful. Taste samples are always successful, though they may be expensive. Building a sustained program of weekly fish preparation features with basic recipes and cooking methods will demonstrate your commitment to the consumer and share your expertise. Restaurants can similarly use samples, specials and even cooking classes to strengthen goodwill and improve business.

## The Time Is Right

More people than ever before are expressing interest in nutrition. For example, the 1984 Food Marketing Institute survey of a national sample of supermarket shoppers reported that 63 percent of respondents were very concerned about the nutritional content of what they ate (313). A total of 95 percent were either very or somewhat concerned. Surveys such as this indicate a strong consumer awareness of and interest in nutrition. Awareness and interest, however, do not always translate directly into selection of healthful foods. Marketing efforts need to develop the connections between consumer interest in nutrition and appropriate food selections.

People are seeking nutrition information to help them follow medical advice for the control of diabetes, high blood pressure, heart disease, body weight and other health conditions. They need more information about how much of certain nutrients like sodium are in foods so that they can control their sodium intake. They need information about the amount and kind of fat present. They can profit from calorie comparisons showing how advantageous seafood is compared with its more popular alternatives. Hence the need for good seafood nutrition labels and point-of-purchase information. But people also need simple, useful guidance about which foods will help them achieve a sound diet without unduly contributing to the health problems they are trying to avoid. Advice about balance and moderation in eating needs continual explanation and repetition.

## Dietary Advice Favors Seafood

Emphasizing the many ways seafood fits in with modern concepts of healthful eating can help meet consumer needs while at the same time increasing interest in using seafood regularly.

The government has become more active in encouraging people to adopt food habits which are more health-promoting. Publication of the Dietary Guidelines for Americans provides a general framework of dietary advice appropriate to virtually everyone (29). Mandatory inclusion of sodium as part of nutrition labeling along with strong encouragement of food manufacturers to use less sodium and salt in foods was designed to help everyone consume less sodium. It should also make it easier for those with high blood pressure to limit their intake of sodium rich foods. Unprocessed seafood's low sodium content fits well with these aims.

The National Cancer Institute (NCI) is promoting food habits designed to discourage the development of some forms of cancer known to be associated with diet (286). Their recommendations are also consistent with the Dietary Guidelines. Promoting seafood consumption, especially because of its low fat content, goes along with the suggestions from NCI too.

Other health organizations like the American Heart Association have been disseminating dietary advice for years. People with heart disease are told to attain desirable body weight, eat less fat and cholesterol, throw out the salt shaker and try to eat polyunsaturated fats instead of saturated ones. Promoting seafood consumption is entirely consistent with all these recommendations because seafood is very low in fat (unless it is deep fried), it has a preponderance of unsaturated fatty acids and most forms are very low in cholesterol and sodium. The latest work on omega-3 (or n-3) fatty acids, covered extensively in Chapter Two, also indicates the strong health benefits of eating seafoods. Seafood is heart healthy food. (See Chapter Seven).

Private groups such as food companies, weight control programs, supermarkets, insurance companies, hospital out-patient clinics and public health departments have conducted nutrition information programs. Their efforts have kept nutrition in front of the public. Yet, in spite of all this work, there is widespread confusion about nutrition and health. Interest in nutrition does not readily translate into knowledge or understanding of basic nutrition principles (314). Given a situation of good intentions but little understanding, a consumer will not be able to distinguish between a false claim, a misleading one and a truthful one, much less detect the errors of omission common to food and health claims. To be useful, information about seafood and health needs to be practical and relevant. To be credible, the presentations must avoid the trappings of faddism or stark commercialism.

## Seafood Fits Today's Lifestyles and Demographics

Seafood fits into today's fast-paced lifestyles too. It is easy and quick to prepare and lends itself to both casual and elegant dining. All forms, whether fresh, frozen or processed are convenient to use and adaptable to any mealtime situation. Promoting seafood as a sensible part of the way people live, offering convenience without loss of nutritive value, is consistent with the needs of most people.

The changing demographic profile of American society has created needs for different kinds, sizes and styles of food. An increasing number of households are headed by one adult. This means that single serving portions are important, especially among the elderly. Multiple single servings in a pack, information on ways of storing and using leftovers as well as guidance on quick ways to prepare seafood are food product needs of the eighties.

Households which devote little time to food preparation need prepared food products that are tasty, easy and fast to heat and eat and make important contributions to nutritional needs. This is critical for single parent households and families where youngsters have a large part of the responsibility for obtaining their own meals. Seafood based products, main dishes and meals can readily be devised to meet these needs.

There is sufficient diversity in seafood to make it a possible choice for all income groups. Both fresh and processed forms are high in nutritional value. Many less familiar species of fish are reasonably priced and offer the same qualities of freshness, flavor and nutrition as more expensive forms. Seafood can also be less costly than red meat, processed meat products and sometimes poultry. Quality frozen fish is often attractively priced and is certainly competitive with its menu alternatives. Microwave ovens are increasingly common in home kitchens making it possible to serve well-prepared seafood in a minimum amount of time. Prepared accompaniments make recipe and serving design simple. Seafood offers greater variety of flavor, form and economy than almost any other menu mainstay.

## Using Nutrition in Seafood Promotion

Nutrition is a concern to most people, but is not the primary or even secondary reason for selecting specific foods. Healthy people take complete freedom of food choice for granted and develop food habits with little regard for the health consequences. When health declines, however, or a catastrophic event like a heart attack occurs, many people become motivated to examine and change their dietary ways.

Changes over recent years in overall food consumption patterns offer some basis for cautious optimism that people are not wholly irrational about their food choices. The popularity of margarine not only for reasons of price but of health is an example. The growing consumption of poultry at the expense of red meats is another. Price is a factor in these trends, but health reasons also guide consumers. The strong market for bran-containing cereals is another example of health considerations influencing food choices on a large scale. The popularity of low fat dairy products, the proliferation of low sodium products and the success of juice-packed fruits over their syrupy counterparts are other examples of health concerns affecting the food marketplace. Another related example of changes in behavior because of health concerns is the decline in smoking among men, in spite of heavy advertising pressures. People can and will change their ways if the inducements are sufficiently important and convincing.

A key question for seafood marketers is whether or not there is a sufficiently strong health benefit associated with seafood consumption to influence its purchase by a large proportion of consumers. The answer is yes. The research evidence is highly indicative of a protective effect from seafoods, especially fatty seafoods, against the risk of heart disease. Both fish and shellfish contain a unique class of highly unsaturated fatty acids called omega-3 fatty acids. These appear to affect blood lipids, platelet metabolism and perhaps other tissues in ways which are consistent with lower chances of heart disease. The omega-3 (or n-3) fatty acids are covered in Chapter Two and their health implications in Chapter Seven.

Studies among Greenland Eskimos, who consume large amounts of seafood and who are virtually free of heart disease, in spite of their high fat intake, have been interpreted to indicate a protective effect attributable to their large intake of marine animals (51). A 20 year epidemiological study in the Netherlands also reported lower mortality rates from heart disease among people who regularly consumed fish than among those who did not. We do not yet know how much fish is needed nor how often one must consume seafood in order to benefit from it, nor even whether everyone's health would be similarly improved. However, the evidence strongly indicates that regular consumption of fish, especially the fattier varieties, gives substantial health advantages.

Should people become convinced that eating fish more often will help them, the seafood industry can anticipate an unprecedented demand for its products. The trade press, some health professionals and others are encouraging the development of this demand. Certainly, greater consumption of seafood is unlikely to be harmful, although it is much less certain whether a single food category can deliver the immense promise expected of it. The outcomes people expect are very long term and this writer is sceptical whether large numbers of people would alter their food habits on a sustained basis solely for health reasons without also developing a fondness for seafood. Inspiring people to acquire a preference for seafood also requires that they learn how to handle and prepare it successfully.

It is in our nature to seek quick solutions to complex problems and a "simple" alternative presents itself in the form of fish oil capsules. Why bother eating seafood if a capsule will do the same thing? Fish oil supplements are already in the marketplace and seafood merchants can expect vigorous competition from those marketing supplements. It is more difficult to market good nutrition but the industry will have to meet the challenge. Quality product and a marketing approach that addresses consumer needs and concerns will be indispensable. Although the omega-3 work is enormously encouraging for anyone who sells seafood products, unless the overall benefits of seafood consumption are properly sold, the opportunity could be missed and the rewards go instead to makers and sellers of fish oil capsules. The rest of this Chapter provides outlines and ideas for marketing seafood and using the nutritional benefits discussed throughout this book in a positive way as promotional tools and advantages.

## Know your products

Find out everything about the handling, processing and distribution of your products so that you can assure your customers of top quality and so that you know what is in your merchandise:

• are dips used? under what conditions?

• what substances remain in the product as a result?

- what ingredients are added during processing or preparation?

- what is the proportion of fish in the final product?

- what is the final yield of your product?

- what is the cooked yield?

- how has processing affected nutrient composition?

- how much sodium, fat or other substances have been added?

- know how your product is best used. Is that the way your customers are using it?

- do you have other products better suited to their circumstances or needs?

- are there other uses for your products that your customers have not tried?

- is your product being served within the recommended freshness period?

- do you provide open dating or a "best if used by" date?

- how is your product different from the competition?

- how can you make it superior to those of your competitors?

- what additional value can you offer that currently is not available, such as portion controlled sizes, calorie-adjusted servings, product with maximum sodium content guaranteed, source and amount of fat guaranteed or different delivery schedules?

## Know Your Customers

- find out what his needs are.

- does what he currently buys suit him best, or do you have other products more suitable?

- could he better use your products in a different way?

- what other items or preparations are appropriate to his operation?

- can you provide information, such as nutrition labeling or health awareness, to help increase sales of your products?

- what problems or concerns do your customers have?

- do they have any problems with deliveries, handling and storage, preparation, consumer acceptance, quality?

- what is on your customers' wish list? Can you fulfil those wishes?

- how can you enhance the results your client has with your product?

- build on client concerns to improve your product line or quality.

- what new directions are your customers exploring? Your users are one of the best sources of ideas for developing new products, improving old lines and identifying new customers. If they are developing new serving styles, new recipes, different flavor combinations or preparation techniques, are your products the best for these uses?

- can you work with your customers to facilitate new developments and expand his product requirements? For example, if stir-fried fish is a new menu item, can you provide the most suitable firm fleshed species for his needs, or is your client going elsewhere for such items?

- conversely, are you promoting a variety of menu or preparation suggestions for your firm fleshed fish?

- consider your client's equipment and facilities. Is he trying to do the impossible with what he has?

- is he making the best choices for the options he has? If you do not think so, have you made appropriate suggestions? Working with him might improve his operation and the way he handles your product and ultimately determine how pleased he is with your service.

## Encourage Trial of Your Products

**Expand the range of products your customers use**    If your client regularly selects one or a few items and not others, find out why the others are not used. Offer incentives to encourage trials and follow up on the results whenever possible. Be sure the client has the information he needs to handle and serve your products properly. That means you must give him the ideas and information he needs and not send him elsewhere. For example, many consumers and restaurants will not try whole or dressed fish because they do not know what to do with it. Tell them how to handle, cook and serve it with suggestions you know are trustworthy. Another way to encourage trial is to offer information comparing the nutrition, preparation and serving advantages with alternate items.

**Expand the number of people trying your products**    If people are unfamiliar with your product, give them plenty of introductory offers: taste samples, price features, recipe and cooking suggestions and comparisons with related items. People may be attracted to an unfamiliar item if it offers convenience and nutrition advantages that were not readily apparent until you pointed them out. Encourage people to see themselves as users of the product through appeals to their needs for healthful foods, the speed and ease of product preparation and, most of all, their enjoyment of its taste.

## Make Seafood the Center of Attraction

In retailing, make the seafood counter boldly attractive, visually appealing and quality assuring. Be sure the staff are friendly and outgoing, willing to talk to shoppers and offer advice freely, even if the advice is unsolicited. Of course, ensure that the seafood staff are knowledgeable and enthusiastic about seafood themselves and be sure they have the back up materials to assist consumers. That means point of purchase displays, take home brochures, recipes, nutrition labels, and open dating. Encourage people to have a fish dish at least once a week. Encourage them to try a different species each week and tell them how many weeks it would take them to try all the varieties you have to offer!

## Have a seafood feature every week.

Retailers can generate traffic in the seafood area by having seafood demonstrations, speakers, manager's specials, raffles, cooking and tasting features (there's nothing like an aroma to attract or a freebie to appeal). When the seafood area becomes established as a center of attraction and innovation in a store, it can be the focus of considerable business and profit.

In the foodservice market, much can be done to increase the frequency with which seafood is served. Part of doing so involves expanding the menu items. The following suggestions may serve as a basis for encouraging expanded use of seafoods:

**Breakfast:**

| | |
|---|---|
| omelettes | seafood/potato combinations |
| hot/cold smoked fish | smoked salmon/seafood and bagels |
| seafood in sauce | seafood pancakes, crepes, seafood hash |

**Lunch/Dinner:**

Soups: chowders, bisques, cioppino, bouillabaisse, creole, curry, oriental

| Lighter Fare: | |
|---|---|
| quiche | ramekins |
| souffle | sandwiches, pockets, open-face |
| mousse | pizza |
| quenelles, terrines, pate | omelette |

Salads:
combinations with grains, pasta
molded
marinated
combinations with vegetables – leafy, cooked, raw, marinated "hot"
salads

Hors d'oeuvres: dips, spreads, canapes, cocktail cups, bouchees, pastries, turnovers, kebabs, fritters, terrines, pate, rolls, marinated, smoked

Entrees:
baked, broiled, grilled, stir-fried, steamed, poached
casseroles, seafood combinations as in paella, seafood fettucine
tempura
fondue oriental, using fish stock or court-bouillon instead of oil
kebabs
sausages
crepes

## Provide Information About Seafood Nutrition

Nutrition information can be communicated in a variety of ways. The more ways you use, the greater awareness you will create, and the better the chance there is that consumers will learn the nutritional advantages of using seafood often. Some ways to provide nutrition information:

## Nutrition labels

Generic information about the nutrient composition of seafood is presented in Chapter Nine. We do not have as extensive or reliable information about the nutrient composition of seafood as we would like, but for the major nutrients, we have a credible basis for making general statements. The basis for devising nutrition labels is the U.S. RDA. Nutrients are expressed in terms of absolute amounts per serving and as a percentage of the U.S. RDA. Full details of nutrition labeling are given in Chapter Six.

As a minimum, nutrition labels must declare the number of calories and the amounts of fat, protein, carbohydrate, and sodium per serving, as well as the percent of the U.S. RDA of vitamins A and C, thiamin, riboflavin, niacin, iron and calcium. Information on cholesterol and other nutrients is optional. Where the nutrient data base is inadequate or the methodology unreliable, it is not advisable to make quantitative statements about nutrient content.

An important issue with nutrition labels is whether to give data for cooked or raw seafood. Most analyses are conducted on raw seafood but most seafood is consumed cooked. Data on raw edible portion can be converted to cooked values by making assumptions about cooking methods and losses and performing the appropriate calculations. This makes the data more useful to consumers, but increases the margin of error. Details of calculations necessary, together with some useful data on yields, is contained in Chapter Five.

Nutrition label information can be presented on seafood packages, by stick-on labels or by means of point-of-purchase (POP) materials. These last have the advantage that explanations of the numbers and additional material can be included. An example of a nutrition label for fish is shown in Chapter Six.

## Point of purchase materials

These include signs, brochures, leaflets, booklets, recipes, fact sheets and resource lists. Shelf signs can highlight the nutritional features of the varieties available, as long as nutrition information is provided on the package label. Remember that POP materials count as labeling. Be cautious about making health claims (see Chapter Six).
For example:

"The following varieties are very lean – less than 2% fat: sole, flounder, cod, haddock, monkfish, sea bass, pollock and halibut."

"Contains 2 servings of less than 150 calories each, when prepared as directed."

"Very low in fat; each serving contains no more than 3 grams fat when prepared as directed."

"Low in sodium; each serving contains less than 100 mg sodium when prepared as directed."

Note that all such statements are regarded as health claims. Proper nutrition labeling is required.

The nutrient content of various species can be compared with that of appropriate meal alternatives to give the consumer a better perspective on how seafood compares with more familiar meal items. Ways in which it excels, like being low in calories, fat, cholesterol and sodium, can be flagged. Bar graphs make the comparisons obvious, as the example in Figure 8.1 illustrates:

Incorporating nutrition information into recipes is helpful for giving people a sense of the relative amounts of major nutrients. If the amounts are further described in a general way, such as low, moderate or high, people can put the numbers into perspective. Graphic representations, such as illustrating fat content in terms of teaspoons rather than grams, clarifies the issue for consumers. For example, 3½ ounces of baked chum salmon might have about 3.6 grams of fat, which is about ¾ of a teaspoon. By contrast, a cooked medium-fat hamburger may have as much as 17 grams of fat – nearly 3½ teaspoons!

Posters comparing different aspects of seafood nutrition can be part of the display in the seafood shop. Comparisons of different varieties of seafood with

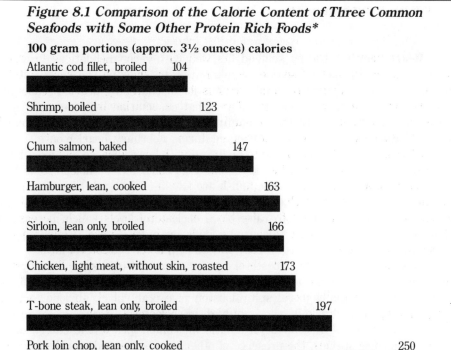

*Figure 8.1 Comparison of the Calorie Content of Three Common Seafoods with Some Other Protein Rich Foods\**

**100 gram portions (approx. 3½ ounces) calories**

Atlantic cod fillet, broiled     104

Shrimp, boiled     123

Chum salmon, baked     147

Hamburger, lean, cooked     163

Sirloin, lean only, broiled     166

Chicken, light meat, without skin, roasted     173

T-bone steak, lean only, broiled     197

Pork loin chop, lean only, cooked     250

*Data from Reference 243 and from Chapters Five and Nine.

respect to various nutrients is one type of display. Comparisons among alternative foods with respect to a single nutrient is another. The point is that if materials focusing on different aspects of seafood and nutrition are an integral part of the seafood department, consumers will be reminded of the seafood/health connection.

Showing which preparation methods best preserve the nutritional value of seafood and are in keeping with the most healthful eating habits is another way to emphasize good nutrition. That means discouraging deep fat frying and emphasizing baking, broiling, stir-frying, steaming, poaching, and microwaving seafood. Recipes should be reviewed not only for flavor and ease of preparation but also for calorie, fat, and sodium content and nutrient retention.

Restaurants can offer a majority of seafood items prepared by baking, broiling, poaching and steaming instead of frying to emphasize the most heart healthy preparation of seafood. Use rich sauces as a garnish rather than as a disguise for seafood and keep added butter to a minimum.

## Links with health themes

**Heart health.** Eating seafood fits well with recommendations for "heart healthy" eating. Promoting seafood consumption by showing the ways in which seafood fits in with dietary recommendations for discouraging heart disease gives seafood a heart healthy image. Reinforce that association by developing heart healthy seafood menus with the remaining meal items also being heart healthy choices. Feature the heart health advantage during February, heart month.

Cholesterol intake is believed to be linked with heart disease and most health professionals urge people to reduce their intake of cholesterol. Cholesterol is found only in foods of animal origin. Most finfish are low in cholesterol. Since most of us consume more cholesterol than is thought to be good for us, and since high cholesterol consumption tends to raise blood cholesterol levels which increase the risk of heart attacks, it is wise to consume foods low in cholesterol. Consuming fish frequently, say twice a week, is an easy way to help lower cholesterol intake.

Shellfish vary in their cholesterol content. Clams, mussels, scallops oysters, American lobster and some varieties of crab are as low in cholesterol as most finfish. Others have substantially more: spiny lobster, blue crab, black abalone, octopus, shrimp and squid. Fish roe is also very high in cholesterol. Because the varieties with more cholesterol also have very little fat, much less of the cholesterol is absorbed. In some species, the presence of other sterols also reduces the uptake of cholesterol during digestion.

Frequent consumption of most seafood can help a person reduce his intake of cholesterol. The only caution relates to the frequent consumption of large amounts of those few cholesterol-rich varieties of seafood. Unless a person eats on a regular basis great quantities of the few seafood products that are high in cholesterol, seafood will not be an important source of dietary cholesterol. Keeping to the low cholesterol varieties is easy to do as there are relatively few species whose intake should be monitored. Seafood can be enthusiastically promoted as a low cholesterol food as long as the exceptional varieties are noted and sweeping generalizations are avoided. There are substantial numbers of people with lipid disorders whose cholesterol intake needs strict monitoring and for whom indulgence in caviar should not be encouraged.

**Discourage cancer** Seafood consumption is consistent with the National Cancer Institute's dietary recommendations to lower total fat intake. High fat intake, such as most Americans have, is associated with some forms of cancer. The vast majority of seafood items are low in fat, and, as long as they are not deep fried, will retain their low fat advantage over other animal protein foods.

**High blood pressure** The excessive intake of sodium is associated with high blood pressure in many people. Because seafood is naturally low in sodium (except for canned, smoked, pickled, dried and some prepared seafood), it is especially appropriate for everyone trying to maintain a sensible sodium intake.

Make sure that suppliers are not adding unwanted sodium through the use of water-retaining dips.

**Reaching desirable body weight**   Because most seafood is very low in fat, it is also very low in calories. This feature is ideal for people trying to limit their calorie intake and lose or maintain weight. You can still have a generous portion and stay within your suggested calorie range.

## Overcome Consumer Concerns

Consumers may not comfortably admit it, but many are hesitant to cook seafood at home, try unfamiliar species, explore new recipes or approach something in a shell. From a marketing standpoint, the more we understand about why people are cautious about seafood, the better able we are to dispel fears and advance the enjoyment of eating fish and shellfish. The following lists some concerns people have about seafood, with suggestions for conquering such worries.

**Determining freshness**   Many consumers cannot tell by appearance or touch whether the seafood they are selecting is at peak freshness; moreover, should doubts be realized, they are even more reluctant to try buying fresh seafood again. For this reason, your seafood reputation depends on having top quality seafood for sale and discarding all merchandise that is less than fresh.

Tell consumers what qualities they should look for to determine freshness. Keep in mind that if your seafood is sold already packaged, the consumer has very few criteria to examine. Even the firmness of the flesh can be distorted by the tightness of the wrap.

Determining the freshness of fish with skin and head is much easier than for fish fillets; however, few varieties are sold in this form. Telling people to check the color of the gills and the brightness of the eye is about as helpful as suggesting they catch the fish themselves. You can, within reasonable limits, suggest using odor as one guide. Tell consumers to open the package, rinse the fish under cold water and then smell it. Packages tend to accumulate and concentrate odors, so that the smell immediately after opening the package may be misleading. After rinsing, fish may have a slight smell, but it should not have an unpleasant odor. Strong "off" odors indicate staleness. Tell consumers that fattier fish normally have stronger odors than leaner varieties. Buyers need to learn not to confuse the characteristic smells of the species with spoilage. At the same time, it is helpful to know that fattier species spoil more readily, too.

Firmness of flesh is another quality consumers can inspect. Top quality fish should have firm flesh that springs back when pressed lightly with the finger. If there is no elasticity in the flesh, pass it by.

Usually a fillet is presented with the skin side down, but if the skin is visible it should look bright and tight. Scaling and washing removes some of the luster from the skin, but truly fresh fish never has dull skin.

Cut fish loses moisture and natural juices. To reduce this "drip", fish is frequently dipped in a polyphosphate solution. Improper dipping conditions leave the fish with a glassy, slimy appearance. The cut surface should appear moist and glistening, not deeply shiny.

The fluid lost from cut fish is another clue to freshness. Tray packed fish often has absorbent material to hold the lost fluid so that it is not visible. If the fluid can be seen it should be clear or slightly translucent, not milky.

**Use open dating on your packages**   If you show a "sell by" date, also include a "best if used by" date to help the consumer take best advantage of the seafood's prime flavor.

**Recognizing quality**   Educating your shoppers to recognize and select top quality means that they will not be disappointed with the seafood you sell them. Happy customers return and bring others with them. Other aspects of quality are not necessarily related to freshness, like absence of bruising or blood spots, cleanly cut edges and so on. These can be presented under the "quality" umbrella, keeping freshness as a separate theme. You can prepare posters, fact sheets and POP materials describing the features of top quality in different seafood items and telling of the steps you take to ensure that you are offering top quality. Go over the checkpoints of quality when you talk to shoppers, during in-store seafood demos and in your advertising. Be sure your customers know that you run a first class seafood business and are willing to guarantee what you sell.

Here are some quality features you may be able to highlight in your operation:

- no bruises, blood, or hook marks;

- USDC inspected;

- clean cut edges on fillets;

- temperature of your seafood case: 31-32°F. (never above 34°F.);

- on-site preparation of retail cuts so that your buyers can inspect and choose only the freshest fish on the market;

- guaranteed customer satisfaction;

- open dating.

Restaurants can create unique presentations of their seafood to show their patrons how fresh their items are. Showing the fish to the diner before preparation, fresh seafood displays and menu and placemat descriptions tell the diner how important top quality is in your establishment. Daily changes of menu items and staff trained to describe the seafood dishes properly to the customer help to give the impression of fresh product at its peak. Training of staff is particularly important. If individuals are not capable of doing this effectively, make sure that they have a senior staff member available to talk to the customers and are instructed to call in this help as soon as they are unable to answer a question. Uninformed or uninformative servers can immediately undermine any reputation you are building for expertise with seafood.

**Choosing frozen fish**    Frozen fish is top quality fish when it has been handled properly in the first place. Fish frozen shortly after catch under good processing conditions has little chance to spoil or lose flavor.

Show consumers how to recognize top quality frozen fish. It should be free of dark spots or dried, discolored, spongy areas where freezer burn may have affected it. Freezer burn occurs when a patch of frozen food becomes exposed to the air and dries out. The flesh may darken as a result. Such dried areas are safe to eat but are greatly inferior in quality and appeal. Freezer burn is mainly the result of improper packaging. Air spaces within the package draw moisture out of the flesh to the wrap and promote freezer burn.

Frozen seafood should be tightly wrapped and have no ice crystals or frost when opened. Consumers and buyers should examine the tightness of the wrap and look for the exclusion of air and intact packaging material. If the temperature of frozen fish fluctuates or is not maintained at a low enough level, the fish may partly thaw and refreeze. This drastically reduces quality and may be evidenced by ice crystals or even lumps of ice within the packet. However, temperature fluctuations that remain well below freezing point may show no external symptoms, but shelf life will be greatly reduced, especially of fat fish.

Glazing prevents losses from the fish, helps retain flavor and texture and prevents drying and freezer burn. While not all frozen fish will be glazed, it is a method that is very effective in preserving moisture, freshness and flavor and can be construed as an indicator of high quality frozen fish. However, watch that the net weight excludes the glaze. Consumers are entitled to receive the weight of product they pay for and the law gives them that protection.

**Use freshness dating on frozen fish**    Indicate when the period of top quality expires for a particular fish. However, this is not easy to determine. Recommendations by consumer organizations, often quoted in press articles by cookery and food writers, give very short periods, designed to ensure that even poorly handled product will be bought when it is still reasonably good. The problem with some of these recommendations is that they barely allow time for some imported product to reach the US from their origins, let alone be placed on sale through the complexities of the distribution system. The best advice is to work with your regular suppliers to determine reasonable expiration dates that fit with the actual handling the product receives. Fat fish have a shorter life than shellfish and shellfish a shorter life than lean fish, though these rules are not invariable. Much depends on the packaging, handling and the quality control at the packing plant.

Remind consumers to check the temperature of their own freezer. Freezing units as part of a refrigerator seldom achieve the very low temperatures required to maintain top quality. If the freezer is above 0°F., storage time should be reduced sharply, probably no more than 8 weeks. Frost free refrigerator-freezers tend to extract moisture from frozen foods more than conventional freezers so that keeping time may be reduced. Frozen fish stored in frost-free freezers should be checked periodically.

Fresh fish that cannot be used immediately can be frozen at home for later use. Tell consumers and buyers how to do this properly. Fish must be well washed and wrapped to exclude as much air as possible. Wrapping materials such as Saran wrap, heavy plastic film, and aluminum foil serve well. Fish can be wrapped first with wax paper and then overwrapped with a snug cover of aluminum foil. Wax paper by itself is neither sufficiently moisture resistant nor pliable to give adequate protection.

Home frozen fish should also be glazed (315). First, wrap and freeze the fish quickly and completely. Then unwrap and immerse the fish in a bowl of ice water. A glaze should form immediately. If it does not, return the fish to the freezer and repeat later. Dip the fish three or four times, then wrap it in moistureproof wrapping and return it to the freezer. Any cracks in the glaze should be sealed by reglazing.

Clams and oysters can be frozen with their juices in freezer containers. Scallops can be handled similarly. Lobster and crab are always cooked before freezing and do not freeze well at home.

**Retail forms**   Experienced consumers and fish lovers are more likely to try an unfamiliar variety or form of seafood than novice fish users. But the latter are the majority and the industry needs to reach them. Many people simply have no idea what to do with a whole or dressed fish. Others are familiar with cod fillets but not cod steak. Will it handle differently? Are the portion sizes right? People fear fish bones, and few realize how simple it is to remove them, when done properly. Explain which fish have large, coarse bones, and which have small fine ones. Where appropriate, guarantee that a piece of fish is boneless.

Shellfish present different challenges. How do you get the meat out of a crab? How much edible meat can you expect from a crab or lobster? Can you eat shrimp shells? Offer simple gadgets for shelling and deveining shrimp; lobster crackers and picks are also needed and not readily available to most shoppers unless they make a special trip to a specialty kitchen store. How do you get clams out of their shells easily? Offer tips on light steaming and microwaving clams and oysters.

Even something as simple as washing the animal or fish is not straightforward to someone on his first adventure with a variety of shellfish or finfish. And many people may not be able to tell from the appearance of the package whether the item is raw or cooked. Tell them. Give "how-to" facts, preferably with illustrations. Some things consumers, especially first time adventurers, need to know are:

- how to cook live seafoods like clams and mussels;

- how to shell cooked shellfish;

- where to find all the meat in cooked shellfish, especially crabs;

- which parts of the animal are inedible (if any);

- cooking time for live seafoods;

- quick tricks for shelling and deveining shrimp;

- what are the most suitable accompaniments – your chance to make more healthful suggestions than melted butter;

- how to tell when fish is done and how to avoid overcooking;

- how to cook uneven thicknesses of fish evenly;

- which varieties of fish hold up best in such cooking methods as stir-frying, shish kebob, stuffed fillets, barbecuing;

- what to do with a whole dressed fish;

- the taste differences between clams and mussels, different types of lean, white fish, less familiar varieties.

Recipes need special attention too. The most important message for any seafood recipe to communicate is "DO NOT OVERCOOK." Short cooking times at high temperatures are preferable to longer times at moderate temperatures. Include instructions for microwave cooking also. Instead of developing a battery of recipes and then giving a general indication about the kinds of fish they suit, custom develop your recipes and serving suggestions for the varieties and retail forms you carry. You can do an entire promotion on whole or dressed fish. Provide a variety of preparation styles for the species you offer ranging from quick preparations for the family to entertaining suggestions. Be sure to emphasize the importance of not overcooking seafood.

Promotions can focus on the retail form, like fish steaks. Use salmon, cod, halibut, swordfish. Challenge your customers to compare steaks – meat versus fish – and show how fish comes out ahead in terms of nutrition, cost and flavor.

**Storage and Handling**  Many people believe that fresh fish needs to be consumed the same day it is purchased. Nevertheless, high quality fish can be stored at home for short periods if the conditions are good. Fish should be rinsed off with very cold water, and loosely wrapped with waterproof paper, aluminum foil or plastic film and set in a container to collect any fluid loss. It should be stored in the coldest part of the refrigerator, away from other foods and then used as quickly as possible. Unfrozen fish will keep at least two days if it is in top quality when purchased. Many varieties will keep longer, although it is seldom advisable under home storage conditions.

Fish can also be stored in the refrigerator surrounded by finely crushed ice. This method is the best for assuring the coldest temperature, but few homes have ready access to the necessary crushed ice. Ice cubes or blocks are not suitable because they permit air pockets, and the sharp edges tear the fish.

Frozen fish should be thawed in the refrigerator the day before it is needed. It is ready to use as soon as the pieces or fillets are easily separated. Whole fish are ready when they become flexible, not necessarily soft. Fish should not be thawed at room temperature because the thawed surface can deteriorate while the frozen center is thawing. Defrosting at room temperature also increases fluid loss (315). Fillets and thin cuts of fish are better cooked from frozen. This is an added convenience for the user and should be stressed. It saves time, planning and fish juices in the kitchen. Thawed seafood should not be re-frozen.

Explain why fish is so perishable: its high moisture content makes it an attractive environment for the growth of spoilage bacteria. The enzyme systems of many fish and shellfish are adapted to work at cold temperatures so that refrigeration slows enzyme degradation but does not stop it completely. Any traces of fish viscera will contaminate the flesh and encourage spoilage. Unsanitary handling conditions anywhere in the distribution system will also promote spoilage.

Fish with a relatively high oil content are more susceptible to spoilage than lean varieties. That is because the fat is highly unsaturated and therefore is easily oxidized. This process is accompanied by an increase in odor quite distinct from that of sour flesh. Fat oxidation proceeds at freezing temperatures, though much more slowly. For this reason, the fattier species have a shorter shelf life in the frozen state as well as in the fresh.

**Price**  Sometimes seafood is expensive. Many circumstances determine the final selling price of seafood, but top quality is always worth paying for. Reassure your customers that your product is worth buying not only because of its quality but also its value. Fish fillets have no waste and steaks have very little. Unlike many meats and poultry, you eat most of what you buy. Seafoods with shells and large bones still offer very good value as their price per pound is usually much lower.

Because the edible yield is high with filleted fish and shelled seafood, a promotion emphasizing "great taste, no waste" implies superb value. Depending on the recommended serving size, seafood may offer superior value to its meat alternatives on a cost per serving basis. Cost per serving is an important distinction from cost per pound and customers may have no idea how to calculate this figure. Most price labels give total price and price per pound. Comparing costs per serving of different meat/fish alternates illustrates the excellent value of seafood.

$$\text{Cost per serving} \quad = \quad \frac{\text{Total cost of package}}{\text{Number of servings in package}}$$

The serving size recommended most often for meat, fish and poultry is 3 ounces of cooked product. To compare cost per serving on an "as purchased" basis, that is, raw, allow 4 ounces per serving. As an example, a food retailer might compare the cost of fish fillets with boneless chicken breast, stew veal, boneless round steak and boneless pork loin. These cuts, like fish fillets, all have similarly high cooked yields.

For more expensive seafood items like lobster or shrimp, suggest ways your customers can use them in small amounts, or extend the servings they can obtain from a package. The most popular ways of stretching these items are mixed seafood main dishes like paella and seafood fettucine, chowders, fish stews, salads, terrines, seafood pates and omelettes. Promote these luxuries by featuring the most appropriate recipes and serving suggestions.

---

### The Canadian Cooking Rule for Fish

Prepare the fish for cooking. Preheat oven to 450°F. Measure the THICKNESS of the fish at its thickest point, as the fish sits on its cooking container.

For every INCH of thickness, cook FRESH fish for 10 minutes. This means that if it is half an inch thick, cook it for 5 minutes; if it is 2 inches thick, cook it for 20 minutes at 450°F.

If the fish is FROZEN, double the cooking time to 20 minutes for each inch at 450°F.

The rule applies to every sort of cooking method used for fish – to baking, broiling, sauteeing, pan-frying, grilling, poaching, steaming or braising.

**Bake** UNFROZEN fish at 450°F. in a preheated oven for 10 minutes per inch of thickness.

**Bake** FROZEN fish at 450°F. in a preheated oven for 20 minutes per inch of thickness.

**Broil** in a preheated oven with the fish 2 to 4 inches from the heat source.

**Poach, boil or steam**, timing from the point the water returns to the boil, for 10 minutes per inch, or 20 minutes per inch if the fish is frozen.

---

**Cooking seafood successfully**    There are hundreds of cookbooks devoted to the art of cooking seafood. They differ substantially in their target audience, practicality, sophistication, and ease of preparation. The overall nutritional merit, especially in the use of fat and salt is also highly variable among recipes, and is a point worth considering. Probably the most comprehensive and enjoyable work on the subject is McClane and deZanger's *The Encyclopedia of Fish Cookery* (315).

Seafood retailers can benefit by providing reliable, appealing seafood cookbooks at fish counters. Failing that, a list of recommended cookbooks available locally is helpful. Distinguish your cookbook list with informative annotations about the contents. Note the level of skill and sophistication required. Include references to free information provided by governments and by people in the fish business. A short annotated list of cookbooks is printed at the end of this Chapter.

Many people feel insecure about their seafood cooking skills. Consumers need to be convinced of the simplicity of seafood preparation. The most important point is to avoid overcooking. Ensure that your customers know how to solve this problem by using the Canadian cooking rule (see BOX). This method works for virtually every fish (NOT for shellfish) and is foolproof.

Overcooking is the main reason for disappointing results with fish. Fish tastes much better slightly undercooked rather than slightly overcooked. Use of the Canadian rule ensures good results, every time. Simple measuring rulers like the "Perfect Fish" make useful additional items for fish counters to sell and can also be used as premiums to attract customers.

Explain in handouts, in POP materials and on package labels how to tell when fish is done:

- flesh has just turned from translucent and shiny to opaque;

- fish separates easily or "flakes" when a fork is inserted in the middle.

**Flavor and texture qualities**   One reason consumers are reluctant to try unfamiliar species is that there is no way of anticipating taste, strong or mild, bland or distinctive. Similarly, with texture – will the fish fall apart when cooked, or will it be very firm? How will it adapt to the buyer's customary cooking methods and recipes.

You can make a customer more comfortable about trying an unfamiliar species by providing flavor and texture charts. Such charts are simplifications of the unique qualities of a particular species, and are bound to exclude some of the distinguishing points of some fish. But general guidelines are more helpful than no information at all. More sophisticated comparisons of different species can be developed based on the usual line of seafood you carry. It is important to do this if you have a sophisticated seafood clientele.

Another way of making comparisons among different varieties is to name the species and retail forms that are best suited to a particular recipe or cooking method being featured. This approach gives the buyer some choice among species and affords the merchant the opportunity to feature different varieties with the same preparation suggestions. A practical example of this suggestion is to indicate which varieties are suitable for the outdoor barbecue. In this example, you might also include those varieties suitable for steaming in foil packets on the outdoor grill, especially if your selection of firm species is limited.

In developing flavor and texture charts there is always a trade-off between simplifying the information too much, thereby sacrificing helpful detail, and providing too much information, thereby losing the reader. In general, consumers relate comfortably to information given in three hierarchies comparable to low, moderate and high. Flavor may be generally described as mild, moderate or strong, but texture varies widely from very delicate to very firm.

A general guide to the flavor and texture of selected species is presented in Table 8.1. The numbers are a subjective rating of flavor and texture on a five point scale where five is the strongest in flavor and firmest in texture. The ratings are entirely subjective and are not based on any measurement criteria. They are intended to be only a general guide, not a precise description of the sensory qualities of the fish. Describing the sensory qualities of food calls for very careful word choices. Clearly a moderate flavor to one person is strong to another and mild to a third. We have to accept a certain amount of subjective disagreement in any simple categorization.

### Table 8.1 Flavor and Texture Characteristics of Selected Finfish

| Species | Flavor* | Texture* | Species | Flavor* | Texture* |
|---|---|---|---|---|---|
| Amberjack | 3 | 3 | Perch, lake | 1 | 3 |
| Black sea bass | 3 | 3 | Perch, ocean | 2 | 3 |
| Striped bass | 4 | 1 | Pike | 1 | 3 |
| Bluefish | 4 | 2 | Pollock, Atlantic | 4 | 4 |
| Bonito | 5 | 4 | Pollock, Pacific | 1 | 2 |
| Butterfish | 2 | 2 | Pompano | 2 | 3 |
| Catfish | 2 | 3 | Scup | 4 | 3 |
| Catfish, ocean | 3 | 4 | Rockfish | 2 | 3 |
| Cod | 3 | 3 | Sablefish | 3 | 3 |
| Jacks | 4 | 2 | Salmon | 5 | 4 |
| Dogfish | 3 | 4 | Sea trout | 2 | 2 |
| Drum, red | 3 | 4 | Shark | 3 | 5 |
| Eel | 3 | 5 | Smelt | 3 | 3 |
| Flounder | 1 | 1 | Snapper | 3 | 4 |
| Grouper | 2 | 4 | Sole | 1 | 1 |
| Hake | 1 | 1 | Swordfish | 4 | 5 |
| Haddock | 2 | 3 | Tilefish | 3 | 5 |
| Halibut | 3 | 4 | Trout | 3 | 3 |
| Herring | 5 | 3 | Tuna | 4 | 5 |
| Mackerel | 5 | 2 | Turbot, greenland | 1 | 1 |
| Mahi-mahi | 2 | 4 | Whitefish | 2 | 2 |
| Monkfish | 3 | 4 | Whiting | 1 | 1 |

* Number ratings: 5 is the strongest flavor and firmest texture.

The main purpose of all such charts is to introduce the unfamiliar, not provide exhaustive palatability profiles. Differences among molluscs and crustaceans are better described by comparing the less familiar species with the most familiar ones, such as rock lobster tails with American lobster or Northern shrimp with tropical white shrimp.

**Unfamiliar Species**   It requires persuasion to convince consumers to try unfamiliar species. The fish merchant and restaurant can both do a great deal to overcome doubts. Provide comparative information about the flavor and texture of the item, using the most familiar (and true) example you have. Be explicit in your suggestions for what to do with the item. Adapt recipes specifically for unfamiliar species. Giving a recipe for stuffed sole with the comment that it will work for "this species" is less than inspiring. Have a recipe on hand with the name of the less familiar species in its title. This is a more convincing way of conveying your knowledge about and experience with the species than using a "make do" approach.

It makes sense that someone seeking information on how to prepare pout is going to look under the name pout, not something else.

**Taste demonstrations work**   They are expensive, generate chaos in the seafood department and require a skilled demonstrator, but they sell seafood and can build your market. They are especially well suited to introducing unfamiliar species, new recipes or flavor combinations and good cooking techniques. Consider investing in their use if your market potential is substantial. Cooking demos that tie in with complementary products may reduce the costs, but may also reduce the promotional benefits of the seafood item.

Educational videos for use in training seafood personnel and in providing information to consumers can be an effective marketing tool in the seafood department. They are especially helpful in communicating information about unfamiliar species, different cooking techniques like steaming or poaching, and detailed presentations like removing the bones from a cooked fish.

## Developing Recipes for Marketing Use

Recipes and cooking techniques are an especially important part of converting non-seafood users into seafood users. The development and review of recipes does not always receive the careful attention needed if recipes are to enhance the promotion of seafood. There are several aspects to consider when developing or selecting recipes:

- appeal, through words and through pictures;

- suggested flavor outcome;

- ease of preparation;

- time required to prepare;

- availability of ingredients;

- cooking skill required;

- legibility;

- nutritional merit, especially concerning the amount and type of fat required and the amount of ingredients containing salt or sodium.*

Many times the worth of a recipe is not in whether the buyer actually follows the preparation, but whether the recipe suggests to the reader that the seafood item

---

\* Determining the caloric value of a recipe is seldom a straightforward procedure. There are nutrient and food losses during preparation and cooking and the yield is difficult to determine. Losses are not uniformly distributed among the food and recipe components so that some assumptions usually have to be made about the final composition of the item. There are fewer data for foods on a cooked basis than on a raw basis. In spite of these difficulties, reasonable estimates of the caloric content of a recipe on a cooked basis can be derived. Caloric values are nearly always approximations and need to be viewed with a certain scepticism. For further discussion, see Chapter Four and Chapter Five.

can be prepared in an appealing or simple way, or that it will turn out well. Sometimes the recipe is a reminder of another item the buyer has on hand which would complement the seafood. Often, the recipe literally determines whether or not the item will be purchased and prepared.

The appeal of a recipe is suggested first in its title and next in the list of ingredients. Curried sole may appeal to as many as it deters and if the notion of using spices with seafood instead of citrus is a new one, the suggestion will have served a useful purpose. Appeal is communicated visually with colored photos. These are expensive and not always necessary, but should be seriously considered where budget permits. As part of a print advertising campaign they can be most communicative.

Recipe titles often suggest the final flavor, which may have nothing to do with the flavor of the seafood. Terms like creole, curry, lemon, creamed or au gratin describe the flavor of the sauce or spice used to add flavor to the seafod. Relying on accompaniment flavors is useful in promoting varieties that have very little flavor themselves. Complementary flavors also help expand the culinary repertoire of the seafood chef.

Ease of preparation is especially important for novice or hesitant cooks. This does not necessarily mean relying on prepackaged or bottled accompaniments, but requires the judicious selection of simple tasty recipes with imaginative variations. Sole or flounder stuffed with thawed, drained, chopped spinach and Parmesan cheese and baked with a sprinkling of dried dill is an example. Cod fillets baked with onions and cheddar is another. Curried yogurt is a third, easy topping for fish and is both fast and easy.

Ease of preparation can be verified by checking the number of ingredients required, the number and kind of utensils (must the cook have a food processor or blender?), and the type of preparation involved (are there five or two vegetables to wash, peel or chop, or is one unpeeled vegetable sufficient? Does the fish require time to marinate?).

Time of preparation is a premium feature for busy households and those where the chief cook has limited skill or culinary interest. Because seafood cooks in just a few minutes, this feature deserves prominence in seafood marketing. Putting the suggestion of time into the recipe title makes it clear. Such wording as "5 minute", "jiffy", "quick", "last minute" etc. If the recipe requires 15 minutes of prior preparation to wash and chop vegetables, prepare a sauce, or marinate, then the title is a misnomer. Watch for inconsistencies between the title and the actual preparation time. Recipes giving the approximate preparation time can be helpful to hurried cooks.

The availability of ingredients is one of the most serious deterrents to trying a recipe. It is not that the ingredients are undesirable, but that preplanning or special trips to the shop may be required for items not normally kept at home. Recipes calling for more than one variety of seafood are particularly liable to be avoided on this account. The basic seafood recipe collection should rely on foods most likely to be on hand. Recipes that include alternatives are also more useful than those with no options. Exotic ingredients can convert the ordinary to the delectable, but have to be used to be appreciated.

The skill of the cook should be kept in mind. New seafood users may be enticed by simple recipes, while those with sophisticated palates may be seeking challenging taste ideas. It is preferable to have a simple, imaginative line of recipes covering all seafood varieties you serve, rather than catering exclusively to the needs of one group. Include a variety of cooking techniques among the recipes offered, limit the number of preparation steps required, and avoid developing recipes for the gourmet market, unless, of course, this is truly your market.

Recipes that are not legible either because the type face is too small or the layout too crowded will not meet anyone's needs. If the instructions are excessively cryptic or vague the recipes will not be understood. Develop recipe texts as if for the simple-minded and you will not go astray.

And finally, nutrition. Consider the nutritional merit of your seafood recipes by reviewing the list of ingredients and the cooking techniques. Be alert for the amount of fat suggested. One guideline to use for evaluating the total amount of fat used is to keep the fat content of one serving of the recipe no more than thirty percent of the total calories of the serving. This level is in keeping with the overall recommendations of the Dietary Guidelines for Americans. More simply, allowing a maximum of 2 teaspoons of added fat per serving will keep recipes from being excessively high in fat. Approximately 5 grams of fat is 1 teaspoonful; 1 ounce is approximately 6 teaspoons. **Most recipes will turn out just as well with only one teaspoon of fat per serving and will have fewer calories.**

The type of fat recommended is another issue. Recipes which use butter as the source of fat are including more saturated fat and cholesterol than necessary. It is true that butter imparts a distinctive flavor but few recipes are dependent upon this. Substitute vegetable oil instead. Bacon fat, lard and hydrogenated vegetable oil should also be replaced with vegetable oil to reduce the contribution of saturated fat. Olive oil is an adequate and flavorful substitute for butter, but does not provide the level of polyunsaturated fat that corn or safflower oils do. The most important point is to keep the total amount of the fat as low as possible.

Deep fat frying should not be recommended as a method of cooking seafood; not because it is unflavorful, but because it is unhealthful. No one needs the additional fat taken up by seafood cooked in this way. Promote the leaner, healthier cooking methods instead.

There are other sources of fat in recipe ingredients which are less obvious than oil, butter and margarine. Examples are salad dressing, mayonnaise, sour cream, other kinds of cream, nuts and nut butters, and cheese. Limit the amounts of these items or use lower calorie substitutes like yogurt and low calorie or oil-free salad dressings.

Recipes should also be reviewed carefully for the amount of sodium. In most cases, the major share of sodium is contributed by salt. There are other sources of sodium in recipes to watch for including sea salt, soy sauce, Worcestershire sauce, baking powder, baking soda, canned or cubed bouillon, canned soups, seasoned salt, liquid from canned seafood, canned vegetable juice, canned tomato juice, commercial seasoning and marinade mixes, teriyaki sauce and seasoning, oyster sauce and dried soup mixes.

Recipes using any of these ingredients should not also suggest adding salt. It is very easy to make the sodium level of a recipe, especially one using prepared sauces and mixes, over 500 mg sodium per serving. The recommended daily intake of sodium is a maximum of 3300 mg per day (13 ). Estimates of the number of servings of food consumed per day range upward of fifteen. If each serving were 500 mg of sodium, intake would be 7500 mg per day, over double the recommended level.

**As a guide for salt content, suggest using no more than an eighth of a teaspoon salt per serving; that is half a teaspoon in total for a recipe serving four**. Most recipes exceed this amount. Reducing the salt level to this amount is barely detectable by taste and is doing a favor to the blood pressures of most of us. Never suggest adding salt to taste. Most people add far too much.

When strong flavored ingredients are part of a recipe, eliminate salt entirely. It will seldom be missed. If need be, increase the amount of herbs and other seasonings used. Make the flavor of a recipe dependent on the seafood, not on the flavor of the sea.

There are other opportunities in recipe development to improve the overall nutritional value of the product, increase the number of nutrients provided or decrease the less desirable dietary substances. Consult a qualified nutritionist or registered dietitian to do this. As an example, instead of using bread crumbs as a coating, devise a blend that might contain whole wheat flour, whole grain cornmeal (not the degermed variety), wheat germ, sesame seeds, poppy seeds, unprocessed bran or rye flour. This is an opportunity to increase not just the crunch but the fiber, vitamins and minerals too.

Many commercially prepared sauces and condiments rely on large amounts of sugar and corn syrup for their flavor. The sweetness may be masked by tomato, vinegar or smoke, but the sugar is there nonetheless. Check the ingredients listing for verification of this unfortunate truth. Seafood recipes that do not rely on these sweetened products will be lower in calories and richer in flavor.

Encouraging the use of vegetables in seafood preparation and serving is another way to enhance the nutritional value as well as the color and flavor of the recipe. The more nutrient-rich vegetables like spinach, chard, carrots, peas and potatoes generally complement many basic seafood preparations.

Suggesting meal accompaniments for a seafood recipe is an opportunity to promote good nutrition indirectly through seafood. Emphasize a variety of vegetables and whole grains like bulgur, brown rice and barley.

Seafood recipes can increase nutrition awareness by including information about calories, protein, fat and sodium. Additional information about cholesterol is also useful to many people. Recipes can flag the presence of substantial amounts of other nutrients like trace minerals but few do this. A minimum of 10 percent of the U.S. RDA must be present in order to suggest the recipe as a "significant source of a nutrient". At the very least, a line or illustration depicting the nutritional highlights of a recipe tells the reader that nutrition was a consideration in developing the recipe. That is a positive message.

## Annotated Bibliography of Seafood Cookbooks

The following list of seafood cookbooks was compiled to give the reader a head start in reviewing some of the available material on seafood cookery. The list is not exhaustive as there are thousands of cookbooks on the market, but the review describes some of the currently available recipe books in terms of their nutritional merit, variety, time and skill required.

In order to simplify the assessment of overall merit, the books are arranged in three groups from the most to the least useful to the general reader. The groupings give priority to ease and variety of seafood preparation and to the nutritional merit of the recipes, especially regarding the limited use of fats and salt. The groupings have all the limitations of subjective evaluation and are intended only as a guide, not a definitive assessment.

### Most Useful

**McClane, A.J.** 1977. *The Encyclopedia of Fish Cookery*. Holt, Reinhart and Winston, New York, $50.00 hardcover, illustrated in color.

• Undoubtedly the most comprehensive and lavish collection of seafood species, recipes and information available

• Recipes vary from very simple to elaborate, with easy creative preparations throughout

• Nutrition is not mentioned but most recipes do not depend on large amounts of butter, bacon or cream; recommended amounts of salt are variable and could readily be reduced.

• An indication of other species suitable for the recipes would make the book much more useful to the general reader.

**Giobbi, E. and Wolfe, R. M.D.,** 1985. *Eat Right, Eat Well – The Italian Way*, Alfred A. Knopf, New York, $19.95, hard cover.

• Primary emphasis is on healthful tasty recipes

• Provides extensive nutrition and health information and applies the principles of sound diet to the development of Italian style recipes.

• Uses only small amounts of vegetable oil; no butter or cream.

• Recipes straightforward, creative, flavorful.

**Pappas, L. S.** 1979. *International Fish Cookery*, 101 Productions, San Francisco, $6.95, soft cover.

• Wide variety of cooking techniques & styles, menu items.

• Uses several different sources of fat; vegetable seasonings.

• International flavors, preparations make recipes distinctive.

• Recipes vary in ease and convenience from simple to complex; clearly written.

• No nutrition information; use of salt discretionary.

    **The Rhode Island Seafood Council,** 1982. *Complete Guide To Seafood Cookery.* Wakefield, R.I. 02879, soft cover. Contact publisher for price information.

• Wide variety of cooking methods and recipes

• Species limited to East Coast varieties but substitutions of other seafoods would work

• Includes nutrition information

• Recipes inconsistent in fat and salt

• Most recipes fast, tasty with readily available ingredients.

    **American Heart Association.** 1984. *The American Heart Association Cookbook* – New Revised 4th Edition. David McKay Company, Inc., New York, N.Y. 10016, $15.95, hard cover.

• Emphasis on healthful and tasty low fat, low sodium seafood preparation

• Nutrition information given

• Primarily traditional cooking methods with familiar flavors and easy preparation

• Limited variety of seafood suggested

• Ample use of vegetables and herbs

• Recipes may lack "excitement" for those seeking more creative seafood presentations.

## Moderately Useful

    **Goodman, H.W. and Morse, B.** 1982. *Just What The Doctor Ordered.* Holt, Rinehart and Winston, New York, $25.00, hard cover.

• Complete cookbook developed primarily for healthful eating for those with specific dietary limitations such as restricted fat and sodium

• Recipes specially developed for the pampered palate, yet fulfil dietary objectives

• Recipes emphasize poaching, boiling, broiling, sauteeing, and casserole cookery

• Avoids fatty fish

• Limited variety of seafood.


**Bjornskov, E. 1984.** *The Complete Book of American Fish and Shellfish Cookery*, Alfred A. Knopf, New York, $18.95, hard cover.

• Most valuable for its extensive coverage of North American species and basic information on cooking and handling seafood

• Variety in ease, time and expense of preparation

• No nutrition information and no attempt made to make recipes particularly healthful

• Generous use of fats and sodium-rich ingredients.


**Ackart, R. 1983.** *The Frugal Fish.* Little, Brown & Company, Boston, $17.95, hard cover.

• Variety of cooking methods with discussion of nutrition

• Includes underutilized species

• Application of nutrition principles to recipes inadequate, with frequent use of butter and cream; amounts of salt unspecified

• Enthusiasm for seafood and nutrition.


**Walker, C. 1984.** *Fish and Shellfish*, HP Books, P.O. Box 5367, Tuscon, Arizona, 85703, $7.95.

• Wide variety of cooking methods; appealing format and illustrations

• Some low fat, low calorie recipes, or alternatives given in addition to richer recipes

• Original ideas and extensive seafood information but no nutrition information.


**Omae, K. and Tachibana, Y.** 1981. *The Book Of Sushi.* Kodansha International Limited/USA, New York, N.Y., 10022, hard cover.

• Little or no cooking but skill and time required to prepare

• Ingredients available only in specialty or oriental shops

• No added fat; sodium only from moderate use of soy sauce

• Describes preparation and presentation of sushi.

## Less Useful

**London, S. and London, M.**   1980. *The Fish Lover's Cookbook*. Rodale Press, Emmaus, PA.

• Wide variety of species, cooking methods and flavor combinations

• Background information about seafood

• Small amount of nutrition information

• Recipes low in sodium but fats, eggs, and cream used as desired

• Omits all shellfish for dubious reasons.


**Rombauer, I.S., Rombauer B. M.**   1975. *The Joy of Cooking*. Bobs-Merrill Company, Inc. Indianapolis, $16.95 hard cover.

• Wide variety of cooking techniques, species, and flavors used

• Great detail, preparation instruction, some unusual ingredients

• Abundant use of sauces, fats, and salt

• Recipes fairly time consuming; more healthful quicker approaches are available.


**Editors of Time-Life Books.**   1984. *The Good Cook/Fish* and *The Good Cook/Shellfish*, by Time-Life Books, Chicago, Illinois 60611, hard cover.

• Aimed at the adventuresome gourmet

• Recipes require time, skill, and sometimes unusual ingredients

• No nutrition information; extensive background information on seafood

• Liberal use of fat and cream.


**Beard, J.**   1954. *James Beard's Fish Cookery*, Little, Brown and Company, hard and soft cover.

• Extensive information and detail, great variety of recipes, species, preparation techniques

• No nutrition information; recipes not developed with healthful eating in mind

• Appeals to the more sophisticated, less health-conscious reader.

*Chapter Nine*

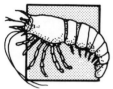

# Nutrient Composition of Seafoods

## General Considerations

This chapter presents quantitative data describing the nutrient composition of finfish and shellfish. The tables are based on the most recent figures in the research and technical literature. Not all the available information has been included. For example, moisture and ash content figures have been omitted but references in the tables provide data sources for the reader seeking more detail.

The tables in this Chapter are:

Table 9.1 Nutrient Composition of Finfish.
Table 9.2 Nutrient Composition of Shellfish.
Table 9.3 Proximate Composition and Sodium Content of Canned Fish.
Table 9.4 Proximate Composition of Selected Hawaiian Finfish.
Table 9.5 Proximate Composition of New Zealand Finfish.
Table 9.6 Vitamin and Mineral Content of Selected New Zealand Finfish.

The information in the tables was selected with a view to its being useful for applied purposes. For example, if you wish to calculate the calorie, fat and protein content of a serving of fish, the information in the nutrient tables in this Chapter, plus the information about yield and nutrient retention in Chapter Five will provide the data and methods for estimating these nutrients.

**Protein and total fat** values are the *means* of values in the literature. Because fat is the most variable component of the flesh, an indication of how large the variation in fat content can be for any given species is shown (where available) as a range just below the average fat content. Any one sample of fish may be quite different in its fat content from the value shown in the tables because of differences due to season, species, age and sex of the fish, geographical location and so on. But people needing an approximation of the nutrient content of a species of fish require an average value and these tables present the best estimate of average nutrient content currently available.

The standard deviation of the measures is not included for two reasons. First, for most practical purposes, the standard deviation is not used. Second, many papers publish average data without a range or standard deviation and without the original observations. Calculation of a meaningful standard deviation (or standard error for data on means) is impossible without the original data.

Another issue in compiling data tables is the number of significant figures to include. By and large, nutrient composition data are not accurate beyond two decimal places, and seldom past one. Many analytical methods are simply not accurate any further. For example, total lipid is often determined by extracting the tissue with solvents and drying the vessel with the extract to constant weight. With errors due to weighing, handling the tissue and glassware, and obtaining one hundred percent recovery of the sample, the final weights are no more accurate than two decimal places. In these tables one decimal figure is given.

When quantities of nutrients are small it may be necessary to carry an additional decimal as has been done with a few of the vitamins. Even so, the figures given should be treated as approximate.

**Kilocalories**   were individually calculated for each item in the following way: for finfish, the calorie equivalent factors for protein of 4.27 calories/gm and for fat of 9.02 calories/gm were used to determine the calories per 100 grams of raw muscle or edible portion. These calorie equivalents are the same as those used by USDA for determining calorie content in its Handbooks of Food Composition (84).

For shellfish (Table 9.2) the same calorie conversion factors were used, plus the carbohydrate equivalent of 4.0 calories per gram.

A final word about the calorie content of seafood concerns the level of accuracy of the final estimate. The numbers shown in the tables in this chapter are those from the direct determination of calorie content as explained. They have not been rounded. When using calorie content data for consumer education purposes, preparing charts about the calorie content of different species and for comparisons with other foods, the numbers should be rounded at least to the nearest five calories. Rounding to the nearest 10 calories for consumer publications is entirely appropriate and avoids giving the impression that small differences in calories are meaningful. The variability in the original data upon which the calculations are based is sometimes substantial. Rounding avoids the appearance of spurious accuracy.

**Carbohydrate**   In Table 9.1 no data are presented for carbohydrate content because most finfish have negligible amounts of carbohydrate, usually less than 2 percent. It makes no meaningful difference in calculations of caloric value to include trace amounts of carbohydrate. A few species have more than two percent carbohydrate according to a 1981 review of the nutrient data on seafood (Table 2.2). There is no consistent agreeement about the carbohydrate content of finfish and so its possible presence in relatively small amounts in a few species was ignored.

Shellfish, on the other hand, sometimes have considerable amounts of carbohydrate. In Table 9.2, carbohydrate content is listed separately and is also included in the calculation of total calorie content. The conversion factor of 4 calories/gm was used in the calculation of total calories.

**Total Fat, Fatty Acids and Cholesterol** Data for the amount of fat in seafood was obtained by averaging the most recent and reliable figures in the literature. Not all studies of proximate and fatty acid composition are based on samples giving an adequate reflection of the differences in composition due to season, life cycle, geographical location, sex etc. so that the original data nearly always leave something to be desired. The limitations in sampling are partially overcome by the large number of observations available, the different time and sources of the studies and the range of values reported. Nevertheless, it is well to be aware that any single sample of fish is apt to be quite different in composition from the values reported here.

The average total fat content in Tables 9.1 and 9.2 was the basis for deriving the quantity of saturated, monounsaturated, polyunsaturated and omega-3 fatty acid content reported. The percentage distribution of fatty acids from the literature was applied to the average values for total lipid to obtain figures different from those appearing in the original literature. The total fatty acids obtained were also corrected for non-fatty acid content according to the method of Weihrauch et al. (356). Correcting for the the non-fatty acid portion of the lipid results in slightly lower figures. Because the total fat content is an average of literature values, the fatty acid content values are also different from those published in the literature.

Omega-3 fatty acid content data were derived in the same way as those for the different types of fatty acids. They are based on the sum of eicosapentaenoic acid and docosahexaenoic acid *only*. The reason for this choice is that not all fatty acid distribution data give values for the small amounts of other omega-3 fatty acids that may be present. EPA and DHA account for almost all the omega-3 fatty acids present in fish. To handle all the data consistently, it was decided to omit trace amounts of other omega-3 fatty acids when they were reported. Omega-3 fatty acid data were also corrected for the non-fatty acid part of the lipid fraction.

Cholesterol data are those obtained from the recent literature and represent only analyses performed by gas liquid chromatography. While this method of analysis does not ensure a true value, when other parts of the determination have been carefully conducted it is the most accurate way of measuring cholesterol content. Cholesterol measurements are notoriously variable and have usually been overestimated in nutrient analyses. On the other hand, if the initial extraction of the sample is incomplete, the resulting cholesterol determination will be low. All values should be viewed as approximate.

**Vitamins and minerals** Vitamin A content in most seafood is very low. Most of the vitamin A in fish is found in the liver with very little in the flesh. The content is somewhat higher in fattier species. In some instances there are widely disparate values in the literature with little reason for selecting or rejecting any of them. Sablefish, swordfish and bluefin tuna are examples where the reported values are highly variable.

The literature values for many of the B vitamins are fairly consistent, although those for vitamin $B_{12}$ showed considerable variation. There are few data on pantothenic acid and pyridoxine content but those available were included.

Seafood is also low in calcium except where the small bones have been included, as in some canned fish (Table 9.3). Most fish are low in sodium and moderate in potassium. Although the content of iron and zinc varies appreciably among species, several varieties are good sources of these minerals.

Many trace minerals were not included in these tables. Two reviews provide comprehensive findings of trace minerals in seafood for those seeking this information (3, 358).

## Canned Fish

The data in Table 9.3 were presented separately from the data on raw seafood for convenience. Sodium content of canned seafood is usually very high, but actual levels differ among brands. Only diet pack fish is low in sodium. Fish packed in sauce also has considerable carbohydrate owing to the presence of vegetables and sometimes sugar. Data on the nutrient content of different brands is usually available directly from the manufacturer and has not been included here.

## Hawaiian and New Zealand Species

Fish consumed in the Hawaiian Islands is sometimes, but not always the same species as those available in the continental United States. The local names, however, are entirely different so that Table 9.4 includes Hawaiian, common and Latin names (357). Only proximate composition and sodium has been included as information about vitamin and mineral content is sparse.

New Zealand species are becoming increasingly available in the U.S. market and much data are available on the nutrient composition of the major New Zealand species. Cholesterol and fatty acid composition data are available for only a few species at the present time. The omega-3 fatty acid content for several species has been calculated as in Table 9.1 but other fatty acids were omitted because of scarcity of data. Total calories were calculated using the same calorie equivalents as in Table 9.1.

The fat content of New Zealand skipjack tuna differs from its tropical relatives. New Zealand skipjack is oily and tropical is not. Moreover, the red muscle is lower in oil than the white muscle, while in tropical skipjack tuna and many other red-fleshed fish, the red muscle is nearly always richer in oil than the white (23).

The available data on vitamin and mineral content of New Zealand species is presented in Table 9.6.

**Table 9.1  Nutrient Composition of Finfish[a]**

| Species: | Calories[f] kcal | Protein gm | Total Fat gm | Fatty Acids Sat'd[b] gm | Mono[b] gm | Poly[b] gm | Omega-3[c] gm | Chole-sterol mg | Refer-ences |
|---|---|---|---|---|---|---|---|---|---|
| Amberjack *Seriola dumerili* | 159 | 18.9 | 8.7 (.8-21.2)[e] | —[d] | — | — | — | — | 3 |
| Anchovy *Engraulis mordax* | 127 | 19.6 | 4.8 (.4-6.4) | 1.3 | 1.2 | 1.7 | 1.4 | 108 | 3, 316 |
| Arctic char *Salvelinus alpinus* | 163 | 21.4 | 7.9 (7.7-8.1) | 1.7 | 5.0 | .9 | — | 27 | 3, 317, 318 |
| Barracuda, Pacific *Sphyraena argentea* | 118 | 21.2 | 3.1 (1.5-4.6) | .7 | .8 | 1.2 | — | — | 3, 44 |
| Bass, black sea *Centropristis striata* | 96 | 18.4 | 1.9 (.8-3.0) | — | — | — | — | — | 3, 251 |
| Bass, striped *Morone saxatilis* | 94 | 17.3 | 2.2 (1.5-2.9) | .5 | .7 | .7 | .7 | 80 | 316, 317 |
| Bluefish *Pomatomus saltatrix* | 112 | 20.1 | 2.9 (1.5-7.4) | — | — | — | — | — | 3, 251 |
| Bonito *Sarda sarda* (Atlantic) | 149 | 23.2 | 5.5 (1.5-11.5) | — | — | — | — | — | 3 |
| *Sarda chiliensis* (Pacific) | 159 | 22.9 | 6.8 (2.6-10.2) | — | — | — | — | 55 | 44 |
| Buffalo or sucker *Ictiobus cyprinellus* (big mouth) | 215 | 15.3 | 16.6 | — | — | — | — | — | 3 |
| Butterfish *Peprilus triacanthus* | 175 | 17.3 | 11.2 (5.1-17.3) | — | — | — | — | 65 | 3, 317 |

**Table 9.1** *Nutrient Composition of Finfish*

| Species | Vit A I.U. | Thiamin mg | Riboflavin mg | Niacin mg | Vit B6 mg | Vit B12 mcg | Pantothenic Acid mg | Calcium mg | Phosphorus mg | Iron mg | Zinc mg | Sodium mg | Potassium mg |
|---|---|---|---|---|---|---|---|---|---|---|---|---|---|
| Amberjack *Seriola dumerili* | — | .18 | .08 | 10.0 | — | 14.3 | — | — | 253 | — | .7 | 52 | — |
| Anchovy *Engraulis mordax* | 490 | .07 | .20 | 3.1 | .14 | 6.3 | — | 150 | 242 | 1.5 | .9 | 148 | 413 |
| Arctic char *Salvelinus alpinus* | — | .31 | .30 | 9.6 | .33 | 7.8 | 1.9 | 20 | 270 | 1.0 | .8 | 65 | 468 |
| Barracuda, Pacific *Sphyraena argentea* | — | .1 | .07 | 4.0 | — | .9 | — | 70 | 258 | .8 | .5 | 46 | — |
| Bass, black sea *Centropristis striata* | — | — | — | — | — | — | — | 10 | 193 | .1 | .4 | 62 | 306 |
| Bass, striped *Morone saxatilis* | — | — | — | — | — | 3.8 | — | 15 | 198 | .8 | .3 | — | — |
| Bluefish *Pomatomus saltatrix* | — | .14 | .12 | 1.6 | — | — | — | 33 | 340 | 2.8 | .8 | 32 | 327 |
| Bonito *Sarda sarda* (Atlantic) | — | — | — | — | — | — | — | — | — | 5.9 | — | — | — |
| *Sarda chiliensis* (Pacific) | — | .01 | .05 | 12.8 | — | — | — | 28 | 246 | 6.0 | .6 | — | — |
| Buffalo or sucker *Ictiobus cyprinellus* (big mouth) | — | — | — | — | — | — | — | — | — | — | — | — | — |
| Butterfish *Peprilus triacanthus* | — | — | — | — | — | — | — | — | — | — | .8 | 81 | 338 |

**Table 9.1 Nutrient Composition of Finfish[a]**

| Species: | Calories[f] | Protein | Total Fat | Fatty Acids | | | | Cholesterol | References |
|---|---|---|---|---|---|---|---|---|---|
| | | | | Sat'd[b] | Mono[b] | Poly[b] | Omega-3[c] | | |
| | kcal | gm | gm | gm | gm | gm | gm | mg | |
| Carp *Cyprinus carpio* | 147 | 16.4 | 8.5 (1.3-15.4) | 1.5 | 4.2 | 1.7 | .5 | 64 | 3, 316-9 |
| Catfish: | | | | | | | | | |
| Freshwater catfish *Ictalurus punctatus* | 115 | 17.6 | 4.4 (.7-11.0) | 1.1 | 1.8 | 1.1 | .6 | 52 | 3, 316, 317, 319 |
| Ocean catfish, wolffish *Anarhichas lupus* | 101 | 17.6 | 2.9 (2.1-3.0) | .4 | 1.0 | 1.0 | .7 | — | 3, 316, 317, 319 |
| Sea catfish *Ariidae* | 108 | 17.6 | 3.6 (.2-16.8) | — | — | — | — | — | 3, 320 |
| Cisco *Coregonus artedii* | 108 | 18.2 | 3.3 (1.5-6.8) | — | — | — | — | 18 | 3, 317, 318 |
| Cod, Atlantic *Gadus morhua* | 75 | 16.4 | 0.6 (.1-1.2) | 0.1 | .1 | .2 | .2 | 42 | 3, 80, 317, 321 |
| Pacific *Gadus macrocephalus* | 80 | 17.3 | 0.7 (.1-2.0) | .1 | .1 | .4 | .1 | 37 | 3, 316, 322 |
| Crevalle jack *Caranx crysos* (blue runner) | 112 | 21.5 | 2.2 (1.2-3.1) | — | — | — | — | — | 3 |
| Croaker, Atlantic *Micropogon undulatus* | 91 | 17.8 | 1.7 (.4-5.8) | .6 | .6 | .3 | — | 61 | 3, 317 |
| Cusk *Brosme brosme* | 84 | 18.5 | 0.6 (.2-1.8) | — | — | — | — | — | 3, 109, 317 |
| Drum, black drum, black croaker *Pogonias cromis* | 87 | 17.3 | 1.5 (.5-2.9) | .5 | .6 | .4 | — | — | 3, 317 |
| Drum, red drum *Sciaenops ocellata* | 90 | 19.0 | 1.0 | — | — | — | — | — | 3 |

**Table 9.1  Nutrient Composition of Finfish**

| Species | Vit A (I.U.) | Thiamin (mg) | Riboflavin (mg) | Niacin (mg) | Vit $B_6$ (mg) | Vit $B_{12}$ (mcg) | Pantothenic Acid (mg) | Calcium (mg) | Phosphorus (mg) | Iron (mg) | Zinc (mg) | Sodium (mg) | Potassium (mg) |
|---|---|---|---|---|---|---|---|---|---|---|---|---|---|
| Carp *Cyprinus carpio* | 29 | .06 | .20 | 2.7 | .19 | 0.9 | .15 | 24 | 188 | 1.0 | 1.4 | 57 | 307 |
| Catfish: Freshwater catfish *Ictalurus punctatus* | 0 | .04 | .11 | 2.1 | — | 0.2 | .47 | 46 | 221 | 1.0 | .8 | 63 | 348 |
| Ocean catfish, wolffish *Anarhichus lupus* | 375 | .18 | .08 | 2.1 | .35 | 2.0 | .57 | 6 | — | .9 | .5 | 76 | — |
| Sea catfish *Ariidae* | 96 | .07 | .08 | 1.8 | — | 2.4 | — | 40 | 176 | — | — | 100 | 456 |
| Cisco *Coregonus artedii* | — | .05 | .38 | 2.5 | — | — | — | 30 | 175 | .4 | — | 55 | 511 |
| Cod, Atlantic *Gadus morhua* | 38 | .12 | .15 | 1.9 | .20 | .8 | .14 | 16 | 265 | .4 | .6 | 67 | 38 |
| Pacific *Gadus macrocephalus* | 28 | .02 | .04 | 2.0 | .22 | .4 | .15 | 10 | 184 | .2 | .3 | 69 | 380 |
| Crevalle jack *Caranx crysos* (blue runner) | — | — | — | — | — | — | — | 72 | 316 | — | — | — | — |
| Croaker, Atlantic *Micropogon undulatus* | — | .08 | .10 | 5.5 | — | — | — | 35 | 180 | — | .4 | 72 | 234 |
| Cusk *Brosme brosme* | 30 | .04 | .14 | 2.7 | .29 | .8 | .20 | 10 | 204 | .4 | .8 | 31 | 392 |
| Drum, black drum/black croaker *Pogonias cromis* | — | — | — | — | — | — | — | — | — | — | .4 | 51 | 226 |
| Drum, red drum *Sciaenops ocellata* | 30[g] | .06[g] | .17[g] | 2.4[g] | — | — | — | — | — | — | — | — | — |

**Table 9.1  Nutrient Composition of Finfish[a]**

| Species: | Calories[f] kcal | Protein gm | Total Fat gm | Fatty Acids Sat'd[b] gm | Mono[b] gm | Poly[b] gm | Omega-3[c] gm | Cholesterol mg | References |
|---|---|---|---|---|---|---|---|---|---|
| Eel, American eel *Anguilla rostrata* | 223 | 18.8 | 15.8 (11.6-18.3) | 3.4 | 7.7 | 2.3 | 1.2 | 10[g] | 3, 316, 319 |
| Flounder, flatfish or sole: | | | | | | | | | |
| Bothidae/ Pleuronectidae | 82 | 16.8 | 1.2 (.1-4.8) | .4 | .5 | .4 | — | 48 | 3, 81, 317, 319, 321 |
| Blackback, winter flounder, lemon sole *Pseudopleuronectes americanus* | 92 | 19.6 | 0.9 (.2-1.4) | — | — | — | — | — | 3, 251, 319 |
| Yellowtail *Limanda ferruginea* | 94 | 20.4 | 0.8 | .3 | .2 | .4 | .2 | — | 316 |
| Summer, fluke *Paralichthys dentatus* | 89 | 20.0 | 0.4 (.1-1.0) | — | — | — | — | — | 3 |
| Starry, rough jacket *Platichthys stellatus* | 86 | 17.1 | 1.5 (.8-3.5) | — | — | — | — | — | 3, 322 |
| Grouper: | | | | | | | | | |
| Black grouper *Mycteroperca bonaci* | 93 | 20.4 | 0.7 | — | — | — | — | — | 3 |
| Jewfish, giant sea bass *Epinephelus itajara* | 96 | 19.8 | 1.3 | .4 | .4 | .5 | — | 49 | 317 |
| Red grouper *Epinephelus morio* | 91 | 19.2 | 1.0 (.2-4.0) | .3 | .2 | .4 | — | — | 3, 317 |
| Hake: see whiting also | | | | | | | | | |
| Red hake *Urophycis chuss* | 70 | 15.2 | 0.6 | .1 | .2 | .2 | — | 35 | 80 |
| Silver hake, Atlantic whiting *Merluccius bilinearis* | 87 | 15.8 | 2.2 (.2-3.8) | .4 | .6 | .7 | .4 | — | 3, 80, 316, 317 |

**Table 9.1**  *Nutrient Composition of Finfish*

| Species | Vit A I.U. | Thia-min mg | Ribo-flavin mg | Niacin mg | Vit B6 mg | Vit B12 mcg | Panto-thenic Acid mg | Cal-cium mg | Phos-phorus mg | Iron mg | Zinc mg | Sodium mg | Potas-sium mg |
|---|---|---|---|---|---|---|---|---|---|---|---|---|---|
| Eel, or American eel *Anguilla rostrata* | 2700[g] | .15[g] | .46 | 2.6[g] | .23 | 1.0 | .15 | 56 | 247 | 2.7[g] | 1.0 | — | — |
| Flounder, flatfish or sole: *Bothidae/Pleuronectidae* | 110 | .11 | .08 | 3.4 | .17 | 2.6 | .85 | 32 | 184 | .6 | .5 | 121 | 332 |
| Blackback, winter flounder, lemon sole *Pseudopleuronectes americanus* | 40 | — | .14 | 3.4 | — | .8 | .30 | 13 | 220 | .1 | .4 | 33 | 595 |
| Yellowtail *Limanda ferruginea* | — | — | — | — | — | — | — | 27 | 203 | — | .5 | 64 | 314 |
| Summer, fluke *Paralichtys dentatus* | — | — | — | — | — | — | — | — | — | — | — | — | — |
| Starry, rough jacket *Platichthys stellatus* | — | .14 | .11 | 3.5 | .13 | 1.0 | — | 4 | 384 | .5 | .5 | 64 | 424 |
| Grouper: Black grouper *Mycteroperca bonaci* | — | — | — | — | — | — | — | 11 | 214 | — | — | — | — |
| Jewfish, giant sea bass *Epinephelus itajara* | — | — | — | — | — | — | — | — | — | — | .6 | — | — |
| Red grouper *Epinephelus morio* | — | .11 | .37 | 1.4 | — | — | — | 40 | 184 | 0.2 | .4 | 80 | 358 |
| Hake: see whiting also Red hake *Urophycis chuss* | — | — | — | — | — | — | — | 20 | — | — | — | — | — |
| Silver hake, Atlantic whiting *Merluccius bilinearis* | — | — | — | — | — | — | — | 45 | 201 | — | .4 | 83 | 308 |

**Table 9.1  Nutrient Composition of Finfish[a]**

| Species: | Calories[f] | Protein | Total Fat | Fatty Acids | | | | Cholesterol | References |
|---|---|---|---|---|---|---|---|---|---|
| | | | | Sat'd[b] | Mono[b] | Poly[b] | Omega-3[c] | | |
| | kcal | gm | gm | gm | gm | gm | gm | mg | |
| Haddock *Melanogrammus aeglefinus* | 83 | 18.2 | 0.6 (.1-1.0) | .1 | .1 | .2 | .2 | 58 | 3, 316, 317, 319 |
| Halibut: Atlantic *Hippoglossus hippoglossus* | 115 | 19.3 | 3.6 (1.1-8.5) | .6 | .6 | 1.4 | 1.3 | 47 | 316, 317 |
| Pacific *Hippoglossus stenolepsis* | 105 | 20.0 | 2.2 (.9-3.8) | .4 | .9 | .8 | .5 | 32 | 3, 80, 316, 317, 319, 322 |
| Herring: *Clupeidae* | 101 | 17.7 | 2.8 (1.3-19.2) | — | — | — | — | 53 | 3, 265 |
| Atlantic *Clupea harengus harengus* | 149 | 18.0 | 8.0 (2.4-20.2) | 2.0 | 3.6 | 2.1 | 1.2 | 53 | 3, 109, 317 |
| Pacific *Clupea harengus pallasii* | 162 | 17.3 | 9.8 (2.6-19.0) | 2.3 | 5.0 | 1.5 | 1.2 | 77 | 3, 316, 317 |
| Thread herring *Opistonema oglinum* | 112 | 20.7 | 2.6 (2.6-19.0) | 1.0 | .5 | .9 | .6 | — | 3, 317, 331 |
| Inconnu *Stenodus leucichthys* | 184 | 18.2 | 11.8 (4.1-18.8) | — | — | — | — | 43 | 317, 318 |
| Lingcod *Ophiodon elongatus* | 86 | 18.2 | 0.9 (.5-1.3) | — | — | — | — | — | 3, 322 |

## Table 9.1  Nutrient Composition of Finfish

| Species | Vit A | Thiamin | Riboflavin | Niacin | Vit B$_6$ | Vit B$_{12}$ | Pantothenic Acid | Calcium | Phosphorus | Iron | Zinc | Sodium | Potassium |
|---|---|---|---|---|---|---|---|---|---|---|---|---|---|
| | I.U. | mg | mg | mg | mg | mcg | mg | mg | mg | mg | mg | mg | mg |
| Haddock *Melanogrammus aeglefinus* | 46 | .04 | .09 | 3.4 | .2 | 1.2 | .13 | 27 | 203 | .8 | .6 | 98 | 357 |
| Halibut: | | | | | | | | | | | | | |
| Atlantic *Hippoglossus hippoglossus* | 155 | .07 | .08 | 5.0 | .3 | 1.0 | .31 | 16 | 364 | — | .3 | 71 | 412 |
| Pacific *Hippoglossus stenolepsis* | — | .12 | .06 | 9.2 | .34 | 1.0 | .28 | 34 | 222 | .1 | .3 | 59 | 434 |
| Herring: *Clupeidae* | — | — | — | — | — | — | — | 58 | 262 | — | — | 105 | 322 |
| Atlantic *Clupea harengus harengus* | 128 | .10 | .25 | 3.8 | .81 | 11.8 | .97 | 38 | 280 | 1.0 | .8 | 89 | 240 |
| Pacific *Clupea harengus pallasii* | 100 | .06 | .20 | 2.2 | — | 1.7 | — | 83 | 228 | 1.4 | .5 | 96 | 420 |
| Thread Herring *Opisthonema oglinum* | — | — | — | — | — | — | — | 166 | 324 | — | .9 | — | — |
| Inconnu *Stenodus leucichthys* | — | .06 | .30 | 4.4 | — | — | — | 16 | 166 | .2 | — | 36 | 329 |
| Lingcod *Ophiodon elongatus* | 25 | .03 | .11 | 1.9 | — | 10.8 | — | 25 | 206 | .4 | .4 | 50 | 424 |

**Table 9.1** *Nutrient Composition of Finfish*[a]

| Species: | Calories[f] kcal | Protein gm | Total Fat gm | Sat'd[b] gm | Mono[b] gm | Poly[b] gm | Omega-3[c] gm | Cholesterol mg | References |
|---|---|---|---|---|---|---|---|---|---|
| | | | | **Fatty Acids** | | | | | |
| Mackerel: *Scombridae* | 173 | 19.5 | 9.9 (.1-17.7) | — | — | — | — | 34 | 3 |
| Atlantic mackerel *Scomber scombrus* | 176 | 18.5 | 10.7 (.7-24.0) | 2.6 | 4.0 | 2.6 | 1.9 | 80 | 3, 316, 319, 323 |
| Pacific mackerel (chub) *Scomber japonicus* | 129 | 20.8 | 4.8 (.3-15.9) | 1.5 | 1.0 | 1.8 | 1.1 | 52 | 3, 264, 317, 319 |
| King mackerel *Scomberomorus cavalla* | 140 | 23.0 | 4.6 | — | — | — | — | — | 3 |
| Spanish mackerel *Scomberomorus maculatus* | 138 | 19.8 | 5.9 (.6-14.4) | — | — | — | — | — | 3 |
| Jack mackerel *Trachurus japonicus* | 98 | 19.1 | 1.8 (.9-3.2) | — | — | — | — | 32 | 3 |
| Mahimahi, dolphin fish *Coryphaena hippurus* | 89 | 18.9 | 0.9 (.2-3.2) | .3 | .2 | .3 | — | 86[h] | 3, 317 |
| Monkfish, goosefish, anglerfish *Lophius americanus* and *L. piscatorius* | 80 | 15.5 | 1.5 (.7-7.5) | — | — | — | — | 35 | 3, 317 |
| Mullet, striped *Mugil cephalus* | 115 | 19.2 | 3.7 (.7-20.2) | 1.1 | 1.1 | .7 | .4 | 35 | 3, 316, 317, 319 |
| Orange roughy *Hoplostethus atlanticus* | 65 | 14.7 | 0.3[i] | 0 | — | 0 | 0 | — | 324 |

**Table 9.1  Nutrient Composition of Finfish**

| Species | Vit A | Thiamin | Riboflavin | Niacin | Vit B$_6$ | Vit B$_{12}$ | Pantothenic Acid | Calcium | Phosphorus | Iron | Zinc | Sodium | Potassium |
|---|---|---|---|---|---|---|---|---|---|---|---|---|---|
| | I.U. | mg | mg | mg | mg | mcg | mg | mg | mg | mg | mg | mg | mg |
| Mackerel: *Scombridae* | 100 | .10 | .19 | 8.6 | — | — | — | 22 | 216 | 1.4 | 0.5 | 94 | 486 |
| Atlantic mackerel *Scomber scombrus* | 132 | .12 | .37 | 8.4 | 1.2 | 6.6 | .85 | 9 | 262 | 1.1 | .6 | 35 | 280 |
| Pacific mackerel (chub) *Scomber japonicus* | 76 | .09 | .44 | 12.0 | .4 | 2.3 | .26 | — | — | 2.0 | .5 | 99 | 372 |
| King mackerel *Scomberomorus cavalla* | — | — | — | — | — | — | — | 9 | 279 | — | .1 | — | — |
| Spanish mackerel *Scomberomorus maculatus* | — | .14 | .18 | 5.5 | — | 1.4 | — | 34 | 208 | 1.0 | .3 | 44 | 234 |
| Jack mackerel *Trachurus japonicus* | 7 | .14 | .14 | 6.5 | — | 3.5 | — | — | — | .4 | .1 | — | — |
| Mahimahi, dolphin fish *Coryphaena hippurus* | 179 | .02 | .07 | 6.1 | — | .6 | — | 15 | 143 | 1.7 | .5 | 128 | 370 |
| Monkfish, goosefish, anglerfish *Lophius americanus* and *L. piscatorius* | 165 | .02 | — | — | — | — | — | 19 | 225 | 1.5 | .5 | 180 | 297 |
| Mullet, striped *Mugil cephalus* | 150 | .08 | .08 | 5.2 | .42 | .22 | .75 | 33 | 228 | 1.2 | .6 | 81 | 308 |
| Orange roughy *Hoplostethus atlanticus* | — | — | — | — | — | — | — | — | — | — | — | — | — |

**Table 9.1  Nutrient Composition of Finfish[a]**

| Species: | Calories[f] | Protein | Total Fat | Fatty Acids | | | | Cholesterol | References |
| | | | | Sat'd[b] | Mono[b] | Poly[b] | Omega-3[c] | | |
| | kcal | gm | gm | gm | gm | gm | gm | mg | |
|---|---|---|---|---|---|---|---|---|---|
| **Perch:** | | | | | | | | | |
| Lake perch, yellow perch *Perca flavescens* | 86 | 18.1 | 1.0 (.5-4.0) | .2 | .2 | .5 | .2 | 90 | 3, 318, 325, 326 |
| Ocean perch, redfish *Sebastes marinus* | 105 | 18.7 | 2.8 (.6-8.4) | .4 | 1.0 | .8 | .4 | — | 3, 80, 319, 321 |
| Pike, northern *Esox lucius* | 87 | 18.5 | 0.9 (.5-1.2) | .2 | .2 | .3 | .1 | 49 | 3, 316, 318, 319 |
| Walleye pike *Stizostedion vitreum* | | 19.2 | 1.4 (.5-2.0) | .2 | .2 | .3 | .2 | 34 | 317, 318, 326 |
| Sauger, sand pike, yellow walleye *Stizostedion canadense* | 83 | 17.1 | 1.1 | — | — | — | — | 58 | 318 |
| Pilchard, California pilchard *Sardinops ocellata* | 167 | 19.2 | 9.4 (3.1-15.6) | 2.4 | 2.3 | 3.4 | 2.9 | — | 3, 316 |
| **Pollock:** | | | | | | | | | |
| Atlantic pollock *Pollachius virens* | 90 | 19.2 | 0.9 (.2-2.0) | .1 | .1 | .4 | .4 | — | 3, 316 |
| Pacific pollock *Theragra chalcogramma* | 78 | 16.7 | 0.8 | — | — | — | — | — | 3, 319, 322, 327 |

**Table 9.1  Nutrient Composition of Finfish**

| Species | Vit A | Thia-min | Ribo-flavin | Niacin | Vit B$_6$ | Vit B$_{12}$ | Panto-thenic Acid | Cal-cium | Phos-phorus | Iron | Zinc | Sodium | Potas-sium |
|---|---|---|---|---|---|---|---|---|---|---|---|---|---|
| | I.U. | mg | mg | mg | mg | mcg | mg | mg | mg | mg | mg | mg | mg |
| Perch: | | | | | | | | | | | | | |
| Lake perch, yellow perch *Perca flavescens* | 40 | .35 | .34 | 1.8 | — | — | — | 95 | 192 | .6 | 1.2 | 61 | 301 |
| Ocean perch, redfish *Sebastes marinus* | 125 | — | — | — | .23 | 1.0 | .36 | 141 | 223 | .8 | .7 | 81 | 307 |
| Pike, northern *Esox lucius* | 70 | .14 | .08 | 1.6 | .12 | — | — | 143 | 183 | .4 | .9 | 48 | 351 |
| Walleye pike *Stizostedion vitreum* | — | .02 | .52 | 1.8 | — | — | — | 60 | 193 | .8 | .7 | 65 | 430 |
| Sauger, sand pike, yellow walleye *Stizostedion canadense* | — | .03 | .39 | — | — | — | — | 8 | 186 | .4 | — | 79 | 318 |
| Pilchard, California pilchard *Sardinops ocellata* | — | — | — | — | — | — | — | — | — | 2.5 | — | — | — |
| Pollock: | | | | | | | | | | | | | |
| Atlantic pollock *Pollachius virens* | — | — | — | — | .12 | — | .30 | — | — | — | — | — | — |
| Pacific pollock *Theragra chalcogramma* | 66 | .17 | .17 | — | .06 | .30 | .33 | 9 | 376 | — | .4 | — | 428 |

**Table 9.1  Nutrient Composition of Finfish[a]**

| Species: | Calories[f] | Protein | Total Fat | Fatty Acids | | | | Chole-sterol | References |
|---|---|---|---|---|---|---|---|---|---|
| | | | | Sat'd[b] | Mono[b] | Poly[b] | Omega-3[c] | | |
| | kcal | gm | gm | gm | gm | gm | gm | mg | |
| Pompano, Atlantic *Trachinotus carolinus* | 165 | 18.5 | 9.5 (3.8-15.6) | 3.8 | 2.8 | 1.2 | — | 50 | 317 |
| *Trachinotus palometus* | 95 | 20.5 | 0.8 | — | — | — | — | — | 3 |
| Pacific *Neptomenus crassus* | 100 | 19.1 | 2.0 (.7-3.3) | — | — | — | — | — | 3 |
| Porgy, scup, sea broom *Stenotomus chrysops* | 109 | 18.8 | 3.2 (1.2-5.9) | — | — | — | — | — | 3 |
| Rockfish *Scorpaenidae* | 78 | 16.2 | 1.0 (.5-1.4) | .2 | .2 | .4 | .3 | — | 3, 319 |
| Black *Sebastodes melanops* | 88 | 17.9 | 1.3 (1.0-1.8) | — | — | — | — | — | 3 |
| Canary, Orange *Sebastodes pinniger* | 96 | 18.8 | 1.8 (.4-6.0) | .4 | .5 | .7 | — | 35 | 317, 322 |
| Yellow *Sebastodes flavidus* | 95 | 18.9 | 1.6 | — | — | — | — | — | 3 |
| Sablefish, black cod *Anoploploma fimbria* | 184 | 13.2 | 14.2 (6.4-23.6) | 3.2 | 8.1 | 2.0 | 1.3 | 49 | 3, 316, 322 |
| Salmon, Atlantic *Salmo salar* | 129 | 18.4 | 5.6 (.2-14.5) | .9 | 2.0 | 2.4 | 1.4 | — | 3, 317 |
| Salmon: Pacific Chinook, king *Oncorhynchus tschawytscha* | 184 | 19.0 | 11.4 (2.2-19.0) | 3.0 | 5.4 | 2.4 | 1.9 | — | 3, 316, 317, 322 |
| Chum, keta *Oncorhynchus keta* | 125 | 20.4 | 4.2 (1.3-7.9) | 1.1 | 2.0 | 1.0 | 0.6 | 74 | 3, 316, 317 |

**Table 9.1** *Nutrient Composition of Finfish*

| Species | Vit A | Thia- min | Ribo- flavin | Niacin | Vit B₆ | Vit B₁₂ | Panto- thenic Acid | Cal- cium | Phos- phorus | Iron | Zinc | Sodium | Potas- sium |
|---|---|---|---|---|---|---|---|---|---|---|---|---|---|
| | I.U. | mg | mg | mg | mg | mcg | mg | mg | mg | mg | mg | mg | mg |
| Pompano, Atlantic *Trachinotus carolinus* | — | .56 | .12 | 3.0 | — | — | — | 22 | 195 | .6 | .7 | 65 | 380 |
| *Trachinotus palometus* | — | — | — | — | — | — | — | 18 | 143 | — | — | — | — |
| Pacific *Neptomenus crassus* | .5 | .09 | .06 | 8.1 | — | — | — | — | — | 2.7 | — | — | — |
| Porgy, scup, sea bream *Stenotomus chrysops* | — | — | — | — | — | — | — | — | — | — | .5 | 63 | 287 |
| Rockfish *Scorpaenidae* | — | .06 | .12 | — | .06 | 3.2 | .08 | — | — | — | .1 | — | — |
| Black *Sebastodes melanops* | — | .05 | .08 | 2.8 | — | — | — | 5 | 204 | .3 | .2 | 49 | 408 |
| Canary, Orange, *Sebastodes pinniger* | 23 | .04 | .06 | 2.7 | — | — | — | 9 | 200 | .4 | .4 | 48 | 359 |
| Yellowtail *Sebastodes flavidus* | 16 | .04 | .08 | 3.4 | — | — | — | — | — | — | .4 | 54 | 382 |
| Sablefish, black cod, *Anoploma fimbria* | 1029 | .10 | .08 | — | — | — | — | 35 | 168 | 1.2 | .3 | 56 | 469 |
| Salmon, Atlantic *Salmo salar* | 40 | .16 | .28 | 8.0 | .82 | 8.2 | 1.9 | 15 | 210 | 1.0 | .5 | 44 | 410 |
| Salmon: Pacific Chinook, king *Oncorhynchus tschawytscha* | 274 | .07 | .16 | 7.8 | — | — | — | 14 | 404 | 1.1 | .6 | 56 | 321 |
| Chum, keta *Oncorhynchus keta* | 73 | .09 | .13 | — | — | .14 | — | 12 | 283 | .5 | 1.0 | 50 | 396 |

**Table 9.1  Nutrient Composition of Finfish[a]**

| Species: | Calories[f] kcal | Protein gm | Total Fat gm | Fatty Acids | | | | Cholesterol mg | References |
| --- | --- | --- | --- | --- | --- | --- | --- | --- | --- |
| | | | | Sat'd[b] gm | Mono[b] gm | Poly[b] gm | Omega-3[c] gm | | |
| Coho, silver *Oncorhynchus kisutch* | 150 | 21.1 | 6.6 (1.3-9.9) | 1.1 | 2.4 | 2.0 | 1.5 | — | 3, 316, 317 |
| Pink, humpback *Oncorhynchus gorbuscha* | 131 | 20.1 | 5.0 (1.8-12.5) | .8 | 1.4 | 2.0 | 1.5 | — | 3, 316 |
| Sockeye *Oncorhynchus nerka* | 158 | 20.3 | 7.9 (1.6-13.2) | 1.6 | 1.3 | 4.2 | 2.7 | 35 | 3, 82, 316, 317, 322 |
| Sardine: *Clupeidae* | 142 | 18.9 | 6.8 (2.3-15.2) | — | — | — | — | 52 | 3, 319 |
| Sardine, Spanish *Sardinella aurita* | 133 | 21.5 | 4.6 (2.3-9.9) | 1.5 | .8 | 1.8 | 1.2 | — | 3, 331 |
| Sauger *Stizostedion canadense* | 83 | 17.1 | 1.1 | — | — | — | — | 58 | 318 |
| Sea trout: Gray, weakfish *Cynoscion regalis* | 106 | 17.5 | 3.5 (0.8-6.0) | 1.1 | 1.0 | .70 | .50 | — | 3, 225, 251, 317 |
| Spotted, speckled *Cynoscion nebulosus* | 97 | 18.8 | 1.9 (1.4-3.2) | .5 | .4 | .4 | — | — | 3, 317 |
| Shad, American *Alosa sapidissima* | 187 | 17.4 | 12.5 (3.0-17.2) | — | — | — | — | — | 3, 317, 322 |
| Shark: Spiny dogfish *Squalus acanthias* | 167 | 15.1 | 114 (3.6-17.9) | 3.8 | 4.3 | 2.4 | 1.9 | 46 | 316, 317, 319, 328 |
| Blue shark *Carcharhinus bracyurus* | 82 | 18.9 | 0.1 | — | — | — | — | — | 3 |
| *Carcharhinus glaucus* | 64 | 12.5 | 1.2 (.5-2.0) | — | — | — | — | — | 3 |

**Table 9.1  Nutrient Composition of Finfish**

| Species | Vit A (I.U.) | Thiamin (mg) | Riboflavin (mg) | Niacin (mg) | Vit B6 (mg) | Vit B12 (mcg) | Pantothenic Acid (mg) | Calcium (mg) | Phosphorus (mg) | Iron (mg) | Zinc (mg) | Sodium (mg) | Potassium (mg) |
|---|---|---|---|---|---|---|---|---|---|---|---|---|---|
| Coho, silver *Oncorhynchus kisutch* | — | .17 | .16 | 7.0 | — | — | — | 36 | 231 | 1.3 | .4 | 38 | 445 |
| Pink, humpback *Oncorhynchus gorbuscha* | 108 | .17 | .06 | 7.0 | — | — | — | 13 | 230 | .9 | .5 | 78 | 330 |
| Sockeye *Oncorhynchus nerka* | 137 | .14 | .13 | — | .19 | .23 | .61 | 6 | 230 | .9 | .4 | 46 | 338 |
| Sardine: *Clupeidae* | 229 | .08 | .23 | 8.2 | — | 11.0 | 1.1 | 73 | 240 | 2.3 | 1.0 | 100 | 55 |
| Sardine, Spanish *Sardinella aurita* | — | — | — | — | — | — | — | — | 331 | — | — | — | — |
| Sauger *Stizostedion canadense* | — | .03 | .39 | — | — | — | — | 8 | 186 | .4 | — | 79 | 318 |
| Sea trout: Gray weakfish *Cynoscion regalis* | — | — | — | — | — | — | — | 14 | 217 | .2 | .5 | 50 | 436 |
| Spotted, speckled *Cynoscion nebulosus* | — | — | — | — | — | — | — | 17 | 250 | .3 | .4 | 55 | 435 |
| Shad, American *Alosa sapidissima* | — | .15 | .24 | 8.4 | — | — | — | 47 | 237 | .8 | .3 | 52 | 384 |
| Shark: Spiny dogfish *Squalus acanthias* | 233 | .06 | .15 | 5.0 | — | 1.4 | .69 | 11 | 266 | — | .5 | 100 | 174 |
| Blue Shark *Carcharhinus bracyurus* | — | — | — | — | — | — | — | — | — | — | — | — | — |
| *Carcharhinus glaucus* | — | — | — | — | — | — | — | 5 | 150 | .4 | — | — | — |

**Table 9.1  Nutrient Composition of Finfish[a]**

| Species: | Calories[f] kcal | Protein gm | Total Fat gm | Fatty Acids Sat'd[b] gm | Mono[b] gm | Poly[b] gm | Omega-3[c] gm | Cholesterol mg | References |
|---|---|---|---|---|---|---|---|---|---|
| Smelt *Osmerus mordax* | 98 | 18.6 | 2.1 | .3 | .4 | .8 | .6 | 70 | 3, 316, 325/6 |
| Snapper: *Lutjanidae* | 90 | 18.8 | 1.1 (.3-2.1) | — | — | — | — | — | 3, 317 |
| Red *Lutjanus campechanus Lutjanus blackfordii* | 110 | 20.2 | 2.6 (.4-7.4) | .5 | .5 | .9 | .6 | 40 | 316, 317 |
| Yellowtail *Ocyurus chrysurus* | 98 | 19.9 | 1.4 (.7-2.5) | — | — | — | — | — | 3, 317 |
| Sole: *Soleidae/Pleuronectidae* | 88 | 17.9 | 1.3 (.3-2.0) | .4 | .3 | .1 | .1 | 43 | 3, 317 |
| Dover sole (Pacific) *Microstomus pacificus* | 73 | 15.1 | 0.9 (.6-1.2) | — | — | — | — | 48 | 3, 322 |
| English sole (Pacific) *Parophrys vetulus* | 87 | 16.8 | 1.7 (1.2-18) | — | — | — | — | — | 3, 322 |
| Petrale sole *Eopsetta jordani* | 92 | 18.2 | 1.6 (.9-3.4) | — | — | — | — | — | 3, 317, 322 |
| Rex sole *Glyptocephalus zachirus* | 76 | 16.4 | 0.7 (.4-3.2) | — | — | — | — | 39 | 3, 317, 322 |
| Rock sole *Lepidopsetta bilineata* | 88 | 18.6 | 1.0 (.7-1.6) | — | — | — | — | — | 3, 317 |
| Sand sole *P. settichthys melanostictus* | 74 | 16.4 | 0.5 | — | — | — | — | — | 3, 317 |
| Yellowfin sole *Limanda aspera* | 84 | 17.4 | 1.1 (.8-1.3) | — | — | — | — | — | 3 |

**Table 9.1  Nutrient Composition of Finfish**

| Species | Vit A | Thia-min | Ribo-flavin | Niacin | Vit B$_6$ | Vit B$_{12}$ | Panto-thenic Acid | Cal-cium | Phos-phorus | Iron | Zinc | Sodium | Potas-sium |
|---|---|---|---|---|---|---|---|---|---|---|---|---|---|
| | I.U. | mg | mg | mg | mg | mcg | mg | mg | mg | mg | mg | mg | mg |
| Smelt *Osmerus mordax* | — | .01 | .13 | 1.2 | — | — | — | 60 | 230 | 1.1 | 1.6 | 60 | 290 |
| Snapper: *Lutjanidae* | — | .07 | .07 | 1.8 | — | .3 | — | 41 | 192 | 4.3 | — | 90 | 323 |
| Red *Lutjanus campechanus* *Lutjanus blackfordii* | — | .12 | .05 | 1.8 | — | — | — | 22 | 134 | .6 | .4 | 96 | 362 |
| Yellowtail *Ocyurus chrysurus* | — | — | — | — | — | — | — | 28 | 217 | — | .4 | — | — |
| Sole: *Soleidae/Pleuronectidae* | 45 | .06 | .05 | 1.7 | — | — | — | 24 | 170 | .4 | .4 | 80 | 440 |
| Dover sole (Pacific) *Microstomus pacificus* | — | .06 | .05 | 1.6 | — | — | — | 29 | 146 | .2 | .2 | 85 | 311 |
| English sole (Pacific) *Parophrys vetulus* | — | .05 | .04 | 2.9 | — | .8 | — | 9 | 176 | .3 | .3 | 68 | 339 |
| Petrale sole *Eopsetta jordani* | — | .07 | .05 | — | — | — | — | 10 | 184 | .2 | .3 | 64 | 343 |
| Rex sole *Glyptocephalus zachirus* | 20 | — | — | — | — | — | — | 10 | 110 | — | .4 | 134 | 287 |
| Rock sole *Lepidopsetta bilineata* | — | .06 | .04 | — | — | — | — | — | — | — | .3 | 80 | 380 |
| Sand sole *Psettichthys melanosticus* | — | — | — | — | — | — | — | — | — | — | — | 56 | 344 |
| Yellowfin sole *Limanda aspera* | — | — | — | — | — | — | — | — | — | — | — | — | — |

**Table 9.1** *Nutrient Composition of Finfish*[a]

| Species: | Calories[f] | Protein | Total Fat | Fatty Acids | | | | Chole-sterol | References |
|---|---|---|---|---|---|---|---|---|---|
| | | | | Sat'd[b] | Mono[b] | Poly[b] | Omega-3[c] | | |
| | kcal | gm | gm | gm | gm | gm | gm | mg | |
| Spot *Leiostomus xanthurus* | 135 | 18.8 | 6.1 (2.7-10.2) | 1.8 | 1.7 | 1.4 | .8 | — | 3, 40, 251, 317 |
| Sturgeon, Atlantic *Acipenser sturio* | 98 | 16.3 | 3.2 (.6-6.2) | .8 | 1.7 | 0.3 | .2 | — | 3, 316 |
| Sturgeon, lake *Acipenser fulvescens* | 169 | 16.8 | 10.8 (9.1-12.5) | — | — | — | — | 18 | 3, 318 |
| Sucker, white *Catostomus commersoni* | 95 | 17.1 | 2.4 (1.1-3.2) | — | — | — | — | 33 | 3, 318 |
| Swordfish *Xiphias gladius* | 122 | 19.4 | 4.4 (2.0-6.7) | 1.3 | 1.9 | 1.1 | .9 | 48 | 3, 329 |
| Tilefish *Lopholatilus chamaelonticeps* | 90 | 18.6 | 1.2 | — | — | — | — | — | 3 |
| Trout: | | | | | | | | | |
| Rainbow *Salmo gairdneri* | 131 | 18.4 | 5.8 (2.1-13.6) | .9 | 1.0 | 2.2 | 1.1 | 56 | 3, 316-318, 325, 326 |
| Brook *Salvelinus fontinalis* | 108 | 20.0 | 2.5 (.7-4.6) | .5 | .6 | .7 | .3 | 68 | 3, 319, 325, 326 |
| Lake trout *Salvelinus namaycush* | 162 | 18.1 | 9.4 (4.6-21.8) | 1.2 | 3.0 | 2.6 | 1.4 | 36 | 3, 318, 325, 326 |
| Tuna:[k] | | | | | | | | | |
| Albacore or longfin *Thunnus alalunga* or *T. germo* | 172 | 25.2 | 7.2 (.7-13.2) | 1.9 | 1.9 | 2.7 | 2.1 | 38 | 3, 316, 317, 319, 322 |

**Table 9.1** *Nutrient Composition of Finfish*

| Species | Vit A | Thia-min | Ribo-flavin | Niacin | Vit B6 | Vit B12 | Panto-thenic Acid | Cal-cium | Phos-phorus | Iron | Zinc | Sodium | Potas-sium |
|---|---|---|---|---|---|---|---|---|---|---|---|---|---|
| | I.U. | mg | mg | mg | mg | mcg | mg | mg | mg | mg | mg | mg | mg |
| Spot *Leiostomus xanthurus* | — | — | — | — | — | — | — | 52 | 203 | .3 | .5 | 29 | 496 |
| Sturgeon, Atlantic *Acipenser sturio* | 700 | — | — | — | — | — | — | — | 466 | — | — | — | 284 |
| Sturgeon, lake *Acipenser fulvescens* | — | .06 | .31 | 2.3 | — | — | — | 14 | 147 | 1.5 | — | 50 | 270 |
| Sucker, white *Catostomus commersoni* | — | 0 | .27 | 1.7 | — | — | — | 42 | 164 | .4 | — | 52 | 678 |
| Swordfish *Xiphias gladius* | 1585j | .05 | .08 | 7.6 | — | 1.4 | .19 | 10 | 316 | .8 | 1.1 | 102 | 342 |
| Tilefish *Lopholatilus chamaelonticeps* | — | — | — | — | — | — | — | — | — | — | — | — | — |
| Trout: Rainbow *Salmo gairdneri* | 65 | .07 | .26 | 3.9 | .69 | 3.0 | 1.95 | 51 | 223 | 1.5 | 1.1 | 39 | 453 |
| Brook *Salvelinus fontinalis* | — | — | .09 | — | — | 3.0 | — | 80 | 258 | 1.4 | 1.2 | 60 | 430 |
| Lake trout *Salvelinus namaycush* | — | .01 | .36 | 3.9 | — | — | — | 44 | 202 | .7 | .7 | 40 | 286 |
| Tuna:k Albacore or longfin *Thunnus alalunga or T. germo* | 20 | .04 | .04 | 15.8 | .44 | .17 | .42 | 8 | 422 | 1.3 | .4 | 51 | 308 |

## Table 9.1  Nutrient Composition of Finfish[a]

| Species: | Calories[f] kcal | Protein gm | Total Fat gm | Fatty Acids Sat'd[b] gm | Mono[b] gm | Poly[b] gm | Omega-3[c] gm | Cholesterol mg | References |
|---|---|---|---|---|---|---|---|---|---|
| Bigeye *Thunnus obesus* | 112 | 22.8 | 1.6 (.9-3.5) | — | — | — | — | 66 | 3, 317, 319 |
| Bluefin *Thunnus thynnus* | 158 | 24.0 | 6.1 (.2-25.0) | 1.6 | 2.2 | 1.8 | 1.5 | 38 | 3, 316, 317, 319 |
| Skipjack *Euthynnus pelamis* | 130 | 24.9 | 2.7 (.2-11.0) | .9 | .5 | .6 | .5 | 32 | 3, 316, 317 |
| Yellowfin *Thunnus albacares* | 124 | 23.8 | 2.5 (.1-11.9) | .6 | .5 | .8 | .6 | 45 | 3, 316, 317 |
| Turbot, greenland: *Reinhardtius hippoglossoides* | 147 | 13.2 | 10.0[n] (8.4-12.4) | 1.9 | 6.3 | 1.0 | .6 | — | 3, 316, 319, 330 |
| Whitefish *Coregonus clupeaformis* | 162 | 18.8 | 9.0 (1.7-16.3) | 1.5 | 3.4 | 3.6 | — | 48 | 3, 318 |
| Whiting, Pacific *Merluccius productus* | 85 | 16.6 | 1.6 | .3 | .3 | .6 | .5 | — | 264, 316, 322 |

a   Data per 100 gm raw fillet
b   Corrected for non-fatty acid portion of the lipid according to Ref 356; sum of saturated, monounsaturated & polyunsaturated is less than total lipid
c   Sum of eicosapentaenoic acid (20:5) and docosahexaenoic acid (22:6)
d   Dashes denote lack of data, not zero values
e   Minimum range of values where data were provided
f   Calculated using the calorie equivalent factors for protein: 4.27 and fat: 9.02. Carbohydrate is not included (see text)
g   Value from closely related species
h   Estimated from data on cooked portion (107 mg/100 gm) assuming 80% yield and 100% retention (Chapter Five)
i   Total lipid is 8.5% of which 3.1% is triglyceride (256)
j   Vitamin A value unusually high & may be questioned
k   Average of light and dark meat
l   Range 1.9-250 mcg
m   Range 7.8-38.0 mcg
n   Fat content unusually high and may be questioned.

**Table 9.1** *Nutrient Composition of Finfish*

| Species | Vit A | Thia-min | Ribo-flavin | Niacin | Vit B$_6$ | Vit B$_{12}$ | Panto-thenic Acid | Cal-cium | Phos-phorus | Iron | Zinc | Sodium | Potas-sium |
|---|---|---|---|---|---|---|---|---|---|---|---|---|---|
| | I.U. | mg | mg | mg | mg | mcg | mg | mg | mg | mg | mg | mg | mg |
| Bigeye *Thunnus obesus* | — | .16 | .12 | 10.8 | .9 | 3.35 | .50 | 7 | 290 | 1.5 | .4 | 31 | — |
| Bluefin *Thunnus thynnus* | 963 | .24 | .26 | 8.6 | .46 | 16.3[m] | 1.1 | 8 | 254 | 1.2 | .6 | 58 | 252 |
| Skipjack *Euthynnus pelamis* | 52 | .06 | .08 | 22.0 | .9 | 66.5[l] | .5 | 24 | 272 | 1.9 | .8 | 37 | 392 |
| Yellowfin *Thunnus albacares* | 59 | .32 | .06 | 11.0 | — | .52 | — | 20 | 232 | 1.7 | .5 | 37 | 444 |
| Turbot, greenland *Reinhardtius hippoglossoides* | 39 | .07 | .06 | 1.0 | — | 1.25 | .25 | 12 | — | 1.0 | — | — | 500 |
| Whitefish *Coregonus clupeaformis* | — | .08 | .12 | 3.0 | — | — | — | 5 | 230 | .3 | 1.3 | 57 | 312 |
| Whiting, Pacific *Merluccius productus* | — | .05 | .06 | 2.2 | — | — | — | 18 | 175 | .4 | .3 | 66 | 328 |

*Table 9.2  Nutrient Composition of Shellfish*

| Species: | Calories | Carbohydrates | Protein | Total Fat | Fatty Acids | | | | Cholesterol | References |
|---|---|---|---|---|---|---|---|---|---|---|
| | | | | | Sat'd | Mono | Poly | Omega-3 | | |
| | kcal | gm | gm | gm | gm | gm | gm | gm | mg | |
| Molluscs: | | | | | | | | | | |
| Abalone | 98 | 5.1 | 17.0 | .5 | .10 | .09 | .12 | .04 | 111 | 3, 83, 332 |
| *Haliotidae*[a] | | | | (.1-1.1) | | | | | | |
| Clams: Whole | | | | | | | | | | |
| Soft shell: | | | | | | | | | | |
| Ipswich, belly, steamer whole: | 65 | 2.1 | 10.7 | 1.2 | .18 | .12 | .44 | .24 | 25[b] | 3, 83, 319, 332 |
| *Mya arenaria* | | | | (1.3-1.4) | | | | | | |
| Hard shell: | | | | | | | | | | |
| Quahog, cherrystone whole: | 60 | 2.8 | 9.2 | 1.0 | .16 | .16 | .33 | .24 | 40[b] | 3, 83, 251 |
| *Mercenaria mercenaria* | | | | (.2-2.0) | | | | | | |
| Razor | 75 | 3.4 | 11.2 | 1.5 | .27 | .21 | .54 | .26 | 107 | 3, 332 |
| *Solenidae* | | | | (1.0-2.4) | | | | | | |
| Surf or sea clams | 70 | 2.1 | 13.5 | 0.5 | .04 | .04 | .16 | .07 | 36[b] | 3, 38, 83, 332 |
| *Spisula solidissima* raw | | | | (.3-.8) | | | | | | |
| Mussels, Atlantic | 89 | 4.5 | 12.0 | 2.20 | .41 | .50 | .75 | .43 | 63 | 3, 83, 332-335 |
| *Mytilus edulis* | | | | (1.2-2.1) | | | | | | |
| Octopus | 77 | 1.7 | 14.8 | .80 | .22 | .08 | .26 | .21 | 122[d] | 3, 333 |
| *Octopus vulgaris* | | | | (.4-1.1) | | | | | | |
| Oysters: | | | | | | | | | | |
| Pacific or Japanese | 90 | 5.8 | 11.1 | 2.2 | .49 | .36 | .90 | .71 | 47 | 3, 86, 322, 333 |
| *Crassostrea gigas* | | | | (.8-2.6) | | | | | | |
| Eastern or American | 74 | 4.8 | 8.2 | 2.2 | .42 | .24 | .86 | .51 | 56 | 3, 251, 319, 333, 336, 337 |
| *Crassostrea virginica* | | | | (1.0-2.7) | | | | | | |

**Table 9.2** *Nutrient Composition of Shellfish*

| Species | Vit A | Thiamin | Riboflavin | Niacin | Vit B6 | Vit B12 | Pantothenic Acid | Calcium | Phosphorus | Iron | Zinc | Sodium | Potassium |
|---|---|---|---|---|---|---|---|---|---|---|---|---|---|
| | I.U. | mg | mg | mg | mg | mcg | mg | mg | mg | mg | mg | mg | mg |
| Molluscs | | | | | | | | | | | | | |
| Abalone *Haliotidae*[a] | 10 | .19 | .10 | 1.5 | — | — | — | 28 | 153 | 2.6 | — | — | — |
| Clams: Whole Soft shell: | | | | | | | | | | | | | |
| Ipswich, belly steamer whole: *Mya arenaria* | 300 | .01 | .14 | 1.8 | .08 | 85.5[c] | .30 | 53 | 152 | — | 1.7 | — | — |
| Hard shell: | | | | | | | | | | | | | |
| Quahog, cherrystone whole: *Mercenaria mercenaria* | — | .01 | .11 | 1.0 | — | — | — | 49 | 107 | 2.8 | 2.3 | 56 | 314 |
| Razor *Solenidae* | 17 | .09 | .49 | 1.5 | — | — | — | 50 | 164 | 11.0 | 6.3 | — | 143 |
| Surf or sea clams *Spisula solidissima* raw | — | — | — | — | — | — | — | 41 | 194 | — | — | — | — |
| Mussels, Atlantic *Mytilus edulis* | — | .16 | .21 | — | — | 12 | — | 20 | 288 | 7.3 | 2.8 | 270 | 273 |
| Octopus *Octopus vulgaris* | 32 | .12 | .11 | 5.3 | .36[e] | — | — | 18 | 96 | 4.8 | — | — | 465 |
| Oysters: | | | | | | | | | | | | | |
| Pacific or Japanese *Crassostrea gigas* | 250 | .07 | .23 | 2.1 | — | 16.0 | — | 36 | 170 | 6.5 | 16.0 | 106 | 168 |
| Eastern or American *Crassostrea virginica* | 300 | .15 | .19 | 2.0 | .05 | 18.0 | .25 | 69 | 148 | 7.1 | 110.4[f] | 112 | 229 |

**Table 9.2  Nutrient Composition of Shellfish**

| Species: | Cal-ories | Carbo-hydrates | Protein | Total Fat | Fatty Acids | | | | Chole-sterol | Refer-ences |
|---|---|---|---|---|---|---|---|---|---|---|
| | | | | | Sat'd | Mono | Poly | Omega-3 | | |
| | kcal | gm | gm | gm | gm | gm | gm | gm | mg | |
| Western or Olympia *Crassostrea lurida* | 85 | 5.4 | 9.6 | 2.5 (1.9-3.6) | — | — | — | — | — | 3 |
| European or French *Ostrea edulis* | 79 | 4.9 | 10.3 | 1.7 (1.3-1.8) | .52 | .21 | .42 | .24 | — | 3, 333, 336 |
| Periwinkles *Littorina littorea* | 114 | 2.3 | 18.2 | 3.0 (1.2-4.5) | .45 | .83 | .90 | .44 | — | 3, 333 |
| Scallops: | | | | | | | | | | |
| Sea scallops *Placopecten magellanicus* | 87 | 2.6 | 16.2 | .81 (.2-1.0) | .10 | .06 | .24 | .18 | 36 | 83, 251, 332, 333 |
| Bay, Cape or Long Island *Argopecten irradians* | 80 | 2.9 | 14.8 | 0.6 (.3-1.5) | .09 | .07 | .22 | .13 | — | 3, 332 |
| Calico scallops *Aequipecten gibbus* | 84 | 2.4 | 16.1 | 0.6 (.2-1.0) | .09 | .05 | .21 | .13 | — | 3, 332 |
| Squid: | | | | | | | | | | |
| Short finned squid *Illex illecebrosus* | 99 | 2.3 | 17.3 | 1.8 (1.4-2.0) | .52 | .16 | .83 | .80 | 260[j] | 3, 332, 333 |
| Long finned squid *Loligo pealei* | 87 | 6.0 | 13.2 | 0.7 (.5-.9) | .16[i] | .04[i] | .25[i] | .24[i] | — | 3, 332 |
| California squid *Loligo opalescans* | 90 | 1.6 | 16.6 | 1.4 (.5-2.2) | — | — | — | — | — | 3, 332 |
| Flying squid *Loligo omnastrephes* | — | 0.7 | 15.3 | 0.8 | — | — | — | — | — | 3 |

**Table 9.2  Nutrient Composition of Shellfish**

| Species | Vit A I.U. | Thia-min mg | Ribo-flavin mg | Niacin mg | Vit B6 mg | Vit B12 mcg | Panto-thenic Acid mg | Cal-cium mg | Phos-phorus mg | Iron mg | Zinc mg | Sodium mg | Potas-sium mg |
|---|---|---|---|---|---|---|---|---|---|---|---|---|---|
| Western or Olympia *Crassostrea lurida* | — | — | — | — | — | — | — | 68 | 178 | — | — | — | — |
| European or French *Ostrea edulis* | — | — | — | — | — | 4.8 | — | 11 | 21 | 3.5 | 38.3[g] | 650 | 258 |
| Periwinkles *Littorina littorea* | — | — | — | — | — | — | — | 165[h] | 277[h] | 1.5 | — | 266[h] | 211[h] |
| Scallops: Sea scallops *Placopecten magellanicaus* | — | — | — | — | — | — | — | 16 | 218 | .6[i] | 1.2 | 87 | 412 |
| Bay, Cape or Long Island *Argopecten irradians* | — | — | — | — | — | — | — | — | — | — | — | — | — |
| Calico scallops *Aequipecten gibbus* | — | — | — | — | — | — | — | 22 | 210 | — | — | — | — |
| Squid: Short finned squid *Illex illecebrosus* | — | — | — | — | — | — | — | — | — | — | — | — | — |
| Long finned squid *Loligo pealei* | — | — | — | — | — | — | — | — | — | — | — | — | — |
| California squid *Loligo opalescens* | — | — | — | — | — | — | — | — | — | — | — | — | — |
| Flying squid *Loligo omnastrephes* | — | .03 | .08 | 3.2 | — | 1.3 | — | 15 | 194 | 20 | – | 176 | 266 |

**Table 9.2  Nutrient Composition of Shellfish**

| Species: | Calories kcal | Carbohydrates gm | Protein gm | Total Fat gm | Fatty Acids | | | | Cholesterol mg | References |
|---|---|---|---|---|---|---|---|---|---|---|
| | | | | | Sat'd gm | Mono gm | Poly gm | Omega-3 gm | | |
| **Crabs:** | | | | | | | | | | |
| Deep sea red crab *Geryon quinquedens* | 79 | 1.6 | 15.0 | 1.0 | — | — | — | — | 78[h] | 3, 85 |
| Blue or soft shelled *Callinectes sapidus* | 81 | 0.6 | 16.2 | 1.0 (.4-2.2) | — | — | — | — | 76 | 3, 251, 321, 337 |
| Dungeness crab *Cancer magister* | 87 | 0 | 17.3 | 1.2 (.8-3.0) | .17 | .22 | .40 | .38 | — | 3, 322, 333 |
| Jonah crab *Cancer borealis* | 95 | 2.2 | 16.2 | 1.9 — | — | — | — | — | 78[h] | 3, 85 |
| King crab *Paralithodes camchaticus* | 74 | .06 | 15.2 | 0.8 (.3-2.5) | — | — | — | — | 60 | 3, 83 |
| Snow crab *Chionoecetes bairdi* | 90 | 0 | 18.4 | 1.3 (1.0-1.5) | .16 | .22 | .52 | .44 | — | 3, 338 |
| Langostinos *Pleuroncodes planipes* | 74 | 6.2 | 8.2 | 1.6 | .32 | .28 | .62 | .58 | — | 3, 338 |
| Crayfish *Astacus spp.* | 76 | 1.0 | 16.0 | .05 | — | — | — | — | — | 3 |
| Lobster *Homarus americanus/vulgaris* | 113 | 5.4 | 18.2 | 1.5 (1.4-2.0) | — | — | — | — | 70 | 3, 85, 319 |
| Lobster, boiled | 93 | — | 20.5 | 0.6 | .08 | .13 | .07 | .06 | 72 | 317 |

**Table 9.2  Nutrient Composition of Shellfish**

| Species | Vit A I.U. | Thiamin mg | Riboflavin mg | Niacin mg | Vit B$_6$ mg | Vit B$_{12}$ mcg | Pantothenic Acid mg | Calcium mg | Phosphorus mg | Iron mg | Zinc mg | Sodium mg | Potassium mg |
|---|---|---|---|---|---|---|---|---|---|---|---|---|---|
| Crabs: | | | | | | | | | | | | | |
| Deep sea red crab *Geryon quinquedens* | — | — | — | — | — | — | — | 46 | 46 | — | — | 406 | 284 |
| Blue or soft shelled *Callinectes sapidus* | 5 | .08 | .04 | 2.7 | — | — | — | 74 | 226 | .6 | 4.0 | 200 | 452 |
| Dungeness crab *Cancer magister* | — | .12 | .10 | 3.1 | — | — | — | 52 | 180 | .4 | 3.8 | 266 | 330 |
| Jonah crab *Cancer borealis* | — | — | — | — | — | — | — | 96 | 120 | — | — | 276 | 279 |
| King crab *Paralithodes camchaticus* | 10 | .09 | .06 | 3.3 | — | — | — | 49 | 186 | 2.0 | — | 70 | — |
| Snow crab *Chionoecetes bairdi* | — | — | — | — | — | — | — | — | — | — | — | — | — |
| Langostinos *Pleuroncodes planipes* | — | — | — | — | — | — | — | — | — | — | — | — | — |
| Crayfish *Astacus spp.* | — | — | — | — | — | — | — | 97 | 226 | 1.8 | 1.8 | — | 260 |
| Lobster *Homarus americanus/ vulgaris* | — | .16 | .10 | — | — | .05 | 1.5 | — | 240 | — | 3.4 | — | — |
| Lobster, boiled | 87 | .01 | .07 | 1.1 | .08 | 3.11 | .28 | 61 | 185 | .4 | 2.9 | 380 | 352 |

**Table 9.2  Nutrient Composition of Shellfish**

| Species: | Cal-ories kcal | Carbo-hydrates gm | Protein gm | Total Fat gm | Fatty Acids | | | | Chole-sterol mg | Refer-ences |
| | | | | | Sat'd gm | Mono gm | Poly gm | Omega-3 gm | | |
| --- | --- | --- | --- | --- | --- | --- | --- | --- | --- | --- |
| Lobster, spiny or rock lobster or crawfish *Panulirus argus* | 100 | 1.7 | 19.2 | 1.2 | .14 | .14 | .59 | .27 | 106[h] | 333 |
| Shrimp: | | | | | | | | | | |
| Tropical: | | | | | | | | | | |
| White shrimp *Penaeus setiferus* | 90 | 0 | 19.4 | 0.8 (.2-1.2) | .20 | .14 | .49 | .34 | 96 | 3, 83, 337, 339, 9 |
| Brown shrimp *Penaeus aztecus* | 100 | 0 | 21.8 | 0.8 (.6-1.1) | .11 | .15 | .23 | .18 | — | 3, 338-340 |
| Pink shrimp *Penaeus durorarum* | 92 | 0 | 20.2 | 0.7 | — | — | — | — | — | 3 |
| Indian White *Penaeus indicus* | 87 | 2.7 | 17.0 | 0.4 | .11 | .05 | .09 | .07 | — | 3, 338 |
| Northern: | | | | | | | | | | |
| Northern pink *Pandalus borealis* | 92 | 0 | 19.4 | .98 (.4-1.5) | .14 | .29 | .20 | .16 | — | 3, 332, 338, 341 |
| Tiger prawn or shrimp *Penaeus monodon* | 95 | 1.8 | 19.2 | 0.6 (.4-.7) | — | — | — | — | — | 3 |
| Shrimp mixed species | 91 | — | 18.7 | 1.2 (.3-3.2) | .28 | .27 | .39 | .20 | 66[k] | 3, 38, 321, 362 |

[a] Includes data for *Haliotidae* and *H. japonica*
[b] Estimated from data on cooked seafood assuming 95% retention
[c] Range 7.1-190.0
[d] Data from *O. ocellatus*
[e] Data from *O. binaculatus*
[f] Range 17.0-217.9

[g] Range 1.7-74.9
[h] Cooked
[i] Data from related species
[j] Range 100-400
[k] Estimated from data on cooked white shrimp assuming 100% retention

**Table 9.2 Nutrient Composition of Shellfish**

| Species | Vit A I.U. | Thiamin mg | Riboflavin mg | Niacin mg | Vit B6 mg | Vit B12 mcg | Pantothenic Acid mg | Calcium mg | Phosphorus mg | Iron mg | Zinc mg | Sodium mg | Potassium mg |
|---|---|---|---|---|---|---|---|---|---|---|---|---|---|
| Lobster, spiny or rock lobster or crawfish *Panulirus argus* | — | — | — | — | — | — | — | 50 | 214 | 0.4[i] | — | — | — |
| Shrimp: | | | | | | | | | | | | | |
| Tropical: | | | | | | | | | | | | | |
| White shrimp *Penaeus setiferus* | — | .05 | .07 | 1.6 | — | — | — | 77 | 206 | — | — | — | — |
| Brown shrimp *Penaeus aztecus* | — | — | — | — | — | — | — | 89 | 258 | 1.8 | 1.6 | 208 | 288 |
| Pink shrimp *Penaeus duorarum* | — | — | — | — | — | — | — | 110 | 215 | 0.2 | — | — | — |
| Indian White *Penaeus indicus* | — | — | — | — | — | — | — | 160 | 295 | 2.5 | — | — | — |
| Northern: | | | | | | | | | | | | | |
| Northern pink *Pandalus borealis* | — | .08 | .19 | — | — | — | — | 54 | 177 | .4 | 1.4 | — | — |
| Tiger prawn or shrimp *Penaeus monodon* | — | .02 | .05 | 4.0 | — | 3.0 | — | 180 | 325 | — | — | 185 | 370 |
| Shrimp mixed species | 189 | .04 | .06 | 2.5 | — | 3.72 | — | — | — | 1.8 | — | — | — |

## Table 9.3 Proximate Composition and Sodium Content of Canned Fish and Shellfish[a]

| Species | Canning Medium | Calories | Carbo-hydrate | Protein | Total Fat | Sodium |
|---|---|---|---|---|---|---|
| | | kcal | gm | gm | gm | mg |
| Finfish:<br>Amberjack, Yellowtail<br>*Seriola quinqueradiata* | smoked, oil | 318 | 0 | 27.2 | 22.4 | — |
| Anchovy, European<br>*Engraulis encrasicolus* | olive oil | 321 | 0 | 19.9 | 26.2 | — |
| Herring, Atlantic | oil | 233 | 2.6 | 17.4 | 16.4 | — |
| *Clupea harengus harengus* | tomato sauce | 184 | 0 | 16.8 | 12.4 | — |
| Herring, Pacific<br>*Clupea harengus pallasi* | not specified | 154 | 1.1 | 19.2 | 7.5 | — |
| *Clupeidae* | not specified | 249 | 0 | 27.9 | 14.4 | — |
| *Clupeidae* | tomato sauce | 192 | 1.2 | 16.7 | 12.8 | — |
| Mackerel, jack<br>*Trachurus trachurus* | not specified | 143 | 2.5 | 23.2 | 3.8 | — |
| Horse mackerel<br>*Carangidae* | not specified | 147 | 0 | 21.4 | 6.2 | — |
| Pacific chub | oil | 232 | 0 | 24.8 | 14.0 | 800 |
| *Scomber japonicus/colias* | not specified | 150 | 0 | 21.3 | 6.5 | — |
| *Scombridae* | oil | 297 | 2.2 | 20.1 | 22.4 | — |
| | tomato sauce | 200 | 1.1 | 16.9 | 13.7 | — |
| | not specifed | 179 | 1.3 | 19.4 | 10.0 | 385 |
| Pilchard, European<br>*Clupea pilchardus* | oil | 300 | 0.9 | 21.7 | 22.6 | — |
| Pilchard, Pacific | tomato sauce | 193 | 0.7 | 18.5 | 12.3 | — |
| *Sardinops caerulea* | not specified | 240 | 1.7 | 16.8 | 17.9 | — |
| *Clupeidae* | not specified | 208 | 1.9 | 17.6 | 13.9 | 585 |
| Salmon<br>Atlantic *Salmo salar* | not specified | 198 | 0.9 | 21.1 | 11.6 | — |
| Chinook/King<br>*O. tshawytscha* | not specified | 222 | 1.6 | 19.3 | 14.8 | — |
| Chum<br>*O. keta* | not specified | 154 | 1.3 | 20.8 | 6.6 | 48 |
| Coho<br>*O. kisutch* | not specified | 163 | 1.5 | 20.7 | 7.6 | 184 |
| Pink<br>*O. gorbuscha* | not specified | 141 | 0.2 | 19.3 | 6.4 | — |
| Sockeye<br>*O. nerka* | not specified | 163 | 1.0 | 20.4 | 8.0 | 417 |

**Table 9.3** *Proximate Composition and Sodium Content of Canned Fish and Shellfish[a]*

| Species | Canning Medium | Calories | Carbo-hydrate | Protein | Total Fat | Sodium |
|---|---|---|---|---|---|---|
| | | kcal | gm | gm | gm | mg |
| Sardine | oil | 252 | 0.3 | 22.3 | 17.3 | 558 |
| *Clupeidae* | tomato sauce | 184 | 2.3 | 17.3 | 11.2 | 321 |
| | not specified | 198 | 0 | 23.9 | 10.6 | — |
| Smelt, lake | not specified | 233 | 5.3 | 21.1 | 13.5 | — |
| *Osmerus mordax* | | | | | | |
| Sprat | oil | 344 | 0 | 19.6 | 29.3 | — |
| *Sprattus sprattus* | tomato sauce | 206 | 1.4 | 16.8 | 14.3 | — |
| Tuna: | oil | 198 | 7.3 | 26.1 | 6.4 | 460[c] |
| Albacore | | | | | | |
| *Thunnus alalonga* | | | | | | |
| Bluefin | oil | 348 | 0 | 22.1 | 28.1 | — |
| *Thunnus thynnus* | | | | | | |
| Skipjack | oil | 175 | 0 | 29.0 | 5.7 | — |
| *Euthynnus pelamis* | brine | 153 | 6.0 | 25.9 | 2.0 | — |
| Yellowfin | oil | 177 | 0 | 27.0 | 6.8 | — |
| *Thunnus albacares* | water | 118 | 0.9 | 22.9 | 1.8 | 1000[b] |
| Tunny | oil | 284 | 0.6 | 23.8 | 20.0 | — |
| *Thunnus vulgaris* | | | | | | |
| Chunk light | | | | | | |
| Shellfish: | | | | | | |
| Crab: | | | | | | |
| Blue | not specified | 91 | 0.9 | 18.4 | 1.0 | — |
| *Callinectes sapidus* | | | | | | |
| Dungeness | brine | 88 | 0 | 18.5 | 1.0 | 844 |
| *Cancer magister* | water | 93 | 0 | 18.8 | 1.4 | 169[c] |
| King | not specified | 96 | 0.6 | 18.5 | 1.6 | — |
| *Paralithodes camtchaticus* | | | | | | |
| Queen | not specified | 82 | 3.0 | 14.2 | 1.1 | 704 |
| *Chionoecetes opilio* | | | | | | |
| Snow | not specified | 92 | 0 | 19.5 | 1.0 | — |
| *Chionoecetes bairdi* | | | | | | |
| Unspecified | not specified | 93 | 0.6 | 17.8 | 1.6 | 750 |
| Lobster, unspecified | not specified | 98 | 1.9 | 18.4 | 1.3 | — |
| Shrimp | | | | | | |
| White | | | | | | |
| *Penaeus setiferus* | brine | 70 | 0 | 15.0 | 0.7 | — |
| Tropical (Gulf) | cooked | 100 | 0.6 | 21.5 | 0.7 | — |
| *Penaeidae* | | | | | | |
| Unspecified | not specified | 99 | 0 | 20.8 | 1.1 | — |

**Table 9.3  Proximate Composition and Sodium Content of Canned Fish and Shellfish[a]**

| Species | Canning Medium | Calories | Carbo-hydrates | Protein | Total Fat | Sodium |
|---|---|---|---|---|---|---|
| | | kcal | gm | gm | gm | mg |
| Abalone *Haliotidae* | not specified | 111 | 9.7 | 16.5 | 0.2 | 990 |
| Clams Razor, *Solenidae* | not specified | 60 | 2.4 | 9.0 | 1.3 | — |
| Softshell *Mya arenaria* | not specified | 96 | 1.7 | 15.6 | 2.5 | — |
| Venus, butter *Saxidomus giganteus* | not specified | 129 | 1.4 | 18.7 | 4.8 | — |
| Venus, little neck, Japanese *Tapes (Venerupis) decussatus* | not specified | 103 | 5.5 | 15.6 | 1.6 | 400 |
| Quahog, cherrystone *Mercenaria mercenaria* | not specified | 71 | 2.0 | 9.7 | 2.4 | — |
| Unspecified | not specified | 80 | 5.1 | 11.1 | 1.3 | 2100[b] |
| Mussels[d] *Mytilus edulis* | brine | 90 | 0.9 | 13.3 | 3.3 | 340 |
| Oysters Eastern *Ostrea virginica* *Ostreidae* | not specified | 75 | 5.0 | 8.6 | 2.0 | — |
| | boiled | 99 | 2.8 | 12.4 | 3.9 | — |
| | smoked/oil | 226 | 10.7 | 15.1 | 13.2 | — |
| | not specified | 65 | 0 | 9.3 | 2.8 | — |

[a] Data from References 3, 81, 265, 318, 322, 333, 334, 343. Data per 100 grams.
[b] Seasoned
[c] Canned without salt
[d] Steamed

**Table 9.4  Proximate Composition of Selected Hawaiian Finfish**

| Local name and Latin name | Common name | Calories | Protein | Fat | Sodium | Ref. |
|---|---|---|---|---|---|---|
| | | | Data per 100 grams raw fillet | | | |
| Ahi (mebachi shibi) *Parathunnus sibi* | Big eye tuna | 171 | 23.6 | 7.8 | 31 | 344 |
| Ahi (maguro) *Thunnus orientalis* | Bluefin tuna | 115 | 24.5 | 1.2 | 39 | 344 |
| Ahi (shibi) *Neothunnus macropterus* | Yellowfin tuna (light) | 119 | 24.3 | 1.6 | 261 | Table 9.1 |
| Aku (katsuo) *Euthynnus pelamis* | Skipjack tuna | 131 | 24.9 | 2.7 | 37 | Table 9.1 |
| Akule *Trachurops crumenophthalmus* | Big eye scad | 125 | 23.7 | 2.6 | 57 | Table 9.1 |
| A'u *Makaira ampla* | Blue marlin | 121 | 23.1 | 3.2 | — | 3 |
| A'u (kajiki) *Makaira audax* | Striped marlin | 109 | 21.1 | 2.7 | — | 3 |
| Aweoweo *Priacanthus cruentatus* | Hawaiian bigeye | 111 | 20.9 | 2.4 | 66 | 344 |
| Kahala *Seriola dumerilii* | Amberjack, yellowtail | 96 | 20.8 | 0.8 | 52 | 344 |
| Kawakawa *Euthynnus yaito* | Little tuna, black skipjack | 129 | 25.5 | 2.2 | 56 | 344 |
| Kumu *Parupeneus porphyreus* | Red goat fish | 120 | 20.4 | 3.6 | 74 | 344 |
| Mahimahi *Coryphaena hippurus* | Dolphin fish | 94 | 19.3 | 1.1 | 170 | 3 |
| Manini *Acanthurus sandvicensis* | Convict tang | 89 | 18.3 | 1.2 | 122 | 344 |
| Moana *Parupeneus multifasciatus* | Goat fish | 99 | 20.1 | 1.5 | 71 | 344 |
| Mullet (uouoa) *Neomyxus chaptalii* | Mullet | 122 | 20.7 | 3.7 | 60 | 344 |
| Oio *Albula vulpes* | Ladyfish | 111 | 22.6 | 1.6 | 80 | 344 |
| Onaga *Etelis carbunculus* | Red snapper | 102 | 20.9 | 1.5 | 62 | 344 |
| Ono *Acanthocybium solandri* | Hawaiian wahoo | 124 | 24.1 | 2.3 | 82 | 344 |
| Opakapaka *Pristipomoides microlepis* | Pink snapper | 102 | 21.9 | 0.9 | 54 | 344 |
| Opelu *Decapterus pinnolatus* | Mackerel scad | 117 | 24.4 | 1.4 | 53 | 344 |
| Tombo *Thunnus alalunga* | Albacore tuna | 158 | 25.2 | 7.2 | 51 | Table 9.1 |
| Taape *Lutjanus kasmira* | Blue-lined snapper | 99 | 18.7 | 2.1 | 120 | Table 9.1 |
| U'u (menpachi) *Myripristis berndti Myripristis argyromus* | Squirrel fish | 118 | 18.6 | 4.2 | 70 | Table 9.1 |
| Weke-Ula *Mulloidichthys auriflamma* | Red goat fish | 107 | 23.0 | 1.0 | 53 | Table 9.1 |

**Table 9.5 Proximate Composition of New Zealand Finfish[a]**

| Species | Cal[b] Kcal | Protein gm | Fat gm | Ash gm | Moisture gm | Omega-3[g] gm | Ref |
|---|---|---|---|---|---|---|---|
| Alfonsino *Beryx splendens* | 151 | 17.8 | 8.3 1.7-19.9[c] | 1.0 | 72.8 | 1.9[e] | 345, 346 |
| Barracouta *Thyrsites atun* | 123 | 20.2 | 4.1 1.0-9.4 | 1.4 | 74.6 | 0.9 | 345, 348 |
| Cardinal fish *Epigonus sp.* | 96 | 19.0 | 1.7 0.9-3.6 | 1.0 | 78.6 | 0.3[e] | 346 |
| Cod: Blue cod *Parapercis colias* | 84 | 18.1 | 0.8 | 1.3 | 79.9 | —[f] | 324 |
| Red cod *Pseudophycis bachus* | 77 | 16.8 | 0.6 .5-.8 | 1.1 | 81.7 | 0.2 | 347, 348, 346 |
| Conger eel *Conger verreauxi* | 100 | 17.6 | 2.8 | 1.4 | 78.2 | — | 324 |
| Dogfish, Baxter's *Etmopterus baxteri* | 84 | 17.5 | 1.0 | 1.0 | 80.6 | — | 324 |
| Dory: John dory *Zeus japonicus* | 95 | 20.6 | 0.8 | 1.1 | 77.5 | — | 324 |
| Lookdown dory *Cyttus traversi* | 100 | 18.1 | 2.5 1.5-3.7 | 0.7 | 78.9 | 0.4[e] | 346 |
| Silver dory *Cyttus novaezelandiae* | 84 | 17.1 | 1.2 .6-3.0 | 0.9 | 80.6 | — | 349 |
| Elephant fish *Callorhinchus milii* | 105 | 22.5 | 1.0 | 1.2 | 75.3 | — | 324 |

**Table 9.5  Proximate Composition of New Zealand Finfish[a]**

| Species | Cal[b] Kcal | Protein gm | Fat gm | Ash gm | Moisture gm | Omega-3[g] gm | Ref |
|---|---|---|---|---|---|---|---|
| Flounder, yellow belly *Rhombosolea leporina* | 92 | 18.9 | 1.2 | 1.2 | 78.7 | — | 324 |
| Frostfish *Lepidopus caudatus* | 92 | 19.2 | 1.1 .9-1.2 | 1.1 | 78.4 | — | 349 |
| Gemfish, Silver kingfish *Rexea solandri* | 150 | 19.6 | 7.4 .9-12.1 | 1.0 | 73.2 | 1.2 | 348 |
| Ghostshark, pale *Hydrolagus spp.* | 84 | 17.4 | 1.1 | 1.3 | 80.2 | — | 324 |
| Gurnard *Cheilodonichthyus kumu* | 93 | 19.8 | 0.9 .8-1.1 | 1.1 | 78.1 | .05 | 345 |
| Hake *Merluccius australis* | 84 | 16.4 | 1.6 .9-2.8 | 1.1 | 81.0 | — | 345 |
| Hapuku *Polyprion oxygeneios* | 100 | 19.7 | 1.8 | 1.5 | 77.0 | — | 324 |
| Hoki *Macruronus novaezelandiae* | 87 | 16.9 | 1.7 | 1.6 | 80.4 | 0.3 | 348, 347, 345 |
| Javelin fish *Lepidorhynchus denticulatus* | 79 | 16.9 | 0.8 .7-.9 | 0.8 | 81.7 | 0.2[e] | 346 |
| Kahawai *Arripis trutta* | 154 | 22.6 | 6.4 | 1.0 | 70.0 | — | 324 |
| Kingfish *Seriola grandis* | 102 | 21.4 | 1.2 | 1.2 | 76.3 | — | 324 |

**Table 9.5  Proximate Composition of New Zealand Finfish[a]**

| Species | Cal[b] Kcal | Protein gm | Fat gm | Ash gm | Moisture gm | Omega-3[g] gm | Ref |
|---|---|---|---|---|---|---|---|
| Leather jacket *Navodon scaber* | 87 | 18.5 | 0.9 .8-1.0 | 1.0 | 79.4 | — | 349 |
| Ling *Genypterus blacodes* | 91 | 19.7 | 0.8 .6-1.0 | 1.0 | 78.3 | — | 349 |
| Mackerel: | | | | | | | |
| Blue mackerel *Scomber australasicus* | 151 | 22.8 | 6.0 2.1-17.7 | 1.4 | 70.7 | 0.2-1.3 | 348, 350 |
| Jack mackerel *Trachurus declivis* | 144 | 21.6 | 5.8 2.3-14.6 | 1.3 | 72.7 | 0.5 | 347, 348 |
| *Trachurus novaezelandiae* | 119 | 21.1 | 3.2 2.0-4.2 | 1.4 | 74.6 | — | 350 |
| Moki, blue *Latridopsis ciliaris* | 103 | 20.7 | 1.6 1.2-2.6 | 1.3 | 76.3 | 0.8 | 349 |
| Monkfish, giant stargazer *Kathetostoma giganteum* | 96 | 17.4 | 2.4 .6-5.5 | 1.2 | 79.3 | 0.1 | 345,348 |
| Mullet: | | | | | | | |
| Grey *Mugil cephalus* | 123 | 21.6 | 3.4 | 1.1 | 73.4 1.3-6.0 | — | 349 |
| Yellow-eye *Aldrichetta forsteri* | 103 | 20.3 | 1.8 1.5-2.1 | 1.3 | 76.4 | — | 349 |
| Oreo dory, black or spiky *Allocytus sp.* | 77 | 17.6 | 0.2[h] | 1.1 | 76.0 | — | 324 |

**Table 9.5  Proximate Composition of New Zealand Finfish[a]**

| Species | Cal[b] Kcal | Protein gm | Fat gm | Ash gm | Moisture gm | Omega-3[g] gm | Ref |
|---|---|---|---|---|---|---|---|
| Oreo dory, smooth *Pseudocyttus maculatus* | 49 | 11.2 | 0.1[h] | 1.0 | 84.2 | — | 324 |
| Orange roughy *Hoplostethus atlanticus* | 65 | 14.7 | 0.3[h] | 0.9 | 75.9 | — | 324 |
| Parore *Girella tricuspidata* | 93 | 19.3 | 1.2 | 1.2 | 78.3 | — | 324 |
| Pilchard *Sardinops neopilchardus* | 126 | 20.8 | 4.1 | 1.8 | 73.3 | — | 324 |
| Porae *Nemadactylus douglasi* | 120 | 20.6 | 3.6 | 1.0 | 74.5 | — | 349 |
| Rattail *Coelorynchus sp.* | 84 | 18.5 | 0.5 | 0.9 | 80.3 | 0.1[e] | 346 |
| Rays bream *Brama brama* | 102 | 20.8 | 1.5 0.9-2.4 | 1.9 | 75.6 | — | 349 |
| Ribaldo *Mora pacifica* | 81 | 17.9 | 0.5 0.5-0.6 | 0.9 | 80.5 | 0.1[e] | 346 |
| Ridge-scaled rattail *Macrourus carinatus* | 80 | 17.4 | 0.6 | 0.9 | 81.2 | — | 324 |
| Rig, spotted dogfish *Mustelus lenticulatus* | 99 | 21.4 | 0.9 | 1.1 | 76.7 | — | 324 |
| Rudder fish *Centrolophus niger* | 223 | 14.1 | 18.1 | 0.8 | 67.0 | — | 324 |

# Table 9.5 Proximate Composition of New Zealand Finfish[a]

| Species | Cal[b] Kcal | Protein gm | Fat gm | Ash gm | Moisture gm | Omega-3[g] gm | Ref |
|---|---|---|---|---|---|---|---|
| Salmon, fresh water *Oncorhynchus tschawytscha* | 110 | 19.7 | 2.9 | 1.6 | 75.8 | — | 324 |
| Salmon, sea pen *Oncorhynchus tschawytscha* | 147 | 19.2 | 7.2 | 1.3 | 72.4 | — | 324 |
| School shark *Galeorhinus australis* | 100 | 21.2 | 1.0 | 1.4 | 76.4 | — | 324 |
| Sea perch *Helicolenus papillosus* | 78 | 17.0 | 0.6 .5-.6 | 0.9 | 81.6 | 0.2[e] | 346 |
| Slickhead, black *Xenodermichthys socialis* | 48 | 9.9 | 0.6 | 1.1 | 88.3 | — | 324 |
| Sole: | | | | | | | |
| Lemon sole *Pelotretis flavilatus* | 90 | 17.9 | 1.5 | 1.0 | 79.6 | — | 324 |
| New Zealand sole *Peltoramphus novaezelandiae* | 94 | 19.4 | 1.2 | 1.1 | 78.4 | — | 324 |
| Snapper *Chrysophrys auratus* | 106 | 20.9 | 1.9 1.8-2.0 | 1.5 | 75.9 | .03 | 368 |
| Spiny dogfish *Squalus acanthias* | 127 | 18.8 | 5.2 | 1.1 | 74.9 | — | 324 |
| Tarakihi *Nemadactylus macropterus* | 113 | 21.0 | 2.6 1.1-4.5 | 1.4 | 76.6 | 1.0 | 368 |

**Table 9.5  Proximate Composition of New Zealand Finfish[a]**

| Species | Cal[b] Kcal | Protein gm | Fat gm | Ash gm | Moisture gm | Omega-3[g] gm | Ref |
|---|---|---|---|---|---|---|---|
| Trevally *Caranx georgianus* | 115 | 21.5 | 2.6 2.5-2.8 | 1.3 | 75.0 | 0.5 | 368 |
| Tuna: | | | | | | | |
| Skipjack *Katsuwonus pelamis* | 183 | 25.6 | 8.2 0.6-18.7[d] | 1.5 | 64.7 | — | 351 |
| Slender *Allothunnus fallai* | 302 | 19.8 | 24.1 16.3-29.1 | 1.4 | 54.7 | — | 352 |
| Warehou: | | | | | | | |
| Blue or common warehou *Seriolella brama* | 125 | 20.6 | 4.1 | 1.3 | 76.8 | 0.3 | 348 |
| Silver warehou *Seriolella punctata* | 195 | 18.8 | 12.7 6.0-16.2 | 1.4 | 68.0 | 1.2 | 345, 348 |
| White warehou *Seriolella caerulea* | 174 | 15.1 | 12.1 9.6-16.3 | 1.3 | 71.5 | — | 345 |
| Whiting, southern blue *Micromesistius australis* | 74 | 15.9 | 0.7 | 0.9 | 82.5 | — | 324 |

[a]Data per 100 gm raw fillet
[b] Calculated using the following calorie equivalent factors: protein: 4.27; fat: 9.02
[c] Range for values when available
[d] Range for 43 other samples in the same reference
[e] Calculated according to Reference 352
[f] Dashes denote lack of data
[g] Calculated from the sum of 20:5 + 22:6 fatty acids
[h] Over 90% of the total lipid is wax esters, which are not metabolized. The fat content shown represents the triglyceride portion (2.5-4.8%) of the total lipid content (354).

**Table 9.6 Vitamins and Mineral Content of Selected New Zealand Finfish[a]**

| | Thiamin | Riboflavin | Niacin | Iron | Zinc | Sodium | Potassium |
|---|---|---|---|---|---|---|---|
| | | | | mg 100/gm raw fillet | | | |
| Barracouta[b] | 0.03 | 0.05 | 2.8 | 1.1 | 0.6 | 70 | 400 |
| Cod, red | 0.02 | 0.01 | 1.6 | 1.0 | 0.3 | 70 | 320 |
| Gurnard | 0.01 | 0.03 | 2.9 | 0.4 | 0.4 | 109 | 466 |
| Hoki | 0.02 | 0.04 | 1.6 | 0.8 | 0.5 | 62 | 355 |
| Kingfish, silver (gemfish) | 0.02 | 0.04 | 1.5 | 0.6 | 0.6 | 50 | 360 |
| Mackerel, blue | 0.11 | 0.24 | 3.6 | 1.8 | 1.3 | 55 | 420 |
| Mackerel, jack | 0.07 | 0.07 | 3.0 | 1.6 | 0.9 | 55 | 390 |
| Moki | 0.18 | 0.10 | 2.9 | 0.5 | 0.4 | 81 | 461 |
| Monkfish | 0.02 | 0.01 | 1.5 | 0.5 | 0.5 | 85 | 390 |
| Snapper | 0.10 | 0.02 | 3.3 | 0.4 | 0.5 | 85 | 465 |
| Tarakihi | 0.02 | 0.02 | 2.2 | 0.5 | 0.4 | 98 | 465 |
| Trevally | 0.18 | 0.06 | 2.9 | 1.0 | 0.5 | 74 | 443 |
| Warehou, blue | 0.09 | 0.06 | 1.6 | 0.4 | 0.4 | 50 | 420 |
| Warehou, silver | 0.07 | 0.03 | 2.8 | 0.8 | 0.3 | 50 | 385 |

[a] Data from References 348 and 353.
[b] Latin species names — same as previous table.

# Appendix I

**Preparation Methods Used in the NFPA Study (205)**


**Baking**  Fish samples were weighed in low sodium pyrex baking pans and placed in an oven preheated to 350°F. Thermocouples were inserted into the fillets and time and temperature were monitored until an internal temperature of 160°F. was reached. Fish were cooled at room temperature for fifteen minutes and weighed.

**Broiling**  Fish samples were weighed on stainless steel broiler pans and placed four inches below the red hot broiling element. Thermocouples were inserted into the fillets and time and temperature monitored until the fillets reached an internal temperature of 160°F. Fish were cooled at room temperature for fifteen minutes and weighed.

**Microwave Baking**  Fish samples were weighed in low sodium pyrex baking dishes and placed in the microwave oven. A temperature probe was inserted into the sample and the oven programmed to reach an internal temperature of 160°F. After the initial cook, the probe was inserted into other areas of the sample to ensure even cooking. The samples were cooled at room temperature for fifteen minutes and weighed.

**Breading and Frying**  The breading procedure used 200 gm flour, 200 gm bread crumbs and 240 gm reconstituted egg. The fish sample was rolled in flour, dipped in egg and rolled in bread crumbs. Weights were recorded before and after frying of the fish sample and each of the breading components. About 1000 gm oil was used to ensure total coverage of the sample during frying. The oil was heated to 350°F. and a single sample was placed in the frying basket and submerged. Temperature was monitored for the oil and fillet with copper wire thermocouples until an internal temperature of 160°F. was reached. The basket was raised and drained for thirty seconds and the sample cooled on paper towels and weighed. The oil was weighed before and after use; the bread crumb residue in the oil and the oil adhering to the paper towels during cooling were also weighed.

**Boiling (Shrimp only)**   500 ml distilled deionized water was added to a saucepan, covered and brought to a boil on high heat. About 200 gm shrimp were added and brought to a second boil. The temperature was reduced to medium and the shrimp cooked for three minutes. The shrimp were stirred twice. After cooking, the shrimp were drained for five minutes and weighed.

**Canning – Salmon and Mackerel**   Skin and bones were removed and about one pound was packed into each can. The cans were sealed and thermally processed at 242 – 245°F. for 72 minutes. Weight of the contents before and after processing was recorded.

**Canning – Shrimp**   Raw, peeled and deveined shrimp were blanched for three minutes in a boiling 10% sodium chloride solution and drained. About 120 gm shrimp were packed in each can and warm 5% sodium chloride brine was used as the packing medium. The cans were sealed and processed at 250°F. for 13 minutes. Weight of the contents before and after processing was recorded.

# Appendix II

## Description of the Seafood Samples in the NFPA Study (205)

Samples of the different species were obtained over a two year period during both summer and winter months so that the effects of seasonal variations could be observed. Data reported are the averages from all the samplings although individual data are presented in the original study. The samples of flounder and shrimp contain more than one species as shown below and the data represent the average of the species sampled.

Samples of flounder, pollock, whiting and salmon were filleted and frozen at −10°F. and maintained frozen until analysis. Atlantic mackerel samples were headed and gutted but not skinned. Shrimp were obtained raw, headless, unpeeled and frozen. They were peeled and deveined prior to analysis.

A summary of the type, number, location and date of purchase of the samples is shown below.

| Species | No. of Samples | Date Purchased | Where Purchased | Where Caught |
|---|---|---|---|---|
| Flounder: (11) | | | | |
| Fluke | 2 | 2/80 | Washington DC | Chesapeake Bay |
| ? | 1 | 3/80 | Washington DC | ? |
| Yellowtail | 3 | 6/8 | Washington DC | Georges Bank, MA |
| Fluke | 2 | 1/82 | Washington DC | NC |
| Fluke | 2 | 2/82 | Washington DC | NC |
| Yellowtail | 1 | 1/82 | Washington DC | Georges Bank |
| Yellowtail | 2 | 6/82 | Northern VA | Georges Bank |
| | | 8/82 | Northern VA | Georges Bank |

252

| Species | No. of Samples | Date Purchased | Where Purchased | Where Caught |
|---|---|---|---|---|
| **Alaska Pollock: (11)** | | | | |
| Alaska Pollock | 3 | 11/80 | Seattle WA | ? |
| Alaska Pollock | 3 | 1-3/81 | Seattle WA | Unimak Pass, AK |
| Alaska Pollock | 3 | 6-8/81 | Seattle WA | Bering Sea |
| Alaska Pollock | 2 | 1-3/82 | Seattle WA | ? |
| **Pacific Whiting: (11)** | | | | |
| Pacific Whiting | 3 | 11/80 | Seattle WA | ? |
| Pacific Whiting | 3 | 3/81 | Seattle WA | Puget Sound WA |
| Pacific Whiting | 3 | 7-8/81 | Seattle WA | North WA/South BC |
| Pacific Whiting | 2 | 3/82 | Seattle WA | Northern W. Coast |
| **Sockeye Salmon: (11)** | | | | |
| Sockeye Salmon | 2 | 9-10/80 | Seattle WA | Southeast Alaska |
| Sockeye Salmon | 1 | 9-10/80 | Seattle WA | Kodiak |
| Sockeye Salmon | 1 | 9-10/80 | Seattle WA | Bristol Bay |
| Sockeye Salmon | 1 | 9-10/80 | Seattle WA | Peninsula |
| Sockeye Salmon | 1 | 9-10/80 | Seattle WA | Prince William Sound |
| Sockeye Salmon | ? | 7/81 | Seattle WA | Bristol Bay |
| Sockeye Salmon | ? | 8/81 | Seattle WA | Bristol Bay (?) |
| **Atlantic Mackerel: (11)** | | | | |
| Atlantic Mackerel | 3 | 3/81 | Washington DC | North Carolina |
| Atlantic Mackerel | 3 | 6/81 | Gloucester MA | ? |
| Atlantic Mackerel | 3 | 3/82 | Washington DC | East Coast |
| Atlantic Mackerel | 2 | 6/82 | Washington DC | East Coast |
| **Tropical Shrimp: (11)** | | | | |
| Tropical Shrimp | | | | |
| Tropical Shrimp | 2 | 1/81 | Washington DC | Alabama |
| Tropical Shrimp | 1 | 1/81 | Washington DC | Louisiana |
| Brown shrimp | 2 | 5/81 | Washington DC | Mexico |
| Pink shrimp | 1 | 5/81 | Washington DC | French Guiana |
| Texas white | 1 | 3/82 | Vienna VA | ? |
| Mississippi white | 1 | 2/82 | Vienna VA | ? |
| Pink shrimp | 3 | 6/82 | Washington DC | British Guyana (sic) |

# Appendix III

## U.S. Definition of an Additive

From the Food, Drug and Cosmetic Act, 1958 Amendment, Chapter II, Section 201(s):

The term "food additive" means any substance the intended use of which results or may reasonably be expected to result, directly or indirectly, in its becoming a component or otherwise affecting the characteristics of any food (including any substance intended for use in producing, manufacturing, packing, processing, preparing, treating, packaging, transporting or holding food; and including any source of radiation intended for any such use), if such substance is not generally recognized, among experts qualified by scientific training and experience to evaluate its safety, as having been adequately shown through scientific procedures (or, in the case of a substance used in food prior to January 1, 1958, through either scientific procedures or experience based on common use in food) to be safe under the conditions of its intended use; except that such term does not include:

1. A pesticide chemical in or on a raw agricultural commodity

2. A pesticide chemical to the extent that it is intended for use or is used in the production, storage, or transportation of any raw agricultural commodity

3. A color additive

4. Any substance use in accordance with a sanction or approval granted prior to the enactment of this paragraph puruant to this Act, the Poultry Products Inspection Act (21 U.S.C. 451 and the following) or the Meat Inspection Act of March 4, 1907 (34 Stat. 1260), as amended and extended (21 U.S.C. 71 and the following)

5. A new animal drug.

# References

1 Suitor, C. W. and Crowley, M. F. 1984. Nutrition. Principles and Application in Health Promotion, 2nd ed. J. B. Lippincott Co., Philadelphia 19105.

2 Watt, B.K. and Merrill, A. 1975. Agriculture Handbook No. 8. Composition of Foods. USDA, Washington, DC.

3 Sidwell, V. D. January 1981. Chemical and Nutritional Composition of Finfishes, Whales, Crustaceans, Mollusks and their Products. NOAA Technical Memorandum. NMFS F/SEC-11 U.S. Dept. of Commerce, Charleston, SC.

4 Krzynowek, J. 1985. Sterols and fatty acids in seafood. Food Tech. 39: 61.

5 Krzynowek, J. 1985. Personal communication.

6 ———— June 1984. Provisional table on the fatty acid and cholesterol content of selected foods. USDA. HNIS.

7 National Research Council 1980. Recommended Dietary Allowances, 9th ed. National Academy of Sciences, Washington, D.C.

8 Guthrie, H.A. July 1985. Recommended Dietary Allowances: 1985 Updates. Society for Nutrition Education Annual Meeting, Los Angeles.

9 O'Dell, Boyd L. 1984. Bioavailability of trace elements. Nutr. Rev. 42: 301-308.

10 Grundy, Scott M., Bilheimer, D., Blackburn, H., et al. 1982. Rationale of the diet/heart statement of the American Heart Association, Circulation 65: 839A-854A.

11 Guthrie, Helen A. 1977. Concept of a nutritious food. J. Am. Diet. Assoc. 71: 14.

12 ———— December 1975. U.S. Senate Committee on Nutrition and Human Needs: Nutrition and Health. U.S. Government Printing Office.

13 ———— Nutrition Labels and the U.S. RDA. Title 21, Food and Drugs. Section 101.9. Nutrition labeling of food.

14 Sorenson, A. W., Wyse, B. W. et al. 1976. An index of nutritional quality for a balanced diet. New help for an old problem. J. Am. Diet. Assoc. 68:236.

15 LaChance, Paul A. 1975. Critique of index of food quality (IFQ). J. Nutr. Ed. 7: 136.

16 Jacobson, M. 1973. Nutrition Scoreboard. Center for Science in the Public Interest. Washington, D.C.

17 Burroughs, A.L. 1975. FTC's proposed food advertising rule. A case of comprehensive complexity. Food Tech. 29: 30.

18 Russo, J. E., Stailin, R., Russel, G. J. and Metcalf, B. L. April 1984. Nutrition information in the supermarket. Working Paper Series. Center for Research in Marketing. Graduate School of Business, Univ. of Chicago, Chicago, IL.

19 _____ 1978. Diet and Coronary Heart Disease. American Heart Association, Dallas, TX.

20 _____ December 1984. Lowering Blood Cholesterol. Nat'l. Inst. of Health Consensus Development Conference Statement.

21 _____ April 1977. Code of Federal Regulations Title 21, Food and Drugs.

22 Aronson, V. 1984. Thirty Days to Better Nutrition. Doubleday, NY.

23 Vlieg, P. 1985. Personal communication.

24 Munro, H.N. and Crim, M.C. 1980. The proteins and amino acids. In: Goodhart, R.S. and Shils, M.E., editors. Modern Nutrition in Health and Disease. 6th ed. Lea and Febiger. Philadelphia, 80.

25 Neuringer, M., Connor, W.E. et al., 1984. Dietary omega-3 fatty acid deficiency and visual loss in infant rhesus monkeys. J. Clin. Invest. 73:272.

26 Holman, R.T., Johnson, S.B. and Hatch, T.F. 1982. Human linolenic acid deficiency. Am. J. Clin. Nutr. 35: 617.

27 Titus, B.G., Kulmacz, R.J. and Lands, W.E.M. 1982. Selective destruction and removal of heme from prostaglandin H Syntase. Arch. Biochem. Biophys. 214: 824.

28 Oliw, E., Granström, E. and Änggard, E. 1983. The prostaglandins and essential fatty acids. In: Pace-Asciak, C. and E. Granström, editors. Prostaglandins and Related Substances. Elsevier, Amsterdam.

29 _____ 1980. Nutrition and your health. Dietary Guidelines for Americans. USDA, USDHHS Home and Garden Bulletin, No. 232. Washington,D.C.

30 _____ 1985. Dietary guidelines and healthy practices. Nutrition Week XV: (21) 4.

31 Ernst, N.D. 1985. NIH Consensus development conference on lowering blood cholesterol to prevent heart disease: implications for dietitians. J. Am. Diet. Assoc. 85: 586-8.

32 Gorbach, S.L., Zimmerman, D.R. and Woods, M. 1984. The Doctors' Anti-Breast Cancer Diet. Simon and Schuster, NY.

33 Thompson, H. 1969. Biochemical composition of fish. In: Firth, Frank E. ed. Encyclopedia of Marine Resources. Van Nostrand Reinhold Co. NY.

34 Exler, J. 1975. Lipids and fatty acids of important finfish: New data for nutrient tables. J. Am. Oil Chem. Soc. 52: 154.

35 Stansby, M.E. 1981. Reliability of fatty acid values purporting to represent composition of oil from different species of fish. J. Am. Oil Chem. Soc. 58:13.

36 Stansby, M.E. 1969. Fats and oils. In: Firth, Frank E. ed. Encyclopedia of Marine Resources. Van Nostrand Reinhold Co. NY.

37 Stansby, M.E. 1969. Nutritional properties of fish oils. World Rev. Nutr. Diet 11:46.

38 Kryznowek, J., Wiggin, K. and Donahue, P. 1983. Sterol and fatty acid content in three groups of surf clams (*Spisula solidissima*), wild clams (60

256

and 120 mm size) and cultured clams (60 mm size). Comp. Biochem. Physiol. 74B: 289.

39 Bannatyne, W.R. and Thomas, J. 1969. Fatty acid composition of New Zealand shellfish lipids. N.Z. J. Sci. 12: 207.

40 Waters, M.E. 1982. Chemical composition and frozen storage stability of spot, *Leiostomus xanthurus*. Mar. Fish. Rev. 44: 14.

41 Hayashi, K., and Takagi, T. 1980. Occurrence of unusually high level of wax esters in deep-sea teleost fish muscle, *Hoplostethus atlanticus*. Bull. Jpn. Soc. Sci. Fish 46: 459.

42 Body, D.R. 1982. The properties of marine wax esters. Chem. in N.Z. 46: 55.

43 Ackman, R.G. 1982. Fatty acid composition of fish oils. In: Barlow, S.M. and Stansby, M.E., editors. Nutritional Evaluation of Long-Chain Fatty Acids in Fish Oil. Academic Press, N.Y.

44 Glomset, J.A. 1985. Fish, fatty acids and human health. New Eng. J. Med. 312: 1253.

45 Goodnight, S.H. Jr., Harris, W.S. et al. 1982. Polyunsaturated fatty acids, hyperlipidermia, and thrombosis. Arteriosclerosis 2: 87.

46 Connor, W. June 1985. Plasma lipid and lipoprotein lowering effects of omega-3 fatty acids from fish. Symposium on Omega-3 Fatty Acids and Human Health. Kingsborough Community College, New York.

47 Bang, H.O., Dyerberg, J. et al. 1976. The composition of food consumed by Greenlandic Eskimos. Acta Med. Scand. 220: 69.

48 Bang, H.O., Dyerberg, J. 1972. Plasma lipids and lipiproteins in Greenlandic West Coast Eskimos. Acta Med. Scand. 192: 85.

49 Dyerberg, J., Berg, H. O. et al. 1978. Eicosapentaenoic acid and prevention of thrombosis and arteriosclerosis. Lancet, ii, 117.

50 Dyerberg, J. and Bang, H.O. 1979. Hemostatic function and platelet polyunsaturated fatty acids in Eskimos. Lancet ii: 433.

51 Dyerberg, J. 1982. Observations on populations in Greenland and Denmark. In: Barlow, S.M. and Stansby, M.E., editors. Nutritional Evaluation of Long-Chain Fatty Acids in Fish Oil. Academic Press, NY.

52 Ahrens, E.H., Insull, W. et al. 1959. The effect on human serum lipids of a dietary fat highly unsaturated but poor in essential fatty acids. Lancet i: 115.

53 Bronte-Stewart, B., Antonis, A. et al. 1956. Effects of feeding different fats on serum cholesterol levels. Lancet ii: 521.

54 Nelson, A.M. 1972. Diet therapy in coronary disease – effect on mortality of high-protein high-seafood, fat controlled diet. Geriatrics 27: 103.

55 von Lossonczy, T.O., Ruiter, A. et al. 1978. The effect of a fish diet on serum lipids in healthy human subjects. Am. J. Clin. Nutr. 31: 1340.

56 Bronsegeest-Schoute, H.C., van Gent, C.M. et al. 1981. The effects of

various intakes of omega-3 fatty acids on the blood lipid composition in healthy human subjects. Am. J. Clin. Nutr.: 34: 1752.

57 Phillipson, B.E., Harris, W.S. et al. 1981. Reduction of plasma lipids and lipoproteins in hyperlipidemic patients by dietary omega-3 fatty acids (abstr). Clin. Res. 29: 628A.

58 Bang, H.O., Dyerberg, J. et al. 1980. The composition of the Eskimo food in north western Greenland. Am. J. Clin. Nutr. 29: 2657.

59 Kagawa, Y., Nishizawa, M. et al. 1982. Eicosapolyenoic acid of serum lipids of Japanese islanders with low incidence of cardiovascular disease. J. Nutr. Sci. Vitaminol. (Tokyo) 28: 441.

60 Hirai, A., Hamazaki, T. et al. 1980. Eicosapentaenoic acid and platelet function in Japanese. Lancet ii: 1132.

61 Kromhout, D. Bosschieter, E.B., et. al. 1985. The inverse relation between fish consumption and 20-year mortality from coronary heart disease. N.E.J.M. 312:1205

62 Harris, W.S., Connor, W.E. et al. 1983. The comparative reductions of the plasma lipids and lipoproteins by dietary polyunsaturated fats: salmon oil versus vegetable oils. Metabolism 32: 179.

63 Nestel, P.J., Connor, W.E. et al. 1984. Suppression by diets rich in fish oil of very low density lipoprotein production in man. J. Clin. Invest. 74: 82.

64 Simons, L.A., Hickie, J.B. and Balasubramaniam. 1985. On the effects of dietary n-3 fatty acids (Maxepa) on plasma lipids and lipoproteins in patients with hyperlipidemia. Atherosclerosis 54: 75.

65 Sanders, T.B., Vickers, M. et al. 1981. Effect on blood lipids and hemostasis of a supplement of cod liver oil rich in eicosapentaenoic acids, in healthy young men. Clin. Sci., London. 61: 317.

66 Connor, W.E., Lin, D.S. et al. 1981. A comparison of dietary polyunsaturated omega-6 and omega-3 fatty acids in humans: Effects upon plasma lipids, lipoproteins and sterol balance (abstr). Arteriosclerosis 1: 363a.

67 Wong, S.H., Nestel, P.J. et al. 1984. The adaptive effects of dietary fish and safflower oil on lipid and lipoprotein metabolism in perfused rat liver. Biochim. Biophys. Acta. 792:103

68 Yang, Y.T. and Williams, M.A. 1978. Comparison of $C_{18}^-$ $C_{20}^-$ and $C_{22}^-$ unsaturated fatty acids in reducing fatty acid synthesis in isolated rat hepatocytes. Biochem. Biophys. Acta. 531:133.

69 Lewis, B. 1977. Plasma-lipoprotein interrelationships. Biochem. Soc. Trans. 9:49.

70 Miller, G.J. and Miller, N.E. 1975. Plasma-high-density-lipoprotein concentration and development of ischaemic heart-disease. Lancet i: 16.

71 Heiss, G., Johnson, N.J. et al. 1980. The epidemiology of plasma high-density lipoprotein cholesterol levels. The Lipid Research Clinics Program Prevalence Study. Circulation 62: Suppl. IV: 116.

72 Goodnight, S.H., Harris, W.S. et al. 1981. The effects of dietary omega-3 fatty acids upon platelet composition and function in man: a prospective, controlled study. Blood 58: 880.

73 Sinclair, H.M. 1953. The diet of Canadian Indians and Eskimos. Proc. Nutr. Soc. 12: 69.

74 Siess, W., Roth, P. et al. 1980. Platelet-membrane fatty acids, platelet aggregation and thromboxane formation during a mackerel diet. Lancet i: 441.

75 Thorngren, M. and Gustafson, A. 1981. Effects of 11-week increase in dietary eicosapentaenoic acid on bleeding time, lipids and platelet aggregation. Lancet ii: 1190.

76 Thorngren, M. and Gustafson, A. 1983. Effects of acetylsalicylic acid and dietary intervention on primary hemostasis. Am. J. Med. June 14, p.66.

77 Foegh, M.L. and Ramwell, P.W. 1983. Physiological implications of products in the arachidonic acid cascade. In: Pace-Asciak, C. and E. Granström, editors. Prostaglandins and Related Substances. Elsevier, Amsterdam.

78 Willis, A.L. 1984. Essential fatty acids, prostaglandins and related eicosanoids. Present Knowledge in Nutrition. 5th ed. The Nutrition Foundation, Inc. Washington, D.C.

79 Lands, W. June 1985. Relationships of eicosanoids and human health. Symposium on Omega-3 Fatty Acids and Human Health. Kingsborough Community College, New York.

80 Kryznowek, J., Peton, D. and Wiggin, K. 1984. Proximate composition, cholesterol and calcium content in mechanically separated fish flesh from three species of the Gadidae family. J. Food Sci. 49: 1182.

81 Weihrauch, J.L. 1984. Provisional table on the fatty acid and cholesterol content of selected foods. USDA, Washington, D.C.

82 Feeley, R.M., Criner, P.E. and Watt, B.K. 1972. Cholesterol content of foods. J. Am. Diet. Assoc. 61: 134.

83 Kryznowek, J. 1985. Personal communication. Unpublished data on cholesterol content of seafood.

84 Mathews, R.H. and Young, J.G. 1975. Food Yields Summarized by Different Stages of Preparation. USDA Agriculture Handbook No. 102. Washington, D.C.

85 Kryznowek, J., Wiggin, K. and Donahue, P. 1982. Cholesterol and fatty acid content in three species of crab found in the Northwest Atlantic. J. Food Sci. 47: 1025.

86 Gordon, D.T. and Collins, N. 1982. Anatomical distribution of sterols in oysters (*Crassostrea gigas*). Lipids 17: 811.

87 Mattson, F.H., Volpenheim, B.A. et al. 1977. Effect of plant sterol esters on the absorption of dietary cholesterol. J. Nutr. 107: 1139.

88 _____ 1984. Serum vitamin and provitamin A levels and the risk of cancer. Nutr. Rev. 42: 214.

89 _____ 1984. Present Knowledge in Nutrition. 5th ed. The Nutrition Foundation, Washington, D.C.

90 Davidson, S. and Passmore, R. 1967. Human Nutrition and Dietetics. 3rd ed. E.S. Livingstone, Ltd., London.

91 Sand, G. 1967. Fish oil industry in Europe. In: Stansby, M.E., editor. Fish Oils. AVI Publishing Co., Westport, CT.

92 Stansby, M.E. and Hall, A.S. 1967. Chemical composition of commercially important fish of the United States. Fish. Ind. Res. 3: 29.

93 McCollum, E.V. 1957. A History of Nutrition. Houghton Mifflin Co., Boston, MA.

94 _____ 1984. The photochemical formation of vitamin D in the skin. Nutr. Rev. 42: 341.

95 Hepburn, F.N. 1984. USDA's nutrient data research. Presentation at the 9th National Nutrient Data Bank Conference. Amherst, MA.

96 McLaughlin, P.J. and Weihrauch, J.L. 1979. Vitamin E content of foods. J. Am. Diet. Assoc. 75: 647.

97 Dubick, M.A. and Rucker, R.B., 1983. Dietary supplements and health aids – a critical evaluation. Part 1 – vitamins and minerals. J. Nutr. Ed. 15:47.

98 Rotruck, J.T., Pope, A.L. et al. 1973. Selenium: biochemical role as a component of glutathione peroxidase. Science 179: 588.

99 Wortzman, M.S., Beskris, H.J., et al. 1980. Effect of dietary selenium on the interaction between 2-acetylaminofluorene and rat liver DNA in vivo. Cancer Res. 40: 2670.

100 Mertz, W. and Schwarz, K. 1959. Relation of glucose tolerance factor to impaired glucose tolerance of rats on stock diets. Am. J. Physiol. 196: 614.

101 Schwarz, K. and Mertz, W. 1959. Chromium (III) and the glucose tolerance factor. Arch. Biochem. Biophys. 85:292.

102 Papavasiliou, P.S., Miller, S.T. et al. 1968. Functional interactions between biogenic amines, 3', 5'-cyclic AMP and manganese. Nature 220:74.

103 Papavasiliou, P.S., Miller, S.T. et al. 1975. Sequential analysis: manganese, catecholamines and L-Dopa induced dyskinesia. J. Neurochem. 25: 215.

104 Tanaka, Y. 1978. Manganese: its neurological and teratological significance in man. Am. Chem. Soc. National Meeting, Chicago, IL.

105 Carlisle, E.M. 1972. Silicon: an essential element for the chick. Science 178: 619.

106 Carlisle, E.M. 1982. The nutritional essentiality of silicon. Nutr. Rev. 40: 193.

107 Jelinek, C.F. and Corneliussen, P.E. 1977. Levels of arsenic in the United States food supply. Environ. Health Perspec. 19: 83.

108 Underwood, E.J. 1973. Trace elements. In: Toxicants Occurring Naturally in Foods. National Academy of Sciences, Washington D.C.

109 Kryznowek, J. 1985. Sterols and fatty acids in seafood. Food Tech. 39: 61.

110 Woodicka, V.O. 1980. Legal considerations of food additives. In: CRC Handbook of Food Additives. 2nd ed. Vol. ll.Furia, T.E., editor. CRC Press, Boca Raton, FL.

111 Middlekauff, R.D. 1984. Risk analysis and the interface of science, law and policy. Food Tech. 38: 97-102.

112 _____ July-Aug. 1958. House Committee on Interstate and Foreign Commerce; Senate Committee on Labor and Public Welfare. 85th Congress, 2nd Sess. U.S. Congress. House Report 2284. Senate Report 2422.

113 Coon, J.M. 1974. Natural food toxicants – a perspective. Nutr. Rev. 32: 321.

114 _____ Moderate aspartame use in pregnancy, FDA says. Nutrition Week April 1985. Community Nutrition Institute. Washington, D.C.

115 _____ December 1983. Briefing materials for the first meeting. Interagency Risk Management Council, Washington, D.C.

116 _____ 1983. Risk assessment in the Federal government: managing the process. NRC/NAS. National Academy Press, Washington, D.C.

117 Ruckelshaus, W.C. 1983. Science, risk and public policy. Science 221: 1026.

118 Kirschman, J.C. 1984. Building an adequate risk assessment data base. Food Tech. 38: 103.

119 _____ 1985. Food safety management: managing risks safely. Nutrition Week XV: (15) 4-5. Community Nutrition Institute. Washington, D.C.

120 Lorentzen, R.J. 1984. FDA procedures for carcinogenic risk assessment. Food Tech. 38: 108.

121 Smith, M.V. 1985. Use of risk assessment in regulatory decision-making. Food Tech. 38: 113.

122 Schramm, A.J. 1984. Future trends in risk analysis. Food Tech. 38: 119-122.

123 Kroger, M. and Smith, J.S. 1984. An overview of chemical aspects of food safety. Food Tech. 38: 62.

124 Wolff, I.A. and Thornbury, M.E. (advisors). August 1981. Report of the Nutrition and Food Safety Research Program Steering Committee for the Northeastern Region. USDA. Vaughn, D.A. and Rasmussen, A.I. (chairpersons).

125 Body, D.R. 1983. The nature and fatty acid composition of the oils from deep-sea fish species from New Zealand waters. J. Sci. Food Agric. 34:388.

126 Licciardello, J.J. 1983. Botulism and heat-processed seafoods. Mar. Fish. Rev. 45: 1.

127 Foster, E.M. 1982. How safe are our foods? Nutr. Rev. Suppl. 40:28-34.

128 _____ Secretariat of the Joint FAO/WHO Food Standards Programme,

General Principles, in Codex Alimentarius Commission Procedural Manual, 4th ed. 1975. Food and Agricultural Organization, Rome.

129 Meyers, T.R. and Hendricks, J.D. 1982. A summary of tissue lesions in aquatic animals induced by controlled exposures to environmental contaminants, chemotherapeutic agents and potential carcinogens. Mar. Fish. Rev. 44: 1.

130 Butler, P.A. 1969. Pesticides in the Sea. Van Nostrand Reinhold Co. NY.

131 Mowatt, F. 1984. Sea of Slaughter. McClelland and Stewart, Ltd. Toronto, Ont.

132 _____ 1978. Report on the chance of U.S. seafood consumers exceeding the current acceptable daily intake for mercury and recommended regulatory controls. National Marine Fisheries Service, Washington, DC.

133 Greig, R.A. and Kryznowek, J. 1979. Mercury concentrations in three species of tunas collected from various oceanic waters. Bull. Environm. Toxicol. 22: 120.

134 FDA. 1984. Action level for methyl mercury in fish; availability of compliance policy guide. Fed. Reg. 49: (224) 45663.

135 Bilton, T.J., Ruppel, B.E., Lockwood, K., et al. 1983. PCBs in selected finfish caught within New Jersey waters 1981-1982 (with limited chlordane data). Office of Science and Research. New Jersey Dept. Environmental Protection.

136 _____ 1980. PCBs . . . a middle chapter. FDA Consumer p. 28.

137 Eisenberg, M., Mailman, R. and Tubiash, H.S. 1980. Polychlorinated biphenyls in fish and shellfish of the Chesapeake Bay. Mar. Fish. Rev. 42: 21.

138 Sloan, R. and Horn, E.G. 1984. PCBs in striped bass from the marine district of New York in 1984. NY State Dept. Environmental Conservation, Albany, NY.

139 _____ April 1985. FDA says data New York used for decision on PCB in fish are inadequate. Food Chem. News.

140 Schaatz, E.J. 1973. Seafood toxicants. In: Toxicants Occurring Naturally in Foods. National Academy of Sciences, Washington, D.C.

141 Ballentine, C.L. and Hernden, M.L. 1982. Who, why, when and where of food poisons (and what to do about them). FDA Consumer (6):26-28.

142 Higashi, G.I. 1985. Foodborne parasites transmitted to man from fish and other aquatic foods. Food Tech 39:69.

143 Bylund, B.G. 1982. Diphyllobothriasis. In: CRC Handbook Series in Zoonoses ed. L.Jacobs and P. Arambulo III, Vol.I, p. 217. CRC Press, Inc., Boca Raton, FL.

144 Dore, Ian 1984. Fresh Seafood - The Commercial Buyer's Guide. Osprey Books, Huntington, N.Y.

145 Margolis, L. 1977. Public health aspects of "codworm" infection: a review. J. Fish. Res. Board Can. 34: 887.

146 Jackson,G.J., Gerding, T.A., and Knollenberg, W.G. 1978. Nematodes in fresh market fish of the Washington, D.C. area. J. Food Protect 41:613.

147 Myers, B.J. 1979. Anisakine nematodes in fresh commercial fish from waters along the United States' Washington, Oregon, and California coasts. J. Food Protect. 42: 380.

148 Mathews, R.A. and Stewart, M.R. 1984. Report summarizes data from food additive surveys. Food Tech. 38: 53.

149 _____ 1981. Food additives: Summarized Data from NRC Food Additive Surveys. NAS/NRC, Washington, D.C.

150 Fulton, K.R. 1981. Surveys of industry on the use of food additives. Food Tech. 35: 80.

151 Murray, C.K. 1967. Polyphosphate dips for fish. Torry Advisory Note No. 31. Torry Research Station, Aberdeen, Scotland.

152 Shimp, L.A. 1985. Food phosphates in seafood processing. Seafood Leader, Spring, p. 114.

153 Gibson, D.M. and Murray, C.K. 1973. Polyphosphates and fish: some chemical studies. J. Food Tech. 8: 197.

154 Daeta, P.K., Frazer, A.C. et al. 1962. J. Sci. Food Agr. 13: 556.

155 _____ 1985. Fish brine, shrimp brine, restructured scallops product sheets. Archer Daniels Midland Co., Chicago, IL.

156 Paquette, G.N. 1983. Fish Quality Improvement. A Manual for Plant Operators. Osprey Books, Huntington NY.

157 McWeeney, D.J. 1979. The chemical behavior of food additives. Proc. Nutr. Soc. 38: 129.

158 Green, L.C. et al. 1981. Nitrate biosynthesis in man. Proc. Nat'l. Acad. Sci. U.S.A. 78: 7764.

159 _____ 1978. Nitrates: an environmental assessment. Coordinating Committee for Scientific and Technical Assessment of Environmental Pollutants. National Academy of Sciences, Washington, D.C.

160 Wagner, D.A. and Tannenbaum, S.R. 1985. In-vivo formation of N-nitroso compounds. Food Tech. 39: 89.

161 Gray, J.I., Reddy, S.K. et al. 1982. Inhibition of nitrosamines in bacon. Food Tech. 36: 39

162 Hotchkiss, J.H. and Vecchio, A.J. 1985. Nitrosamines in fried-out bacon fat and its use as a cooking oil. Food Tech. 39: 67.

163 _____ 1985. USDA considers options to cut nitrite levels. Nutrition Week XV: (17) 7. Community Nutrition Institute, Washington, D.C.

164 Havery, D.C. and Fazio, T. 1985. Human exposure to nitrosamines from food. Food Tech. 39: 80.

165 _____ April 1984. Standards of Identity for Fish and Shellfish. Code of Federal Regulations 21 Part 161 - Fish and Shellfish. Food and Drugs.

166 Kramer, D. 1982. Storage characteristics of major seafood groups and the maintenance of quality. In: Proc. First Nat'l. Conf. Seafood Packaging and Shipping. Martin, R.E. NFI, Washington, D.C.

167 Jacober, L.F. and Rand, A. G. Jr. 1982. Biochemical Evaluation of Seafood. AVI Publishing, Westport, CT.

168 Martin, R.E. 1982. Proc. First Nat'l. Conf. Seafood Packaging and Shipping. NFI, Washington, D.C.

169 Matches, J.R. 1982. Microbial changes in packages. In: Proc. First Nat'l. Conf. Seafood Packaging and Shipping. Martin, R.E. NFI, Washington, D.C.

170 Regenstein, J.M., Schlosser, M.A., et al. 1982. Chemical changes of trimethylamine oxide during fresh and frozen storage of fish. AVI Publishing, Westport, CT.

171 Stansby, M.E. 1967. Fish Oils. AVI Publishing, Westport, CT.

172 Sims, R.J. and Fioriti, J.A. 1980. Antioxidants as stabilizers for fats, oils and lipid-containing foods. CRC Handbook of Food Additives. 2nd ed. Vol. II. Furia, T.E., Editor CRC Press, Inc. Boca Raton, FL.

173 Sidwell, V.D. 1980. Effects of cooking on composition. In: Proc. First National Seafood Nutrition Symposium, NFI, Washington D.C.

174 Manohar, S.V., Rigby, D.L., et al. 1973. Effect of sodium tripolyphosphate on thaw drip and taste of fillets of some fresh-water fish. J. Fisheries Res. Bd. Can. 30: 685.

175 Botta, J.R., Richards, J.F., et al. 1973. Flesh, pH, color, thaw drip, and mineral concentration of Pacific halibut (*Hippoglossus stenolepsis*) and Chinook salmon *(Oncorhynchus tshawytscha)* frozen at sea. J. Fisheries Res. Bd. Can. 30:71.

176 Rechcigl, M. Jr., Ed. 1982. Handbook of Nutritive Value of Processed Food. Vol I Food for Human Use. CRC Press, Inc., Boca Raton, FL 33431.

177 Pottinger, S.R., Kerr, R.G., et al. 1949. Effect of refreezing on quality of sea trout. Commer. Fish. Rev. 11: 14.

178 March, B.E. 1982. Effect of processing on nutritive value of food: fish. In: Handbook of Nutritive Value of Processed Food. Vol. I. CRC Press, Inc., Boca Raton, FL 33431.

179 Regier, L. 1980. Composition of seafood – a survey. Proc. First National Seafood Nutrition Symposium, NFI, Washington DC.

180 Dore, I. 1982. Frozen Seafood - the Buyer's Handbook. Osprey Books, Huntington, N.Y.

181 Ronsivalli, L.J. and Baker, D.W. II. 1981. Low temperature preservation of seafoods: a review. Mar. Fish. Rev. 43: 1.

182 Karmas, E. 1975. Nutritional aspects of food processing methods. In: Nutritional Evaluation of food Processing. Harris, R.S. and Karmas, E. editors. AVI Publishing, Westport, CT.

183 Stansby, M.E. 1967. Misconceptions about nutritional properties of fish oils. In: Stansby, M.E. Fish Oils. AVI Publishing, Westport, CT.

184 Keay, J.N. and Hardy, R. 1978. Fish as food part I. The fisheries resource and its utilization. Process Biochem. 13: 2.

185 Wheeler, J.D. and Hebard, C.E. 1981. Seafood Products Resource Guide. Sea Grant Program, VA Polytechnic Institute, Hampton, VA.

186 Bilinski, E., Jomas, R.E.E., et al. 1979. Control of rancidity in frozen Pacific herring *Clupea harengus pallasii*: use of sodium erythorbate. J. Fish. Res. Bd. Can. 36: 219.

187 Licciardello, J.J., Ravesi, E.M. and Allsup, M.G. 1982. Stabilization of the flavor of frozen minced whiting. 1. Effects of antioxidants. Mar. Fish. Rev. 44: 15.

188 Eklund, M.V. 1982. Effect of $CO_2$ modified atmospheres and vacuum packaging on *Clostridium botulinum* and spoilage organisms of fishery products. In: Proc. First Nat'l. Conf. Seafood Packaging and Shipping. Martin, R.E., ed. NFI, Washington, D.C.

189 Ravesi, E.M. 1976. Nitrite additives – harmful or necessary? Mar. Fish. Rev. 38: 24.

190 Liston, J. 1982. The function of packaging – an overview. In: Proc. First Nat'l. Conf. Seafood Packaging and Shipping. Martin, R.E., ed. NFI, Washington, D.C..

191 Karel, M. and Heidelbaugh, N.D. 1975. Effects of packaging on nutrients. In: Nutritional Evaluation of Food Processing. Harris, R.S. and Karmas, E. editors. AVI Publishing, Westport, CT.

192 Anderson, D.C. 1983. Vacuum packaging of frozen and fresh fisheries products. W.R. Grace and Co., Duncan, SC. Presented at Institute of Food Technologists Convention.

193 de Masi, T.W. 1985. Personal communication. Cryovac Division, W.R. Grace Co., Duncan, SC.

194 Coyne, F.P. 1932. The effect of carbon dioxide on bacterial growth with special reference to the preservation of fish. I. J. Soc. Chem. Ind. 51: 119T.

195 Coyne, F.P. 1933. The effect of carbon dioxide on bacterial growth with special reference to the preservation of fish. II. J. Soc. Chem. Ind. 52: 19T.

196 Parkin, K.L. and Brown, W.D. 1982. Preservation of seafood with modified atmospheres. In: Chemistry and Biochemistry of Marine Food Products. Martin, R.E., Flick, G.J. et al., editors. AVI Publishing, Westport, CT.

197 Finne, G. 1982. Research update on controlled and modified atmosphere packaging. In: Proc. First National Conf. Seafood Packaging and Shipping. Martin, R.E. ed. NFI, Washington, D.C.

198 Veranth, M.F. and Robe, K. 1979. $CO_2$-enriched atmosphere keeps fish fresh more than twice as long. Food Process. 40: 76.

199 Brown, W.D., Albright, M., et al. 1980. Modified atmosphere storage on rockfish (*Sebastes miniatus*) and silver salmon *(Oncorhyrchus kisutch)*. J. Food Sci. 45: 93.

200 Lindsay, R.C. 1982. Sorbate and botulism safety aspects for modified atmosphere packaging. Proc. First Nat'l. Conf. Seafood Packaging and Shipping. Martin, R.E., ed. NFI, Washington, D.C.

201 Fitzgerald, D. 1985. Personal communication. Ducktrap Farm, Maine.

202 Chung, Y.M. and Lee, J.S. 1982. Potassium sorbate inhibition of microorganisms isolated from seafood. J. Food Prot. 45: 1310.

203 Ampola, V.G. and Keller, C.L. 1985. Shelf life extension of drawn whole cod and cod fillets by treatment with potassium sorbate. Manuscript in preparation, courtesy of V. Ampola.

204 Eklund, M.W., Pelroy, G.A., Paranjpye, R., et al. 1982. Inhibition of *Clostridium botulinum* types A and E toxin production by liquid smoke and NaCl in hot-process smoke-flavored fish. J. Food Protect. 45: 935.

205 Dudek, J.A., Berman, S.C. et al. 1982. Determination of effects of processing and cooking on the nutrient composition of selected seafoods. National Food Processors Association, Washington, D.C.

206 Deutsch, H.F. and Hasler, A.D. 1943. Distribution of vitamin $B_1$ destruction enzyme in fish. Proc. Soc. Exp. Biol. Med. 53: 63.

207 Lamb, F.C., Farrow, R.P., et al. 1980. Effect of processing on nutritive value of food: canning. In: Handbook of Nutritive Value of Processed Food, Vol I. Rechcigl, M. Jr. ed. CRC Press, Inc., Boca Raton, FL 33431.

208 _____ 1981. Wholesomeness of Irradiated Food. Report of a Joint FAO/ IAEA/WHO Expert Committee, Geneva, 27 Oct. - 3 Nov., 1980 WHO Technical Report Series, No. 659. Geneva, Switzerland.

209 IFT Expert Panel on Food Safety and Nutrition. 1983. Radiation preservation of foods. Food Tech. 37: 55.

210 Giddings, G.G. 1984. Radiation processing of fishery products. Food Tech. 38: 60.

211 Grecz, N., Rowley, D.B., et al. 1983. The action of radiation on bacteria and viruses. Preservation of Food by Ionizing Radiation. Vol. III. Ed. E.S. Josephson and M.S. Peterson. CRC Press, Boca Raton, FL.

212 Licciardello, J.J. and Ronsivalli, L.J. 1982. Irradiation of seafood. In: chemistry and Biochemistry of Marine Food Products. Martin, R.E., Flick, G.J., et al., editors. AVI Publishing, Westport, CT.

213 Faub, I.A., Angellini, P., et al. 1976. Irradiated food: validity of extrapolating wholesomeness data. J. Food Sci. 41: 942.

214 Josephson, E.S., Thomas, M.H., et al. 1978. Nutritional aspects of food irradiation: an overview. J. Food Proc. and Preserv. 2: 299.

266

215 Reber, E.F., Bert, M.H., et al. 1968. Biological evaluation of protein quality of radiation-pasterurized haddock, flounder and crab. J. Food Sci. 33: 335.

216 Brooke, R.O., Ravesi, E.M. et al. 1966. Preservation of fresh unfrozen fishery products by low-level radiation. V. The effects of radiation pasteurization on amino acids and vitamins in haddock fillets.

217 Kraybill, H.F. 1982. Effect of processing on nutritive value of food: irradiation. In: Handbook of Nutritive Value of Processed Food. Vol I. Rechcigl, M. Jr., ed. CRC Press, Inc., Boca Raton, FL.

218 Ronsivalli, L.J., King, F.J., et al. 1971. Study of irradiated pasteurized fishery products. Isot. Rad. Technol. 8: 321.

219 Josephson, E.S., Thomas, M.H., et al. 1975. Effects of treatment of foods with ionizing radiation. In: Nutritional Evaluation of Food Processing. Harris, R.S. and Karmas, E. editors. AVI Publishing Co., Westport, CT.

220 Nawar, W.W. 1972. Radiolytic changes in fats. Radiat. Res. Rev. 3: 327.

221 Underdal, B., Nordal, J., et al. 1976. The effect of ionizing radiation on the nutritional value of mackerel. Lebensm. Wiss. Technol. 9: 72.

222 Nickerson, J.T.R., Licciardello, J.J., et al. 1982. Radurization and radicidation. A. Fish and shellfish. In: Preservation of Food by Ionizing Radiation. Josephson, E. and Peterson, M. editors. CRC Press Inc., Cleveland, OH.

223 Ader, G.A., Babbitt, J.K. and Crawford, D.L. 1983. Effect of washing on the nutritional quality characteristics of dried minced rockfish flesh. J. Food Sci. 48: 1053.

224 Crawford, D.L., Law, D.K. and Babbitt, J.K. 1972. Yield and acceptability of machine separated flesh from some marine food fish. J. Food Sci. 37: 551.

225 Waters, M.E. 1983. Chemical composition and frozen storage of weakfish, *Cynoscion regalis*. Mar. Fish. Rev. 45: 27.

226 Lee, C.M. 1984. Surimi process technology. Food Tech. 38: 69.

227 Miyauchi, D., Kudo, G. and Patashnik, M. 1973. Surimi a semi-processed wet fish protein. Mar. Fish. Rev. 35: 7.

228 ⸻ Brief history of surimi. Kibun Products International Inc., Pasadena, CA.

229 Okada, M., Miyauchi, D. and Kudo, G. 1973. "Kamaboko" the giant among Japanese processed fishery products. Mar. Fish. Rev. 35: 1.

230 Iwata, K., Okada, M., Fujii, Y. et al. 1968. Influences of storage temperatures on quality of frozen Alaska pollock surimi. Reito (Refrigeration) 43: 1145.

231 ⸻ June 1985. Compliance Policy Guides. Chapter 8, Fish and Seafood. FDA. Guide 7108.16.

232 ⸻ 1984. Final report and recommendations. The case for and against

regulating the protein quality of meat, poultry and their products. Am. J. Clin. Nutr. 40: 675.

233 Anderson, M.L. and Mendelsohn, J.M. 1972. A rapid salt-curing technique. J. Food Sci 37: 627.

234 Daun, H. 1975. Effects of salting, curing and smoking on nutrients of flesh foods. In: Nutritional Evaluation of food Processing. Harris, R.S. and Karmas, E. editors. AVI Publishing, Westport, CT.

235 Kryznowek, J. In press. Fish and Shellfish. In: Nutritional Evaluation of Food Processing. 3rd ed. Karmas, E. and Harris, R.S. ed. AVI Publishing, Westport, CT.

236 Burgess, G.H.O. and Bannerman, A.M. 1963. Fish Smoking. A Torry Kiln Operator's Handbook. Torry Research Station, Aberdeen, Scotland.

237 Root, W. 1980. Food. Simon and Schuster, New York.

238 Scanlan, R.A. and Reyes, F.G. 1985. An update on analytical techniques for N-nitrosamines. Food Tech. 39: 95.

239 Connell, J.J., Gibson, D. et al. 1981. Possible toxic compounds in smoked fish products. In: Nahrung aus den Meer. Springer-Verlag, Germany.

240 Larsson, B.K. 1982. Polycyclic aromatic hydrocarbons in smoked fish. Z. Lebensm. Unters. Forsch. 174: 101.

241 Fishery Products Inc. 1985. New England style bake or broil. 86% fish 14% topping. Seafood Business Report 4: 30.

242 Learson, R.J. 1969. Breaded fishery products. In: Encyclopedia of Marine Resources. Firth, F.E. ed. Van Nostrand Reinhold Co. NY.

243 Pennington, J.A.T. and Church, H.N. 1985. Bowes and Church's Food Values of Portions Commonly Used. 14th ed. Harper and Row, New York.

244 Beacham, L.M., Dudek, J.A., et al. 1984. Labeling stategy for surimi-based food products. Final Report. National Food Processors Assoc. Washington, D.C.

245 Marsh, A.C. and Weihrauch, J.L. 1984. Provisional table on the nutrient content of fast foods. USDA, Washington, DC.

246 Borenstein, B. 1980. Effect of processing on the nutritional value of foods. In: Modern Nutrition in Health and Disease. 6th ed. Goodhart, R.S. and Shils, M.E., editors. Lea and Febiger, Philadelphia.

247 Krampitz, L.O. and Woolley, D.W. 1944. The manner of inactivation of thiamine by fish tissue. J. Biol. Chem. 152: 9.

248 Neilands, J.B. 1947. Thiaminase in aquatic animals of Nova Scotia. J. Fish. Res. Bd. Canada 7: 94.

249 _____ 1985. Vitamin losses in food preparation. Vitamin Nutrition Information Service, Hoffman-LaRoche, Inc. Nutley, NJ.

250 Borenstein, B. 1975. Stability of nutrients in food. In: Nutritional Evaluation

of Food Processing, Harris, R.S. and Karmas, E., editors. AVI Publishing, Westport, CT.

251 Anthony, J.E., Hadgis, P.N., Milan, R.S. et al. 1983. Yields, proximate composition and mineral content of finfish and shellfish. J. Food Sci. 48: 313.

252 Mathews, R.H. and Garrison, Y.J. 1975. Food Yields Summarized by Different Stages of Preparation. Agriculture Handbook No. 102. USDA, Washington, DC.

253 Garland, S.L. and Mathews, R.H. 1984. Provisional table on percent retention of nutrients in food preparation. USDA, Washington, D.C.

254 _____ 1980. Common and Scientific Names of Fishes from the U.S. and Canada. American Fisheries Society. Special Publication No. 12, Bethesda, MD.

255 _____ January 1973. Food Labeling Regulations. Nutrition Labeling and U.S. RDA Federal Register 38: 2131.

256 Stephenson, M. 1975. Making food labels more informative. FDA Consumer 9: 13-17.

257 Lands, W.E.M., 1982. Biochemical observations on dietary long chain fatty acids from fish oils and their effect on prostaglandin synthesis in animals and humans. In: Nutritional Evaluation of Long-Chain Fatty Acids. Barlow, S.M. and Stansby, M.E., editors. Academic Press, N.Y.

258 Witney, E.N. and Hamilton, E.H.N. Understanding Nutrition. 2nd ed. West Publishing Co. St. Paul, MN.

259 Ross, M.L. 1974. What's happening to food labeling? J. Am. Diet. Assoc. 64: 262.

260 _____ June 1977. A consumer's guide to food labels. FDA Consumer. HHS Publication No. (FDA) 77-2083.

261 _____ 1984. Seafood Retail Training Manual. National Fisheries Education and Research Foundation, Inc., Chicago.

262 _____ September 1983. Position on Open Dating. FMI, Washington, DC.

263 _____ 1984. The Safe Food Book. Your Kitchen Guide. Home and Garden Bulletin No. 241 USDA. Write: Consumer Info. Center, Pueblo, CO 81009.

264 _____ Thumbs Up. Consumer Affairs. Giant Food Inc. P.O. Box 1804, Washington, DC.

265 _____ Crack the Codes: A Guide to Understanding the Codes on the Foods You Buy. Rockville, MD.

266 _____ 1981. Blind dates: How to Break the Codes on the Foods You Buy. State Consumer Protection Board, Albany, NY.

267 _____ October 1982. Regulations Governing Processed Fishery Products and U.S. Standards for Grades of Fishery Products. Code of Federal Regulations 50, Wildlife and Fisheries.

268 _____ 1980. Proposed Grading Standards for Fresh and Frozen Groundfish Products. Dept. of Fisheries and Oceans, Ottawa, Canada.

269 Johnson, M. 1985. UPC Update: Shaping Up the Symbol. Progressive Grocer, March.

270 _____ Uniform Code Council, 7051 Corporate Way, Dayton, OH 45459.

271 Regenstein, J.M. and Regenstein, C.E. 1979. An introduction to the kosher dietary laws for food scientists and food processors. Food Tech. 33: 89.

272 _____ April 1984. Food Labeling; Declaration of Sodium Content of Foods and Label Claims for Food on the Basis of Sodium Content; Final Rule. Federal Register. 21 CFR. Parts 101 and 105.

273 _____ January 1983. cited in: Produce Marketing Association. Nutrition Marketing Task Force. Nutrition Marketing. Federal Food, Drug and Cosmetic Act 21 USC Section 102(m) 321(m).

274 Perry, Susan. 1978. What Are Those Labels Really Telling Us? Nutrition Action, February.

275 Heimbach, J.T. and Stokes, R.C. 1982. Nutrition labeling and public health: survey of American Institute of Nutrition members, food industry and consumers. Am. J. Clin. Nutr. 36: 700.

276 _____ December 1982. Nutrition label formats unveiled. CNI Weekly Report. XII (49). Community Nutrition Institute, Washington, D.C.

277 _____ November 1984. Citizen's Petition of Public Voice for Food and Health Policy to Require Fat Content Labeling on Hot Dog and Bologna Products (Cooked Sausage Standard). Public Voice for Food and Health Policy. Washington, D.C.

278 Morris, J.N., Marr, J.W. et al. 1977. Diet and heart, a postscript. Br. Med. J. 2: 1307.

279 Connor, W.E. and Lin, D.S. 1982. The effect of shellfish in the diet upon the plasma lipid levels in humans. Metabolism 31: 1046.

280 Kritchevsky, D. and Story, J.A. 1977. In: Nutrition and Cancer. M. Winick, Editor. John Wiley and Sons, N.Y.

281 Trowell, H. 1974. Definitions of fiber. Lancet i: 503.

282 Anderson, J.W., Chen, W. J.L. et al. 1980. Plant Fiber in Foods. HCF Diabetes Research Foundation, Inc. Lexington, KY.

283 Jenkins, D.J.A., Leeds, A.R. et al. 1976. The cholesterol lowering properties of guar and pectin. Clin. Sci. Molec. Med. 51: 8.

284 Kirby, R.W., Anderson, J.W. et al. 1981. Oat-bran intake selectively lowers serum low-density lipoprotein cholesterol concentrations of hypercholesterolemic men. Am. J. Clin. Nutr. 34: 824.

285 Anderson, J.W. and Chen, W.J.L. 1979. Plant fiber, carbohydrate and lipid metabolism. Am. J. Clin. Nutr. 32: 346.

286 _____ 1984. Cancer prevention. U.S. Dept. Health and Human Services. NCI Dietary Guidelines. NIH Publication No. 84-2671.

287 _____ 1982. Five-year findings of the Hypertension Detection and Follow-up program. III – Reduction in stroke incidence among persons with high blood pressure. Hypertension Detection and Follow-up program Cooperative Group. J.A.M.A. 247: 633.

288 _____ 1979. Reduction in mortality of persons with high blood pressure, including mild hypertension. Hypertension Detection and Follow-up Program Cooperative Group. J.A.M.A. 242: 2562.

289 Reisin, E., Abel, R. et al. 1978. Effect of weight loss without salt restriction on the reduction of blood pressure in overweight hypertensive patients. N. Engl. J. Med. 298: 4.

290 Stamler, J., Farinaro, E. et al., 1980. Prevention and control of hypertension by nutritional-hygienic means. J.A.M.A. 243: 1819.

291 Sidwell, V.D., Buzzell, D.H., et al. 1977. Composition of the edible portion of raw (fresh or frozen) crustaceans, finfish, and mollusks. II. Macroelements: sodium, potassium, chlorine, calcium, phosphorus and magnesium. Mar. Fish. Rev. 39: 1.

292 Committee on Diet, Nutrition and Cancer. 1982. Diet, Nutrition and Cancer. National Academy of Sciences, Washington, D.C.

293 _____ Diet Nutrition and Cancer Prevention. National Cancer Institute. Washington, D.C.

294 van Eys, J. 1982. Nutrition and neoplasia. Nutr. Rev. 40: 353.

295 Davis, J.M. 1985. Diet and breast cancer. National Fisheries Institute, Washington, D.C.

296 May, C.D. 1984. Food sensitivity: facts and fancies. Nutr. Rev. 42: 72-78.

297 Am. Academy of Allergy and Immunology. Committee on Adverse Reactions to Foods 1984. Adverse Reactions to Foods. National Institutes of Health. NIH Publication No. 84-2442.

298 Taylor, S.L. 1985. Food allergies. Food Tech. 39:98-105.

299 Atkins, F.M. 1983. The basis of immediate hypersensitivity reactions to foods. Nutr. Rev. 41.

300 Metcalfe, D.D. 1984. Diagnostic procedures for immunologically-mediated food sensitivity. Nutr. Rev. 42: 92.

301 Aukrust, L., Apold, J. et al. 1978. Crossed immunoelectrophoretic and crossed radioimmunoelectrophoretic studies employing a model allergen from codfish. Intl. Arch. Allergy Appl. Immunol. 57: 253.

302 Aas, K. 1984. Antigens in food. Nutr. Rev. 42: 85-91.

303 Aas, K. 1966. Studies of hypersensitivity of fish. Allergological and serological differentiation between various species of fish. Intl. Arch. Allergy Appl. Immunol 30: 257-267.

304 Aas, K. and Elsayed, S. 1969. Characterization of a major allergen (cod). Effect of enzymic hydrolysis on the allergenic activity. J. Allergy 44: 333.

305 Elsayed, S. and Aas, K. 1971. Characterization of a major allergen (cod). Observations on effect of denaturation on the allergenic activity. J. Allergy 47: 283.

306 Hoffman, D.R., Day, E.D. et al. 1981. The major heat stable allergen of shrimp. Ann. Allergy 47: 17.

307 Gaddie, J., Legge, J.S. et al. 1980. Pulmonary hypersensitivity in prawn workers. Lancet 2: 1350.

308 Beck, H. I. and Nissen, B.K. 1983. Contact urticaria to commercial fish in atopic persons. Acta Dermatovenereology 63: 257.

309 Hoffman, D.R. 1983. Immunochemical identification of the allergens in egg white. J. Allergy Clin. Immunol. 71: 481.

310 Kolbye, A.C. Jr. 1985. Diet and adverse reactions: scientific and regulatory considerations. Food Tech. 39: 106.

311 _____ 1985. Sulfite labeling approved in spite of HHS delays. Nutrition Week XV (14): 7. Community Nutrition Institute, Washington, D.C.

312 _____ 1985. Sulfite ban considered, fresh produce affected. Nutrition Week XV (15): 3. Community Nutrition Institute, Washington, D.C.

313 _____ 1984. Food Marketing Institute Trends. Consumer attitudes and the supermarket. FMI, Washington, D.C.

314 Grivetti, L.E. 1984. Food fact, food myth – the scientific dilemma. Food Tech. 38: 14.

315 McClane, A.J. and deZanger, A. 1977. The Encyclopedia of Fish Cookery. Holt, Rinehart and Winston, NY.

316 Exler, J. and Weihrauch, J.L. 1976. Comprehensive evaluation of fatty acids in foods. VIII. Finfish. J. Am. Diet. Assoc. 69: 243.

317 Exler, J. 1985. Personal communication.

318 Iredale, D.G. and York, R. 1983. A Guide to Handling and Preparing Freshwater Fish. Dept. of Fisheries and Oceans. Freshwater Institute, Winnipeg, Manitoba, Canada.

319 Orr, M.L. 1969. Pantothenic acid, vitamins $B_6$ and vitamin $B_{12}$ in foods. Home Economics Research Report No. 36. USDA, Washington, D.C.

320 Sidwell, V.D., Loomis, A.L., Foncannon, P.R., et al. 1978. Composition of the edible portion of raw (fresh or frozen) crustaceans, finfish and mollusks. IV. Vitamins.Mar. Fish. Rev. 40: 1.

321 Exler, J. 1983. Iron content of food. Home Economics Research Report No. 45. USDA, Washington, D.C.

322 Gordon, D.T. and Martin, R.E. 1982. Vitamins and minerals in seafoods of the Pacific Northwest. In: Chemistry and Biochemistry of Marine Food

Products. Martin, R.E., Flick, G.J. et al., editors. AVI Publishing, Westport, CT.

323 Leu, S.S., Jhaveri, S.N., et al. 1981. Atlantic mackerel *(Scomber scombrus, L)*: seasonal variation in proximate composition and distribution of chemical nutrients. J. Food Sci. 46: 1635.

324 Vlieg, P. 1985. Personal communication. Proximate analysis of New Zealand finfish.

325 Kinsella, J.E., Shimp, J.L., et al. 1977. Sterol, phospholipid, mineral content and proximate composition of fillets of select freshwater fish species. J. Food Biochem. 1: 131.

326 Kinsella, J.E., Shimp, J.L. and Mai, J. March. 1978. The proximate and lipid composition of several species of freshwater fishes. Food Science No. 2.

327 Yanase, M. 1956. The vitamin $B_6$ content of fish meat. Bull. Jpn. Soc. Sci. Fish. 22: 51.

328 Jhaveri, S.N. and Constantinides, S.M. 1981. Chemical composition and shelf life study of grayfish *(Squalus acanthias)*. J. Food Sci. 47: 188.

329 Gruger, E.H. Jr. 1967. Fatty acid composition of fish oils. In: Fish Oils. Stansby, M.E., ed. AVI Publishing, Westport, CT.

330 Ackman, R.G., Eaton, C.A. and Ke, P.J. 1967. Canadian marine oils of low iodine value: fatty acid composition of oils from Newfoundland turbot (greenland halibut), certain Atlantic herring and a sablefish. J. Fish. Res. Bd. (Canada) 24: 2563.

331 Hale, M.B. and Brown, T. 1983. Fatty acids and lipid classes of three underutilized species and changes due to canning. Mar. Fish. Rev. 45: 45.

332 Joseph, J.D. 1982. Lipid composition of marine and estuarine invertebrates. Part II: Mollusca. Prog. Lipid Res. 21: 109.

333 Exler, J. and Weihrauch, J.L. 1977. Comprehensive evaluation of fatty acids in foods. 7. Shellfish. J. Am. Diet. Assoc. 71: 518.

334 Slabyj, B.H. and Carpenter, P.N. 1977. Processing effect on proximate composition and mineral content of meats of blue mussels *(Mytilus edulis)*. J. Food Sci. 42: 1153.

335 Kryznowek, J. and Wiggin, K. 1979. Seasonal variation and frozen storage stability of blue mussels. J. Food Sci. 44: 1644.

336 Paradis, M. and Ackman, R.G. 1977. Potential for employing the distribution of anomalous non-methylene-interrupted dienoic fatty acids in several marine invertebrates as part of food web studies. Lipids 12: 170.

337 Krishnamoorthy, R.V., Venkataramiah, A. et al. 1979. Effects of cooking and of frozen storage on the cholesterol content of selected shellfish. J. Food Sci. 44: 314.

338 Joseph, J. 1985. Personal communication.

339 Bonnet, J.C., Sidwell, V.D. and Zook, E.G. 1974. Chemical and nutritive

values of several fresh and canned finfish, crustaceans and mollusks. Part II. Fatty acid composition. Mar. Fish. Rev. 36: 8.

340 Johnston, J.J., Ghanbari, H.A., Wheeler, W.B., et al. 1983. Characterization of shrimp lipids. J. Food Sci. 48: 33.

341 Krzeczkowski, R.A. 1970. Fatty acids in raw and processed Alaska pink shrimp. J. Am. Oil Chem. Soc. 47: 451.

342 Chanmugam, P., Donovan, J., et al. 1983. Differences in lipid composition of fresh water prawn *(Macrobrachium rosenbergii)* and marine shrimp. J. Food Sci. 48: 1440.

343 Kovacs, M.I.P., Ackman, R.G. and Ke, P.J. 1978. Important lipid components of some fishery-based convenience food products: fatty acids, sterols and tocopherols. J. Can. Diet. Assoc. 39.

344 Walker, M., Wenkam, N.S. and Miller, C.D. 1958. Composition of some Hawaii fishes. Hawaii Med. J. 18: 144.

345 Vlieg, P. 1984. Proximate analysis of 10 commercial New Zealand fish species. N.Z. J. Sci. 27: 99.

346 Vlieg, P. 1982. Proximate composition of the flesh of 7 less common New Zealand deep water fish species. N.Z. J. Sci. 25: 233.

347 Vlieg, P. 1982. Proximate fatty acid composition of the flesh of New Zealand red cod, hoki and jack mackerel. N.Z. J. Sci. 25: 155.

348 Pickston, L., Czochanska, Z. and Smith, J.M. 1982. The nutritional composition of some New Zealand marine fish. N.Z. J. Sci. 25: 19.

349 Vlieg, P. 1984. Proximate analysis of commercial New Zealand fish species. 2. N.Z. J. Sci. 27: 427.

350 Vlieg, P. 1982. Compositional analysis of jack mackerel and blue mackerel. N.Z. J. Sci. 25: 229.

351 Vlieg, P., Habib, G. and Clement, G.I.T. 1983. Proximate composition of skipjack tuna *Katsuwonus pelamis* from New Zealand and New Caledonia waters. N.Z. J. Sci. 26: 243.

352 Vlieg, P. 1984. Proximate composition of New Zealand slender tuna *Allothunnus fallai*. N.Z. J. Sci. 27: 435.

353 Hughes, J.T., Czochanska, Z., Pickston, L., et al. 1980. The nutritional composition of some New Zealand marine fish and shellfish. N.Z. J. Sci. 23: 43.

354 Buisson, D.H., Body, D.R. et al., 1982. Oil from deep water fish species as a substitute for sperm whale and jojoba oils. J. Am. Chem. Soc. 59: 390.

355 Hile, J.P. 1985. Health Claims in Food Labeling and Advertising. Food and Drug Law Institute, seminar. Washington, D.C.

356 Weihrauch, J.L., Posati, L.P. et al. 1977. Lipid conversion factors for calculating fatty acid contents. J. Am. Oil Chem. Soc. 54: 36.

357 Gosline, W.A. and Brock, V.E. 1971. Handbook of Hawaiian Fishes. Univ. of Hawaii Press, Honolulu, HI.

358 Hall, R.A., Zook, E.G. and Meaburn, G.M. 1978. NMFS Survey of Trace Elements in the Fishery Resource. NOAA Tech. Report NMFS. SSRF-721. Washington, D.C.

# Index